The Radiological Diagnosis in Canine and Feline Emergencies

An Atlas of Thoracic and Abdominal Changes

STEN-ERIK OLSSON, D.V.M., Vet. med. dr., M.D.

Professor and Head, Department of Clinical Radiology
Veterinärhögskolan; Docent, Karolinska Institutet, Stockholm, Sweden;
Special Consultant, Hospital for Special Surgery,
New York, New York

Lea & Febiger Philadelphia • 1973

ISBN 0–8121–0265–7

Library of Congress Catalog Card Number 71–146031

PRINTED IN THE UNITED STATES OF AMERICA

Preface

The dependence upon diagnostic radiology in small animal practice has made veterinary radiology an acknowledged specialty. A number of textbooks and journals bear witness of the progress as well as of the interest in this specialty.

The cornerstones of diagnostic radiology are good radiographic technique and correct interpretation of the films. It is usually not the x-ray machine but lack of knowledge and experience that limits the usefulness of radiology. In the hands of a trained radiologist a small diagnostic unit is a more valuable tool than a more sophisticated machine not being skillfully operated. Proper positioning and good darkroom work are equally important.

Nothing can substitute for experience in film reading. Nor is it possible to interpret films or to use any guide without knowledge of the normal radiographic anatomy. There is, however, an obvious need for a handy reference book that can give the student and practitioner some advice and direction in interpreting radiographs. The present atlas should meet this need. Its place is near the view box, within easy reach when guidance is needed in interpreting radiographs in emergency cases.

The scope of the atlas is limited to canine and feline emergency cases with thoracic and abdominal soft-tissue changes. These changes lend themselves less easily to interpretation than do skeletal lesions such as luxations and fractures.

All radiographic changes in the thorax and abdomen could not be included. This would have made the atlas too large. Emergency cases were chosen because they are important in practice and also because little attention has been paid to this subject in previous literature.

Three groups of emergency cases are included in this atlas:

1. Acute diseases and lesions commonly seen by practitioners.
2. Less common acute diseases and lesions with characteristic radiographic signs.
3. Exacerbating chronic diseases requiring emergency treatment.

Emphasis is on illustrations, which are large reproductions of radiographs. The legends are short. Each case is briefly described and data pertinent to the interpretation of the radiographs are given.

Most of the illustrations are plain radiographs—recumbent lateral and ventrodorsal views—made with an overhead tube. Some cases are illustrated by only one radiograph if this is considered sufficient to demonstrate all pertinent details. Only a few cases are illustrated by a lateral radiograph of the subject in standing or erect position. In these cases horizontal beams are used.

All the radiographs are reproduced with the head of the animal to the left of the picture. The ventrodorsal radiographs are reproduced in conventional manner, that is, with the animal's head up and his left side to the right of the picture. Several animals were fluoroscoped either before or after the radiographs were made; in these instances the fluoroscopic findings are recorded in the case histories. Besides plain films, gastrointestinal contrast series (GI series), barium enema radiographs, intravenous pyelographs (IVP), and retrograde urocystographs are included.

The majority of the radiographs were made at the Department of Clinical Radiology of the Royal Veterinary College in Stockholm. The Section of Radiology of the Animal Medical Center, New York, contributed twelve radiographs and two originated from the Department of Radiology, School of Veterinary Medicine, Colorado State University, Fort Collins, Colorado.

After a seminar on the radiologic diagnosis in emergency cases given at the A.A.H.A. annual congress in New York City in 1967, I was approached by Lea & Febiger, publishers, with a request for a book on the subject. After considerable hesitation I undertook the task. A heavy work load delayed the writing of the atlas and it is with a sense of gratitude for the publisher's patience that the work on the atlas is now being completed. For help in compiling the cases and encouragement, I am indebted to my friends and colleagues, Gunnela Ljunggren, Lars-Erik Kängström, Peter Suter, and Joe Morgan. Börje Nilsson, who made the photographs, and Colette Carmeris, who typed the manuscript, merit acknowledgment.

Stockholm, Sweden STEN-ERIK OLSSON

Part 1

The Thorax

Chapter 1

The Heart and the Pericardium

This brief chapter is devoted to the radiologic changes in dogs and cats with heart failure of emergency nature. Severe circulatory problems such as congestion and edema of the lungs and cyanosis can be insidious or sudden in onset. Animals with these problems may sooner or later become so severely affected that emergency treatment will be required.

There are a large number of diseases of the heart which may lead to heart failure, but these are beyond the scope of this book. By the time heart failure has developed it may not be possible to diagnose the underlying condition because of advanced secondary changes. In heart failure the heart is usually enlarged and a change in shape has taken place. The lungs, the pleural cavity, or the abdomen is sometimes the site of very severe changes.

Mitral insufficiency is a common cause of enlargement of the left atrium and increased pressure in the pulmonary veins. Radiographically, the dorsocaudal part of the heart is enlarged and the vascularity of the lungs is increased. Stasis and edema of the lungs often complicate the picture. Left ventricular enlargement is less commonly seen in dogs and cats than in humans.

Enlargement of the right side of the heart may be due to an increased pulmonary venous pressure, to a left-to-right shunt, or to a pulmonary artery stenosis. Very marked enlargement of the right atrium is seen in association with bicuspidal stenosis. Stasis in the caval veins with secondary stasis in the liver and other abdominal organs with or without ascites is a common complication of increased pressure in the right side of the heart.

Pericardial disease of inflammatory or neoplastic nature may cause pericardial effusion. This gives rise to enlargement of the heart shadow, in many instances without obvious stasis of the lungs. In advanced pericardial effusion, heart movements cannot be seen fluoroscopically.

Herniation of bowel loops and other abdominal organs into the pericardial sac may have a radiographic appearance similar to that of pericardial effusion.

Case 1

Standard poodle, male, 1 year old. Four months prior to admission to the clinic this dog suffered an acute attack of respiratory distress. It recovered and remained normal until the day of admission when the signs suddenly recurred. On examination, all signs of lung edema were noted. Severe dyspnea with foamy discharge from the nostrils and the mouth was present. The animal was somewhat anemic and cyanotic. Its heart rate was 150 per minute and a marked systolic and diastolic murmur could be heard on the left side.

The dog was hospitalized. After 2 days in an oxygen tent and treatment with digitoxin and diuretics considerable improvement was noted. However, because the prognosis was believed to be poor, the animal was euthanatized at the owner's request.

Necropsy: Fibrous endocarditis of the mitral valve. General cardiac enlargement with the left atrium relatively more enlarged than the right atrium and ventricles. There was chronic stasis of the lungs and the liver.

Differential Diagnosis: Because of the typical clinical and radiographic picture, no differential diagnostic problem was presented.

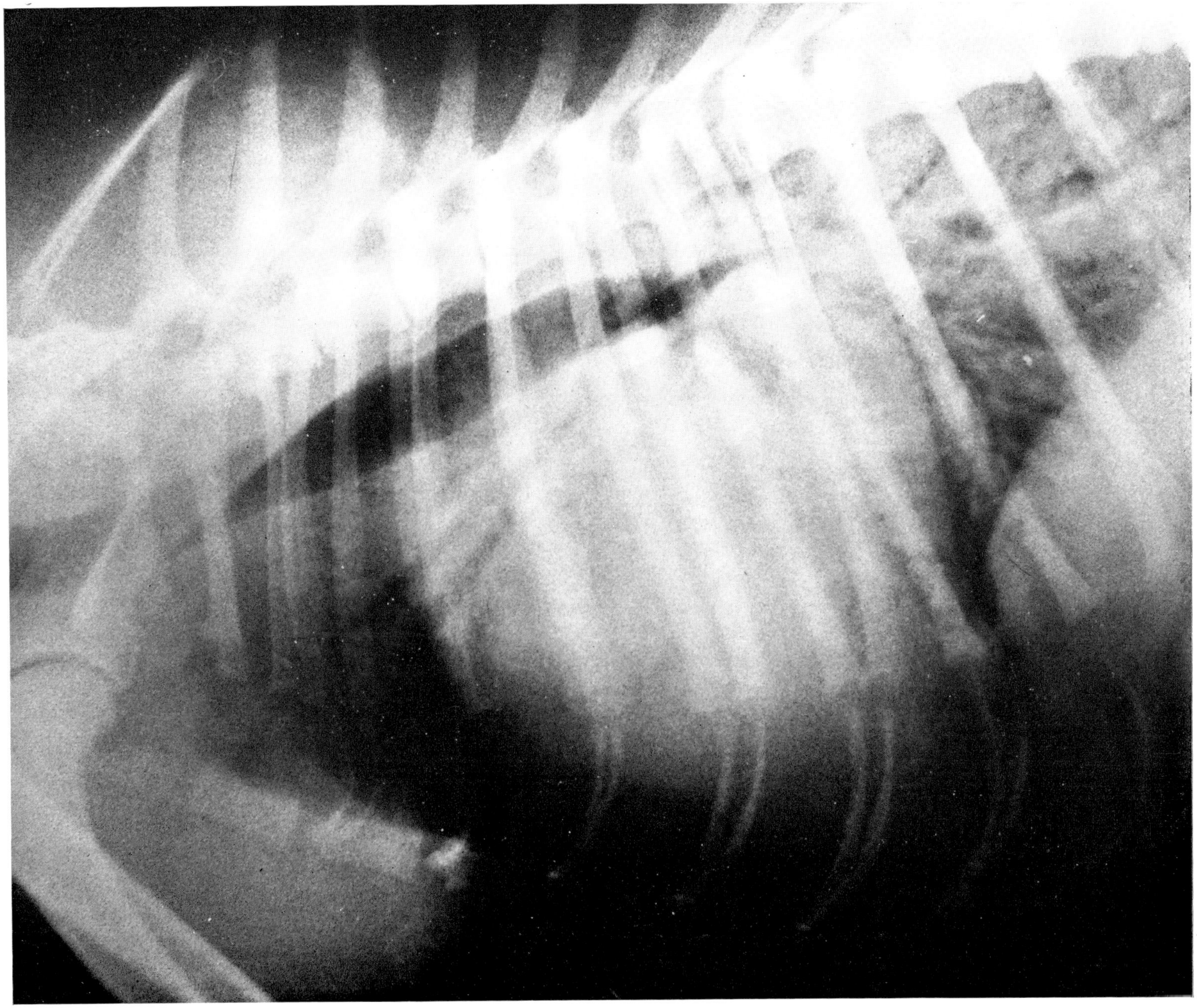

Case 1. **A,** The heart is very enlarged. The trachea is pushed dorsally and the dorsocaudal portion of the heart (the left atrium) is bulging. The lung vessels are very marked, especially near the base of the lungs. The caudal caval vein is elevated. There are coalescing densities in the lung parenchyma. These densities are primarily affecting the central areas near the base of the heart, but they are spread diffusely over the whole lung field. Air-filled bronchi stand out as translucent areas against the consolidated parenchyma, especially in the apical lobes (so-called air bronchogram).

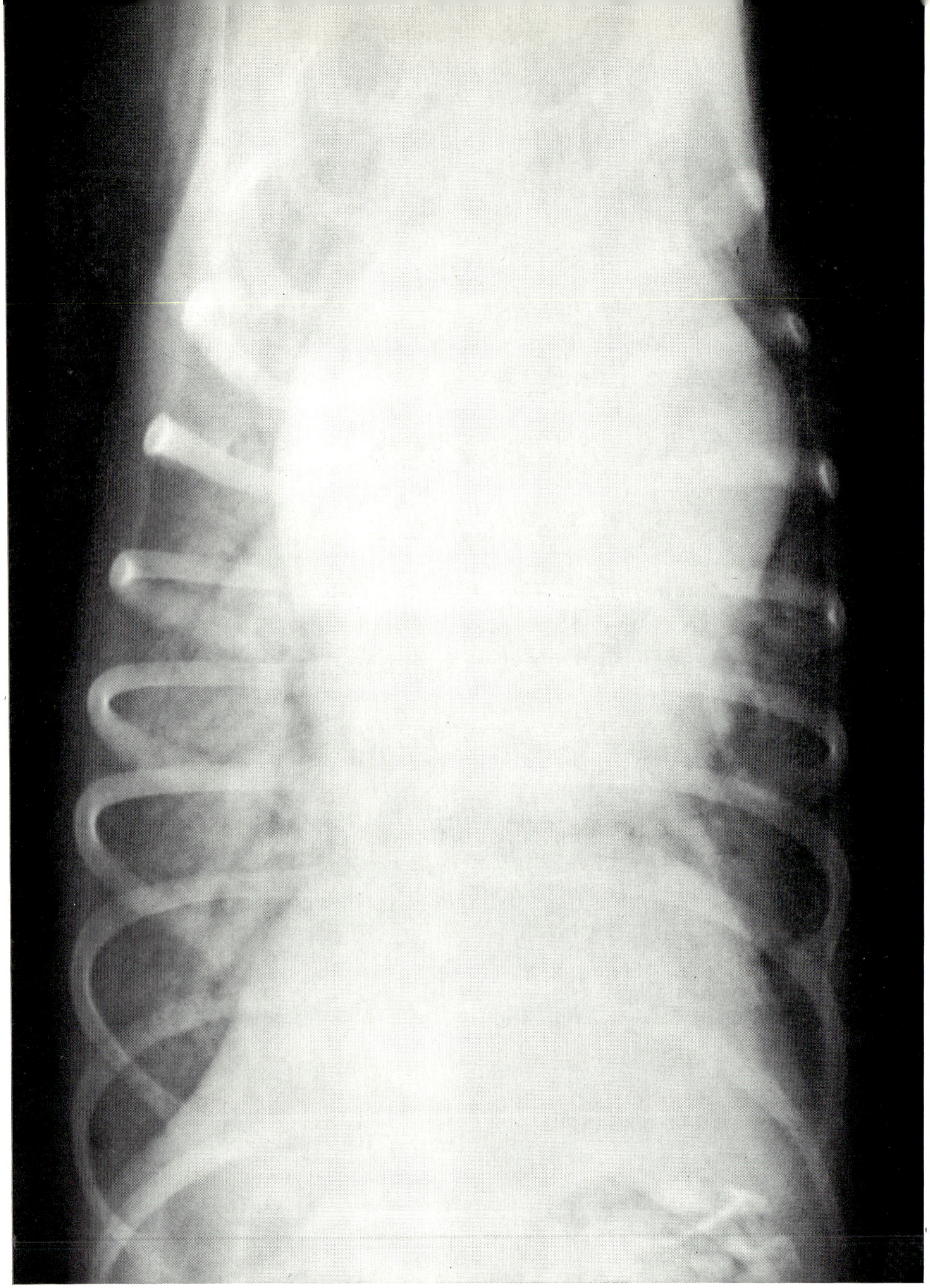

Case 1. **B,** The changes seen in **A,** such as the enlargement of the heart, the densities in the parenchyma, and the air bronchogram, are clearly demonstrable also in the ventrodorsal view. The bulging of the left side of the heart (the left atrium) is especially noteworthy.

Diagnosis: Mitral insufficiency causing enlargement primarily of the left atrium and secondarily of the entire heart. Congestion and edema of the lungs.

Case 2

Old English sheepdog, female, 4 months old. Since weaning, the dog showed signs of circulatory failure, becoming dyspneic after light exercise. The animal was admitted to the clinic in an acute attack of moderate dyspnea and cyanosis. Radiographic examination including angiocardiography revealed a marked stenosis of the tricuspid valve and a right-to-left shunt on the atrial level. An operation was contemplated but the owner requested the release of the dog. A month later the dog suddenly developed signs of acute heart failure with lung edema. It was euthanatized on the owner's request.

Necropsy: The clinical and radiologic diagnosis was confirmed. The tricuspid stenosis was congenital and there was an open foramen ovale.

Differential Diagnosis: There was little question that the dog's problem was primarily of cardiac origin. The involvement of the right atrium pointed to the tricuspid valve as the cause of the circulatory disturbance. The specific nature of the cardiac disease was revealed by angiocardiographic examination.

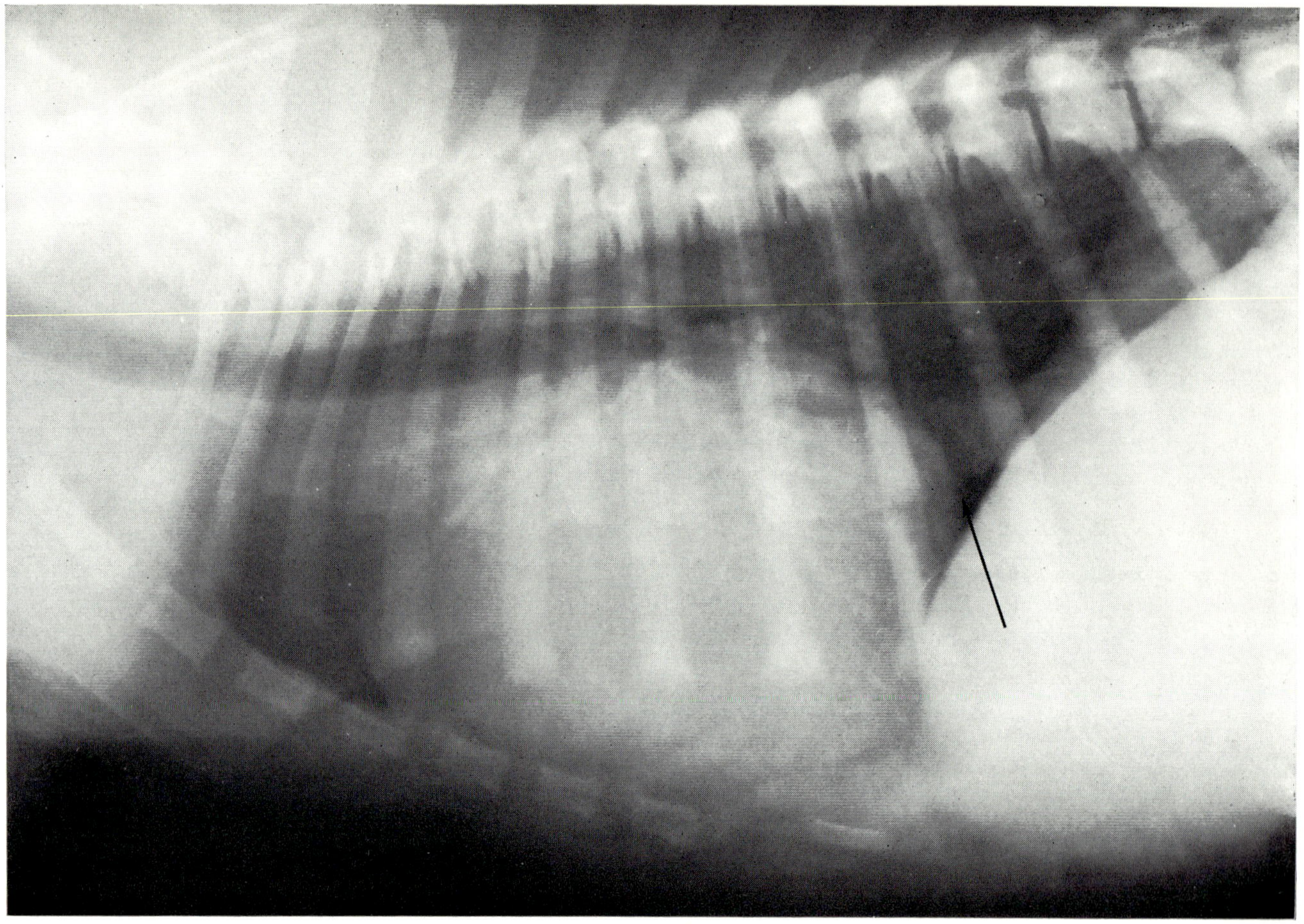

Case 2. **A,** The heart is enlarged. The cranial portion of the cardiac silhouette (the right atrium) is responsible for most of the enlargement. There is no increase in vascularity of the lungs. The caudal caval vein (arrow) is wider than normal, indicating stasis.

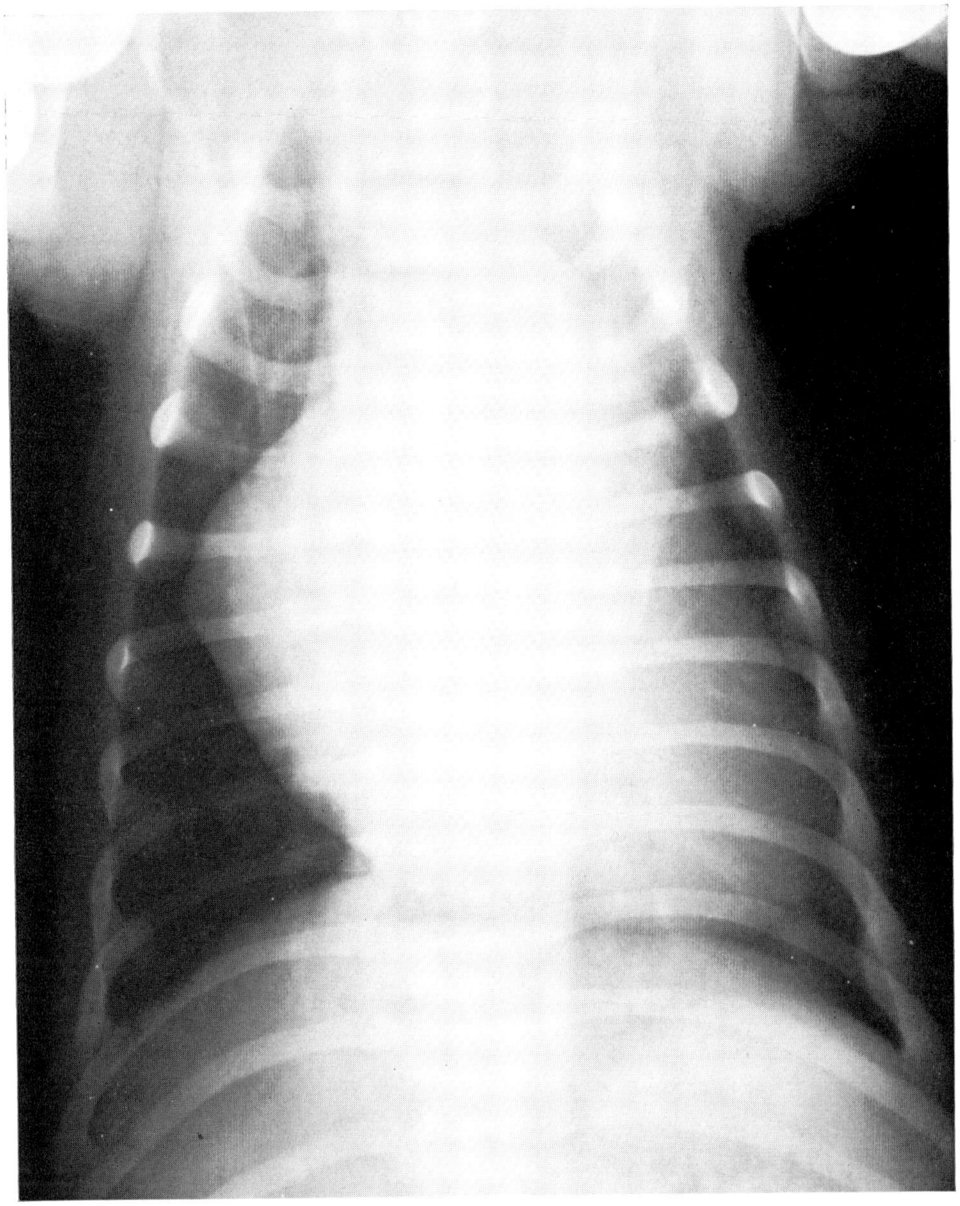

Case 2. **B,** In ventrodorsal view the bulging of the right side of the heart is obvious. The left and caudal part of the heart (the left ventricle) is pushed over to the left side of the thorax.

Diagnosis: Stenosis of the tricuspid valve. Right-to-left shunt through an open foramen ovale.

Case 3

Standard poodle, female, 14 years old. This dog had had difficulties in breathing for several days. It was admitted to the clinic and hospitalized as an emergency patient with very severe dyspnea. The dog was pale, its breathing was wheezing in character, and the heart sounds were weak and rapid. Immediate radiographic examination of the thorax revealed a very large heart shadow. The trachea was pressed against the thoracic spine. The lungs appeared normal with the exception of an area of increased density close to the heart. The low vascularity of the lungs combined with a very large and round heart shadow provided an indication for electrocardiographic and fluoroscopic examinations. As suspected, the ECG showed a low-voltage pattern. No heart movement could be seen at fluoroscopic examination. The diagnosis of pericardial effusion was made. By paracentesis of the pericardial sac, 600 ml of a grayish opaque fluid were withdrawn. On a subsequent radiograph made with the subject in standing lateral position a fluid level was demonstrated in the pericardial sac, thus substantiating the diagnosis of pericardial effusion. The dog was euthanatized.

Necropsy: Pericarditis was found to be the cause of effusion.

Differential Diagnosis: General enlargement of the heart could be the cause of the enlargement of the heart shadow. This was unlikely, however, because of the lack of stasis in the lungs. Definite diagnosis was obtained by fluoroscopy, withdrawal of fluid, and subsequent demonstration of a fluid level. As the cause of pericardial effusion, pericarditis or a heart base tumor was suspected. (The latter is a common cause of pericardial effusion.)

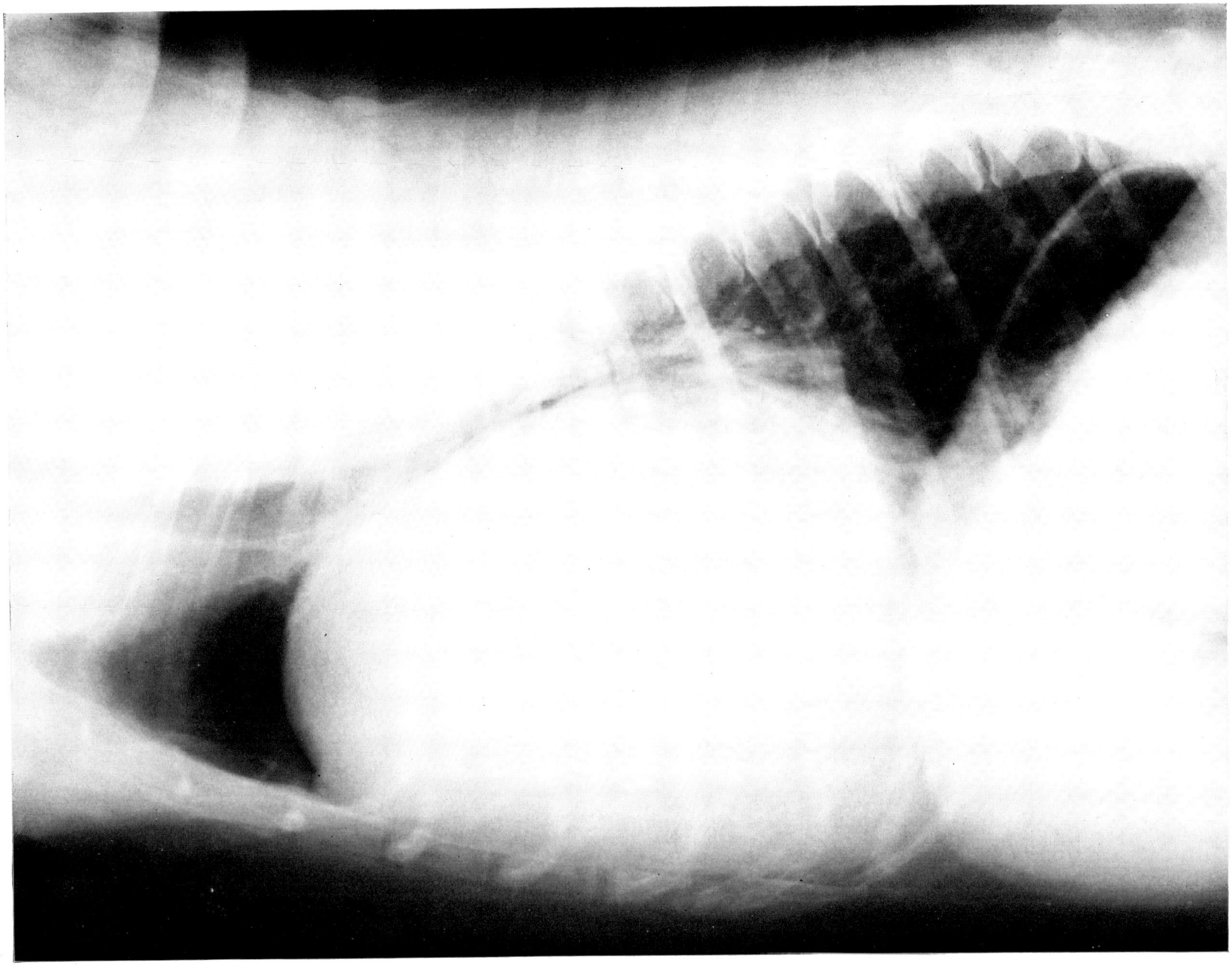

Case 3. **A,** The heart shadow is very large and round. There is no stasis in the lungs, only a slight increase in density, probably due to atelectasis, at the base of the lungs.

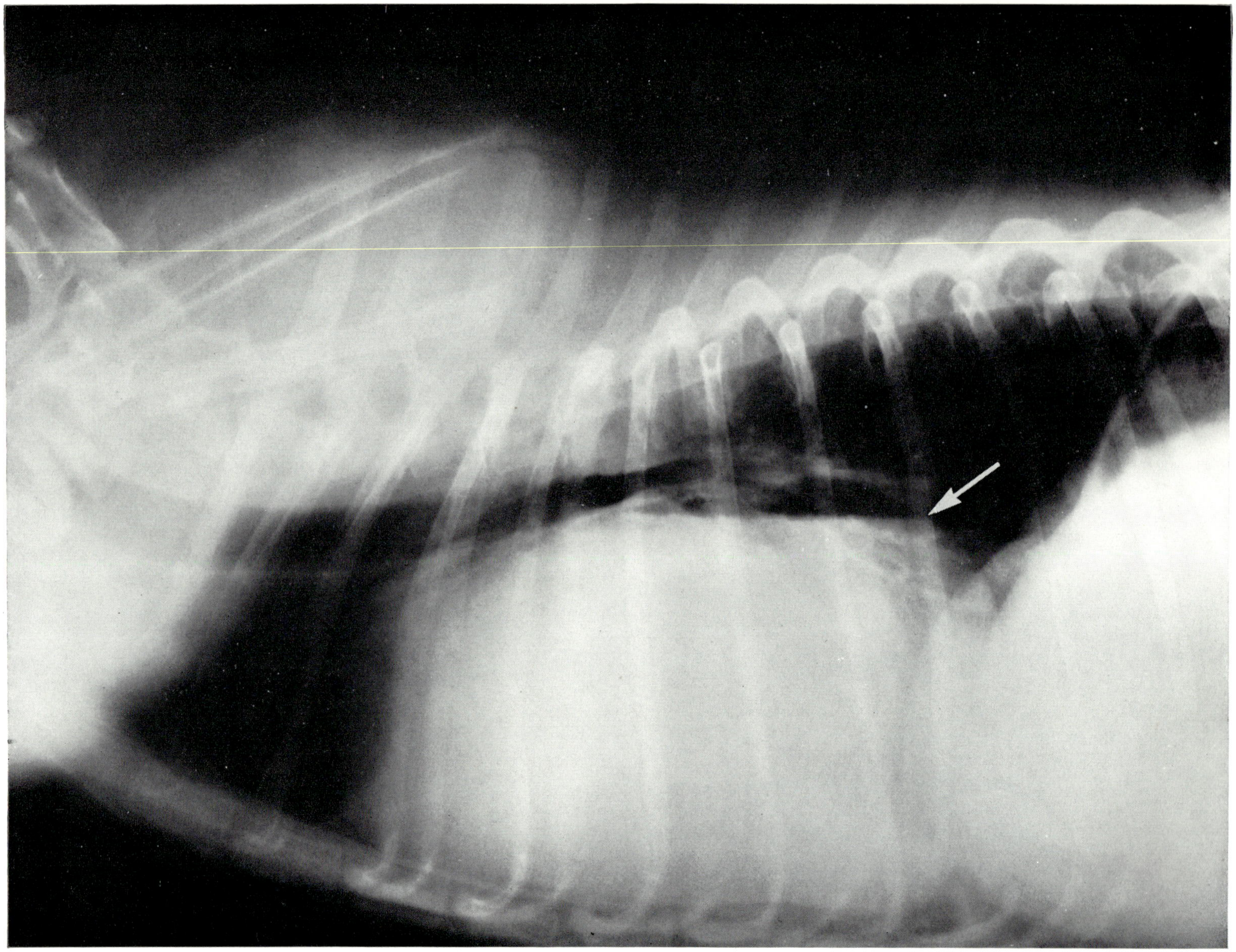

Case 3. **B,** This radiograph was made with the subject in standing lateral position after withdrawal of 600 ml of fluid. A fluid level can be demonstrated in the pericardial sac (arrow). The heart shadow is only slightly smaller than on the radiograph made before paracentesis. A large amount of flu'd remains in the pericardial sac.

Diagnosis: Pericarditis causing pericardial effusion.

Case 4

Dachshund, male, 4 weeks old. This puppy, one of a litter of four, was normal in development and weight gain. One day it suddenly became listless and dyspneic. On admission to the clinic it was in severe respiratory distress.

Immediate radiographic examination revealed changes in the thoracic cavity. There was an enlarged heart shadow and stasis in the lungs. A GI series revealed that many loops of bowel were lodged in the pericardial sac. The diagnosis of peritoneo-pericardial diaphragmatic hernia was made and the puppy was operated upon the following day. Recovery was uneventful.

Differential Diagnosis: The enlarged heart shadow could be a sign of congenital malformation of the heart. The sudden onset and the finding of a gas-filled bowel loop in the thoracic cavity indicated a hernia. The GI series then made the differential diagnosis easy to make.

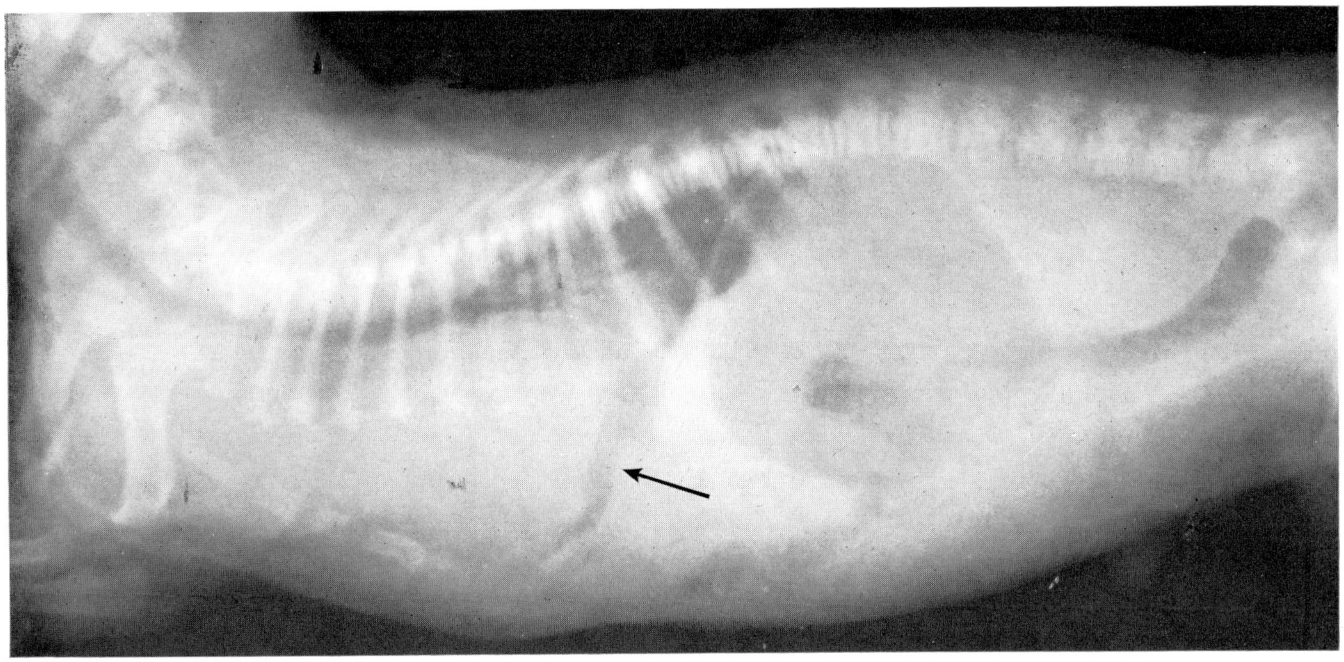

Case 4. **A,** There is a large, somewhat diffuse heart shadow with increased vascularity (stasis) of the lungs. A gas-filled structure (arrow), suggestive of a bowel loop, is located within the thoracic cavity along the diaphragm.

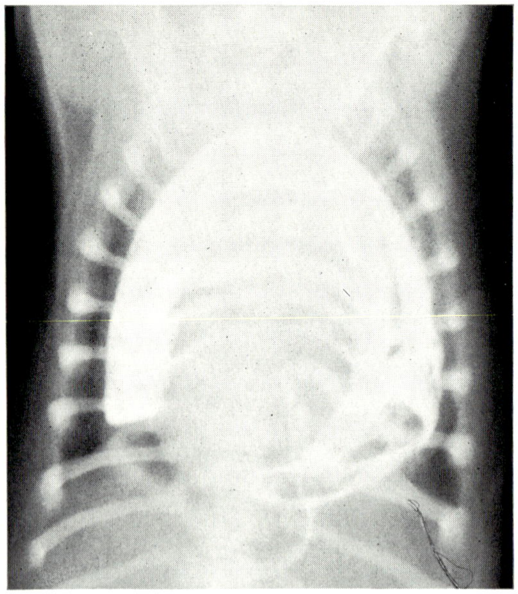

Case 4. **B,** Ventrodorsal radiograph made 10 minutes after administration of a small barium swallow. Loops of the small intestine encircle the heart.

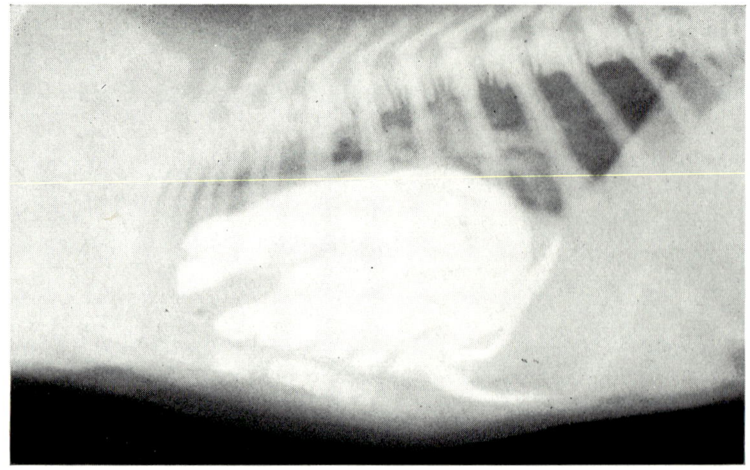

Case 4. **C,** On this lateral radiograph the barium-filled bowel loops cover the heart. The entrance to the pericardial sac from the abdomen is in the midline of the diaphragm on the ventral side, as can be seen here and on radiograph **B**.

Diagnosis: Congenital peritoneo-pericardial diaphragmatic hernia. (Direct communication between the abdominal cavity and the pericardial sac.)

Chapter 2

The Lungs, the Pleura, the Esophagus, and the Diaphragm

The radiographic appearance of pneumonia, pulmonary edema and hemorrhage, mediastinal emphysema and pneumothorax, foreign body in the esophagus, pleural effusion, hemothorax, and diaphragmatic hernia is illustrated in this chapter.

When making radiographs of the chest of animals in respiratory and/or circulatory distress it is necessary to employ a short exposure time (less than 0.05 second) and to use as little restraint as possible.

It is sometimes difficult to differentiate clinically between diseases of the lungs and those of the heart. Differential diagnosis is facilitated by radiograhic examination.

For correct interpretation of radiographs of the lungs it is fundamental to keep in mind that in the normal lung only the vessels and the larger bronchi are visible on the radiographs. The fluid-filled vessels and the walls of the larger bronchi stand out against the air-filled lung parenchyma, which appears dark on the radiograph. When the lungs become consolidated the difference in density between the parenchyma and the vessels disappears. Instead, the air-filled bronchi stand out against the fluid-filled alveoli of the parenchyma, producing a so-called air bronchogram.

Pneumonia is usually bilateral and in most cases localized to the ventral part of the lungs. One or several lobes may be involved. The borders between the normal (air-filled) and consolidated (fluid-filled) lobes are usually very distinct and therefore easy to demonstrate on radiographs. Aspiration of food or foreign bodies gives rise to a circumscript, often unilateral pneumonia, frequently localized to one of the diaphragmatic lobes. In aspiration pneumonia, abscesses sometimes complicate the picture.

Pulmonary hemorrhage may occasionally be difficult to differentiate radiographically from pneumonia. In these cases only the clinical history can give the clue to the correct diagnosis.

Pulmonary edema can occur with or without involvement of the heart, i.e., it can be circulatory or pulmonary in origin. The main features of edema are basically the same as those of pneumonia, but edema is usually more patchy in appearance than pneumonia, without lobar localization, and as a rule is bilaterally symmetric. Hence, distinct lobar borders are not seen. If edema is of cardiac origin, it is usually preceded by and combined with severe stasis of the lungs.

Under normal conditions, negative pressure in the thoracic cavity keeps the lungs expanded. If air leaks into the pleural cavity or if there is pleural effusion or hemorrhage, the lungs become partially collapsed. The poorly expanded lungs are more radiopaque than normally expanded lungs. The lung lobes are also separated by air or fluid. In pneumothorax the space between the thoracic wall and the lungs and the space between the lobes are filled by air, i.e., they look "empty" on the radiograph. If there is hemorrhage or effusion, these spaces are more radiopaque than are the atelectatic lung lobes. In doubtful cases, standing lateral radiographs are useful for demonstration of fluid levels. It has to be remembered, however, that air or fluid in the thoracic cavity can be demonstrated on radiographs made with a vertical beam with the subject in the lateral or dorsal recumbent position.

A foreign body in the esophagus is usually easy to diagnose radiographically. In most cases it has enough radiopacity to stand out clearly against the air-filled lungs. A foreign body of little radiopacity lodged in the esophagus dorsal to the heart may, however, be difficult to detect. Special attention should be paid to the soft-tissue structures surrounding a foreign body in the esophagus. Increased density of these structures indicates severe injury with necrosis and inflammation of the wall of the esophagus involving the mediastinum and pleura.

A diaphragmatic hernia is easier to diagnose radiographically than clinically and is seldom overlooked if the animal is radiographed. It is more common that pleural effusion or tumors are misdiagnosed as a diaphragmatic hernia. If bowel loops are herniated, GI series will, however, reveal the true nature of the condition.

Diseases of the lungs, such as primary and metastatic tumors, bronchiectasis, and emphysema, run a chronic course. Many animals are first seen in the clinic as emergency cases having extreme respiratory and circulatory signs when in the final stages of these diseases. This should be kept in mind when radiographs of pulmonary emergency cases are being interpreted.

Case 5

Poodle, female, 6 years old. Two weeks prior to admission to the clinic this dog developed tonsilitis and was treated with penicillin without any obvious effect. Instead of improvement a violent cough developed. Tetracycline was administered, but the dog's condition continued to deteriorate. It was referred to the clinic a few hours after severe dyspnea had complicated the picture. On admission the animal was in marked respiratory distress and could not lie down. Rales and ronchi could be heard in both lungs. Radiographs revealed areas of increased density in both lungs and the bronchial pattern was more marked than normal. The dog was hospitalized. A serologic test showed a high titer for toxoplasmosis. This prompted a change in therapy from tetracycline to spiramycine.

The dog improved. Radiographs made a week later showed disappearance of the densities in the parenchyma.

Differential Diagnosis: The radiologic picture is typical of that of bronchitis and pneumonia. There is nothing in the radiograph that indicates a specific cause such as toxoplasmosis, mycosis, or tuberculosis. These diseases are usually characterized by more disseminated, often miliary, infiltrates in the parenchyma. In tuberculosis the lymph nodes at the base of the lungs are enlarged.

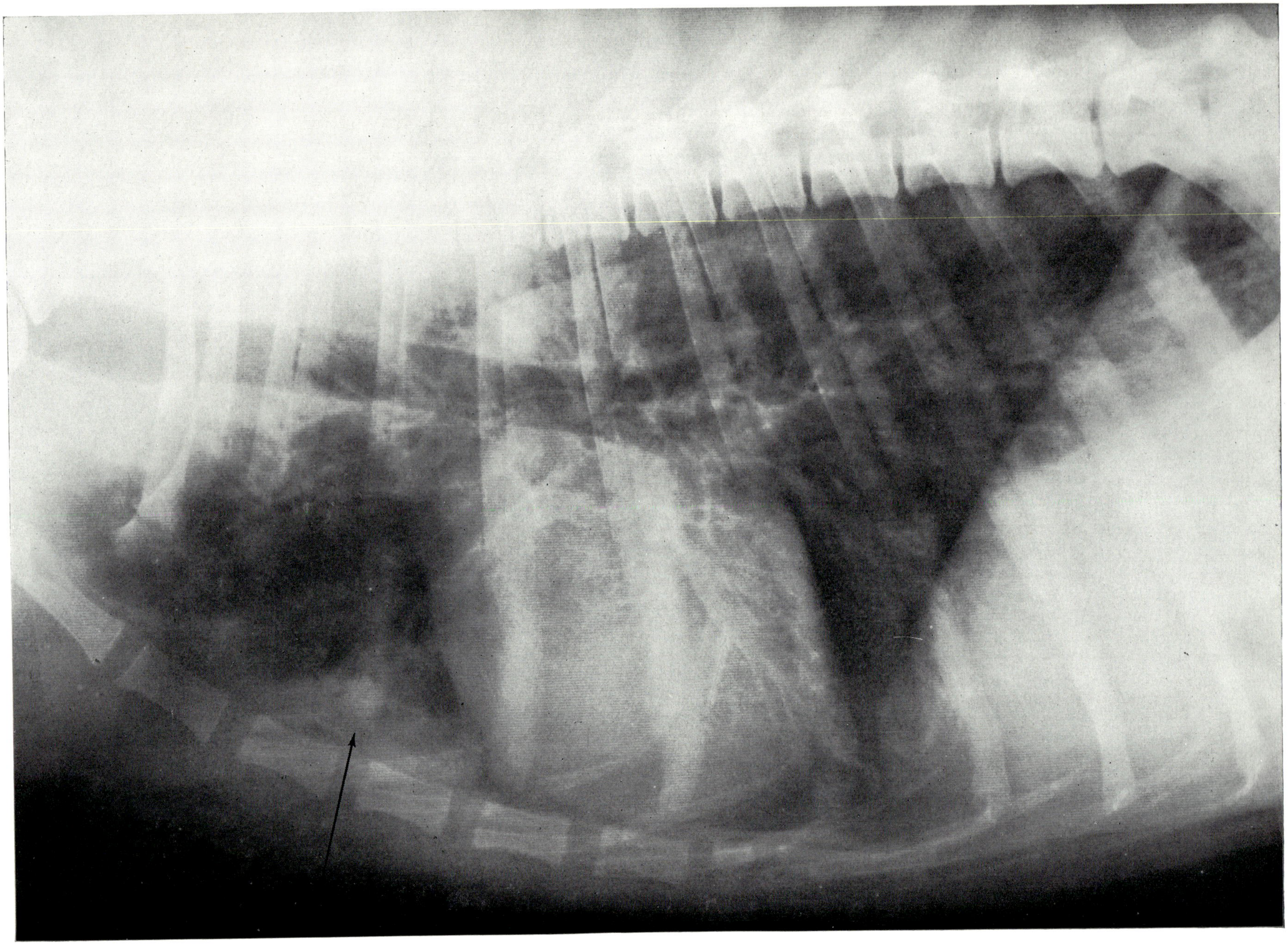

Case 5. **A,** The bronchial pattern is more marked than normal in the entire lung field owing to an increased density of the bronchial walls. There are several diffuse, partly confluent parenchymatous radiopacities most marked in the apical lobes (arrow).

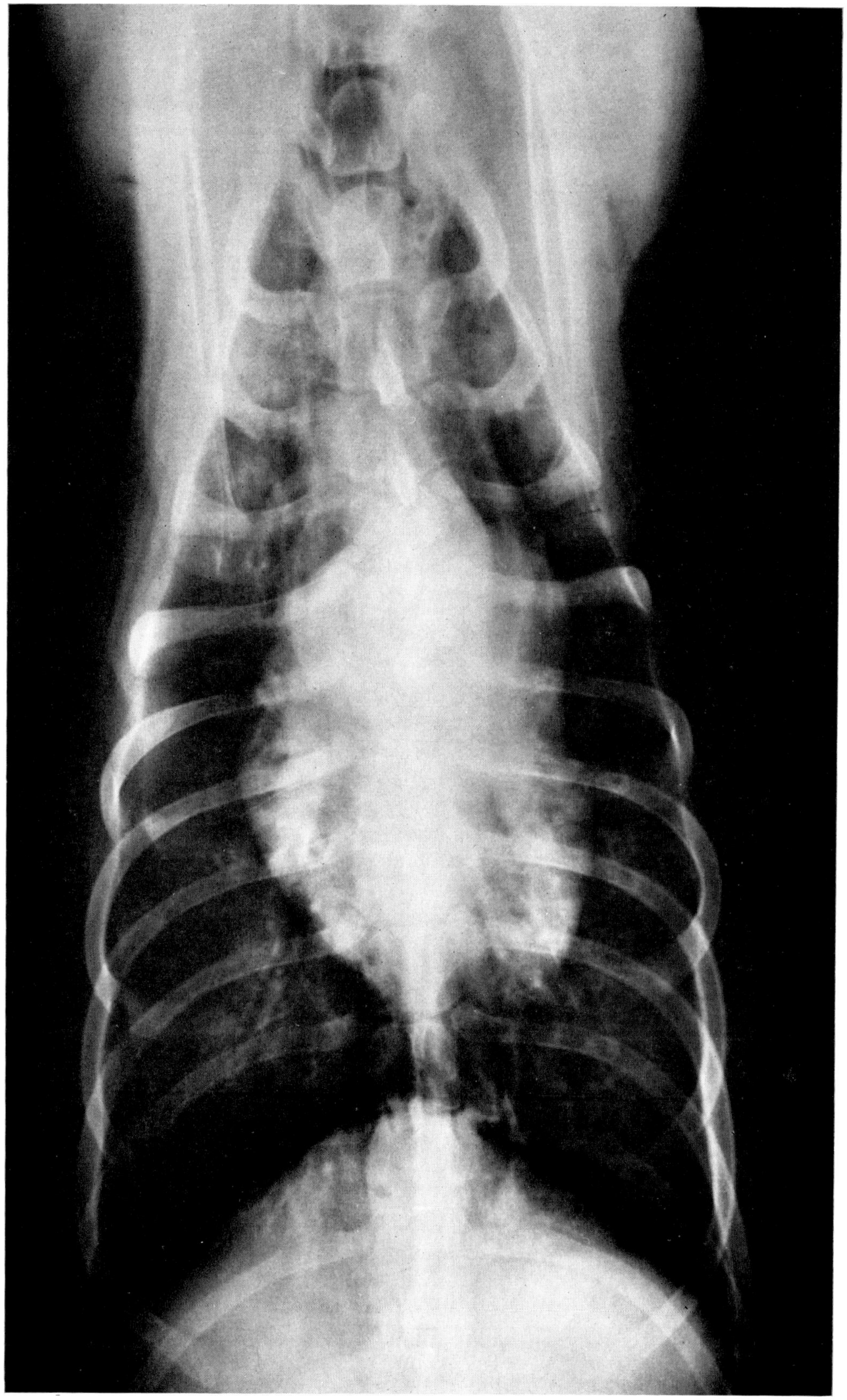

Case 5. **B,** As is seen in this ventrodorsal radiograph, there are marked consolidations in the apical lobes. There are some densities in the cardiac and diaphragmatic lobes with obvious increase of the bronchial pattern.

Diagnosis: Bronchitis and pneumonia.

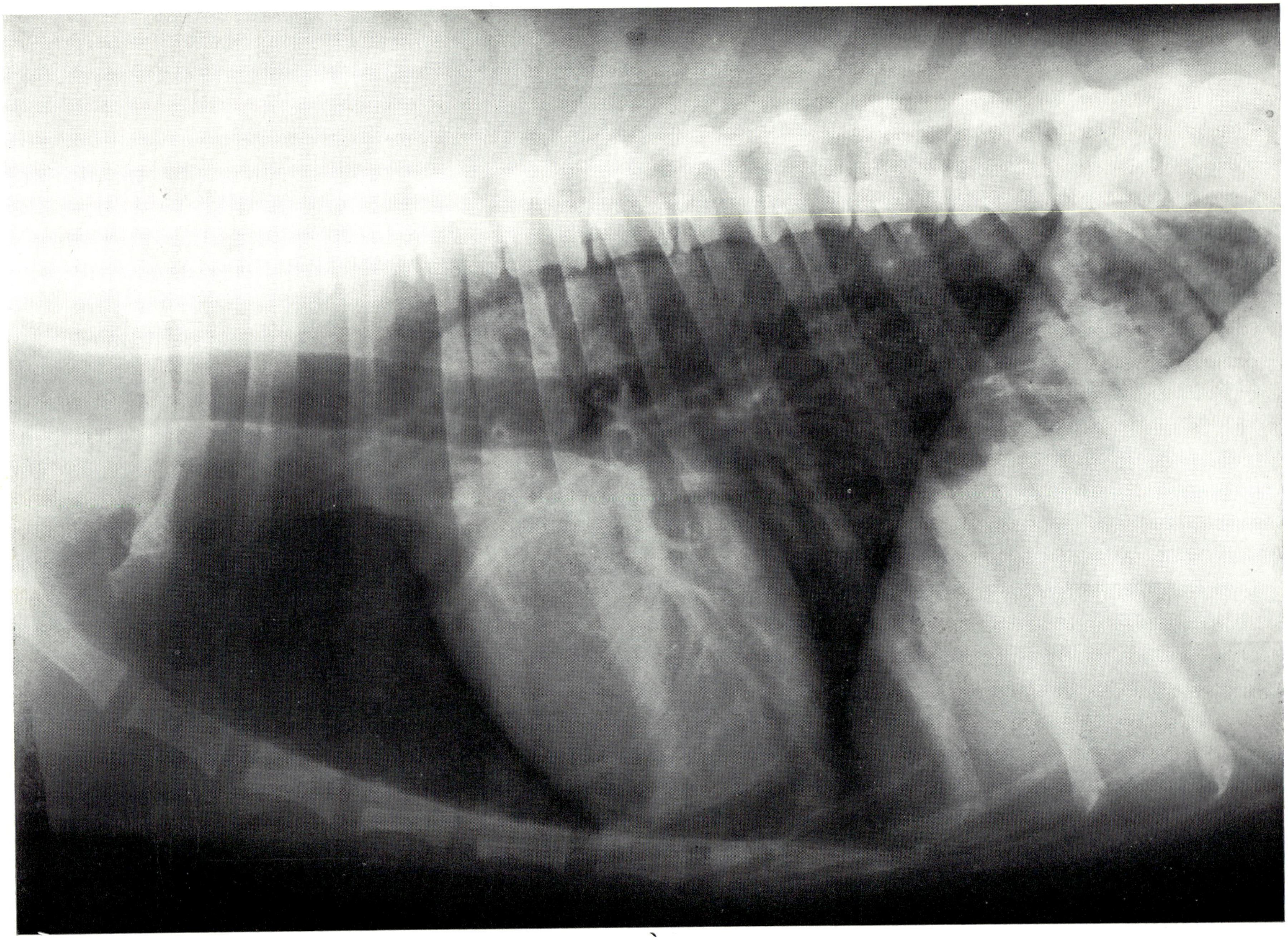

Case 5. **C**

Case 5. **C** and **D,** The densities seen in **A** and **B** have been resolved. The bronchial pattern is nearly normal.

Diagnosis: Disappearance of pathologic changes. Normal lungs with the exception of some remaining slight increase in thickness of the bronchial walls.

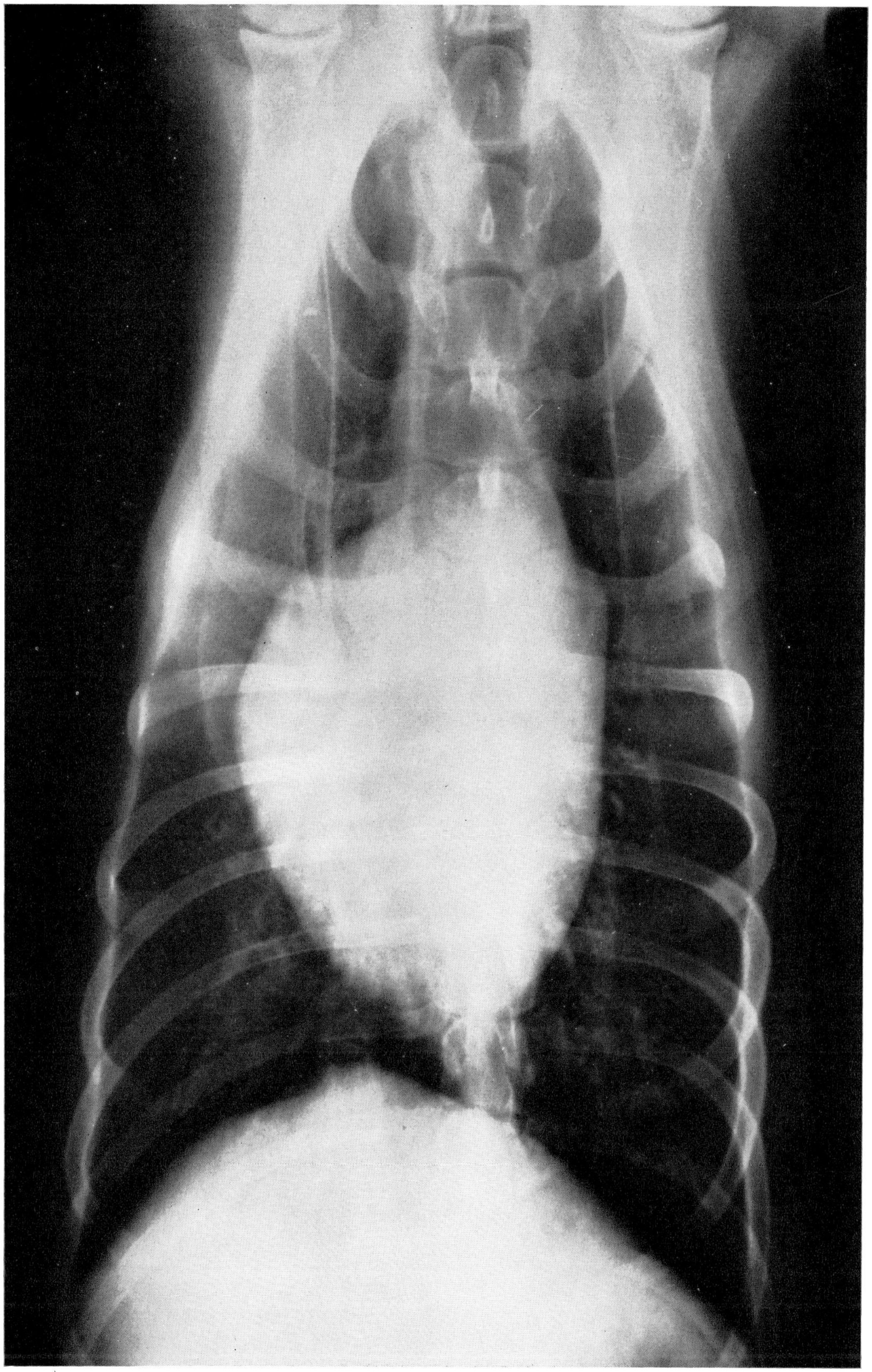

D

Case 6

Cat, male, 3 years old. During the course of one day this cat developed high fever, cough, and dyspnea. On admission it was in poor general condition and slightly cyanotic, and had marked dyspnea. Rales and ronchi could be heard in both lungs. Radiographs revealed mottled densities in the lung parenchyma. These densities were confluent in the apical and cardiac lobes. The diagnosis of pneumonia was made. The animal was treated with chlortetracycline for one week. Recovery was uneventful.

Differential Diagnosis: On the radiographs there were all the characteristic changes of pneumonia and no diagnostic problem arose.

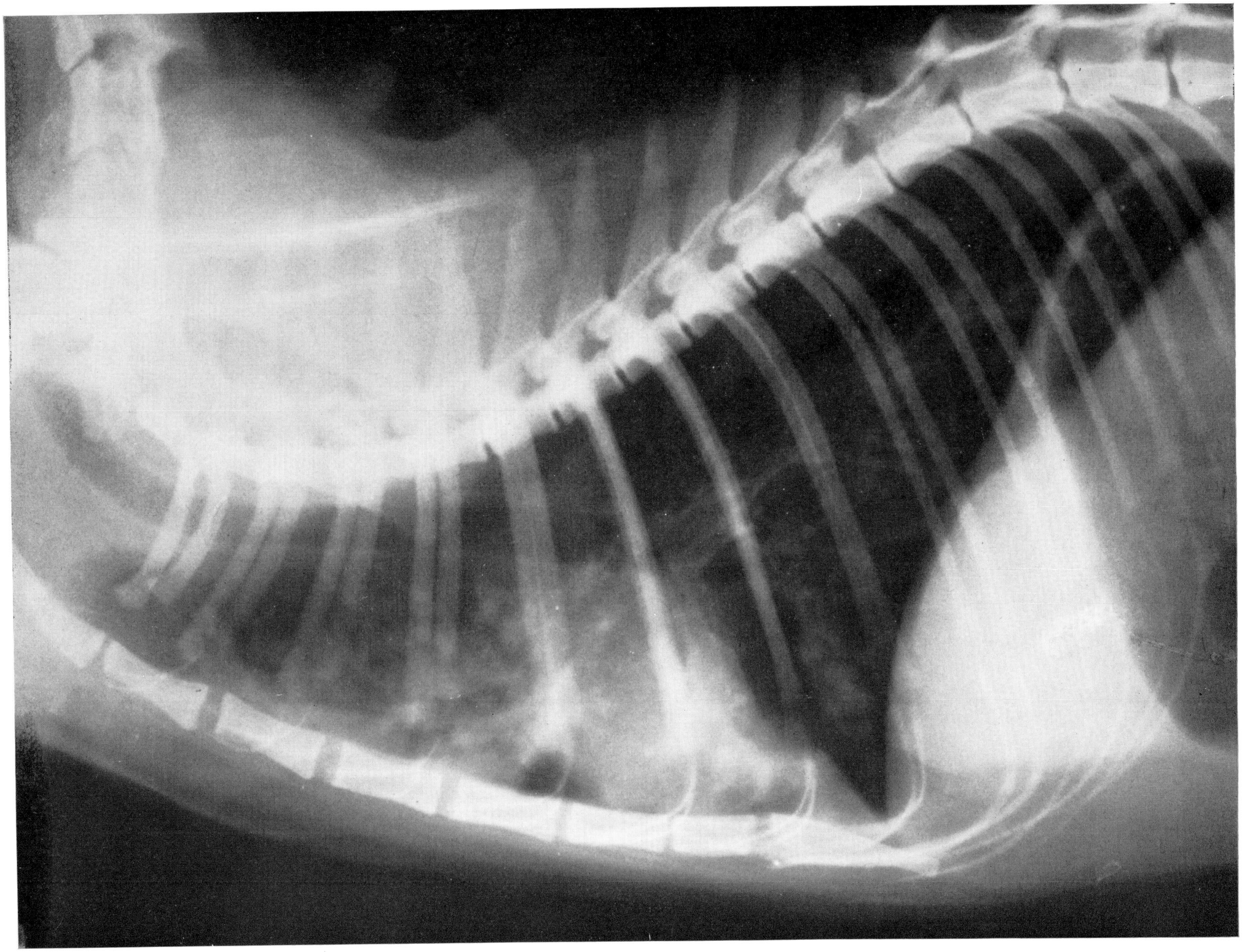

Case 6. **A,** Mottled densities in the ventral parts of the lungs. The apical, the cardiac, and the diaphragmatic lobes are involved.

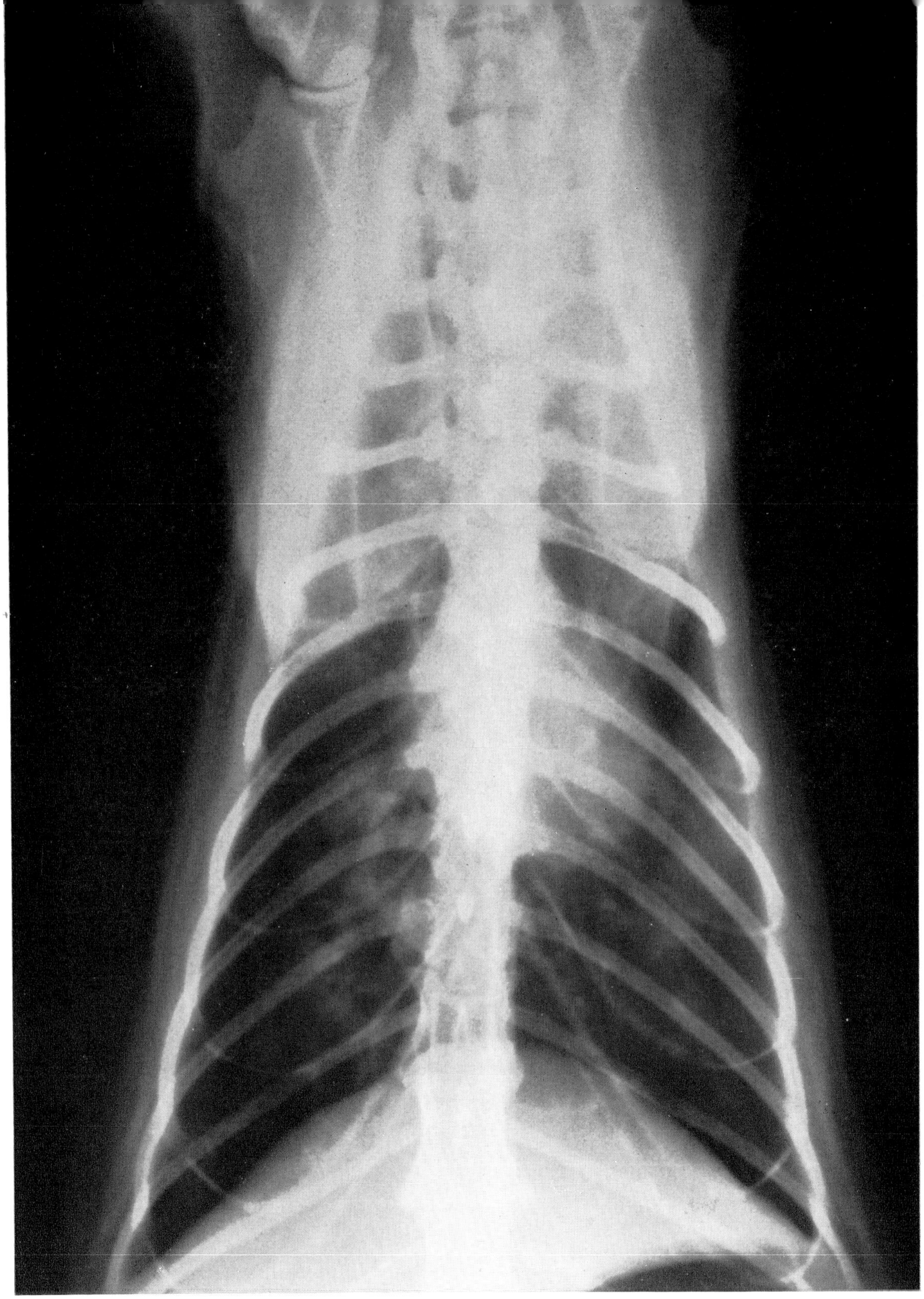

Case 6. **B,** In this ventrodorsal radiograph the densities in the cardiac lobes and in the right diaphragmatic lobe are easily recognized. Similar changes in the apical lobes are partially hidden by the scapulae and the muscles.

Diagnosis: Pneumonia.

Case 7

Dachshund, male, 10 years old. This dog had been listless for several days. Twenty-four hours prior to admission to the clinic it developed a deep cough and dyspnea. On admission it was afebrile but had severe dyspnea. Rales and ronchi could be heard in the right lung. Radiographs revealed a circumscript density in the parenchyma of the right cardiac lobe. The diagnosis of pneumonia was made. Chloramphenicol and prednisolone were given to the dog for a week. Recovery was uneventful.

Differential Diagnosis: Pneumonia may not be diagnosed radiographically if it is only affecting the cardiac lobes. Slightly oblique radiographs are necessary for detection. Once the isolated density in the right cardiac lobe of the present patient was found, there was little question about the diagnosis.

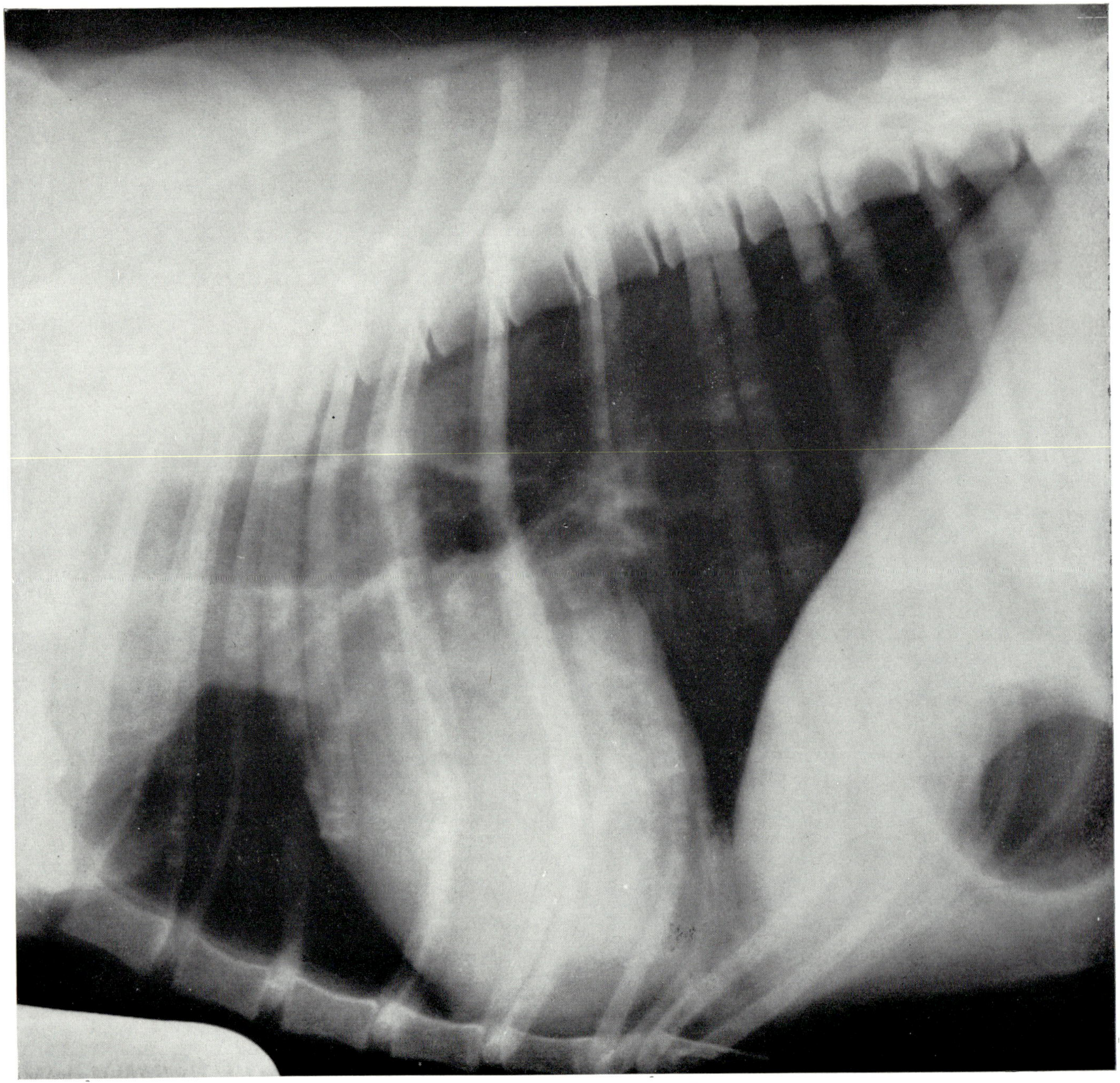

Case 7. **A,** The heart shadow is of normal size and shape, but appears more dense than normal (compare with radiograph **C,** Case 5). The vascular pattern of the cardiac lobes overlapping the heart cannot be seen; instead, on close inspection, a few air-filled bronchi can be seen (so-called air bronchogram).

Case 7. **B,** On this radiograph, made in slightly oblique projection, a consolidation is seen in the parenchyma (arrow). It is located in the right cardiac lobe close to the heart. This consolidation is more or less obscured by the heart shadow both in the lateral view and in the straight ventrodorsal view. A "transverse section" of a bronchus stands out as a dark, round area against the consolidation.

Diagnosis: Pneumonia localized to part of the right cardiac lobe.

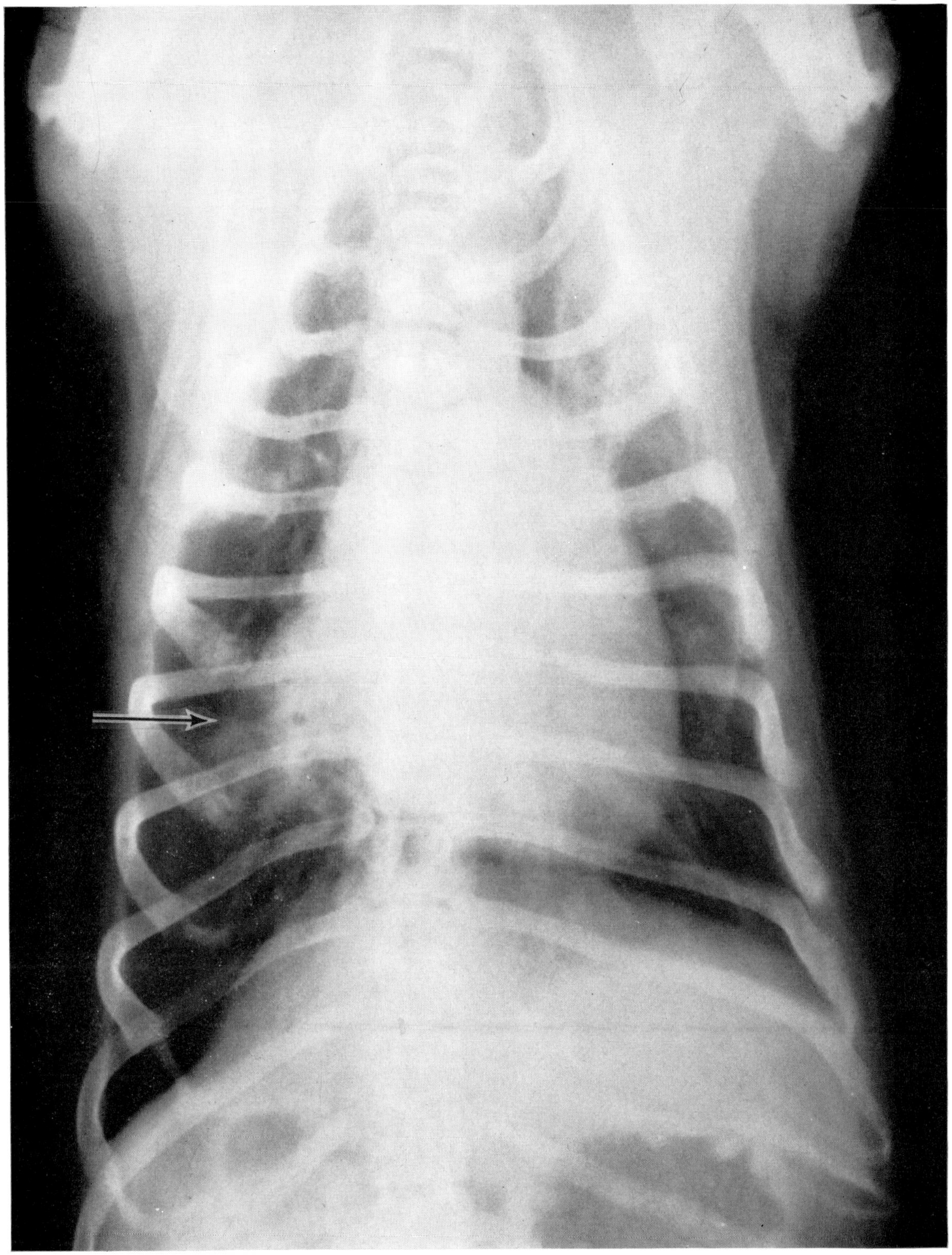

Case 8

Standard poodle, female, $2\frac{1}{2}$ years old. A few days prior to admission to the clinic this dog started to vomit. After a day it developed a severe cough. On admission, cough, slight dyspnea, increased respiratory sounds, and dehydration were noted. The temperature was 39.7° C. Radiographs of the lungs revealed an increased vascular pattern and a well-delineated consolidation in the left diaphragmatic lobe. The diagnosis of aspiration pneumonia was made. Saline and glucose solutions were given parenterally and the dog was hospitalized and treated with chloramphenicol. Recovery was complete within a week.

Differential Diagnosis: The radiographic appearance of the density was typical for pneumonia. On the other hand, the site was atypical for regular bronchopneumonia which usually is localized ventrally in the lungs. The location of the parenchymatous density in this case indicated aspiration as the cause of pneumonia.

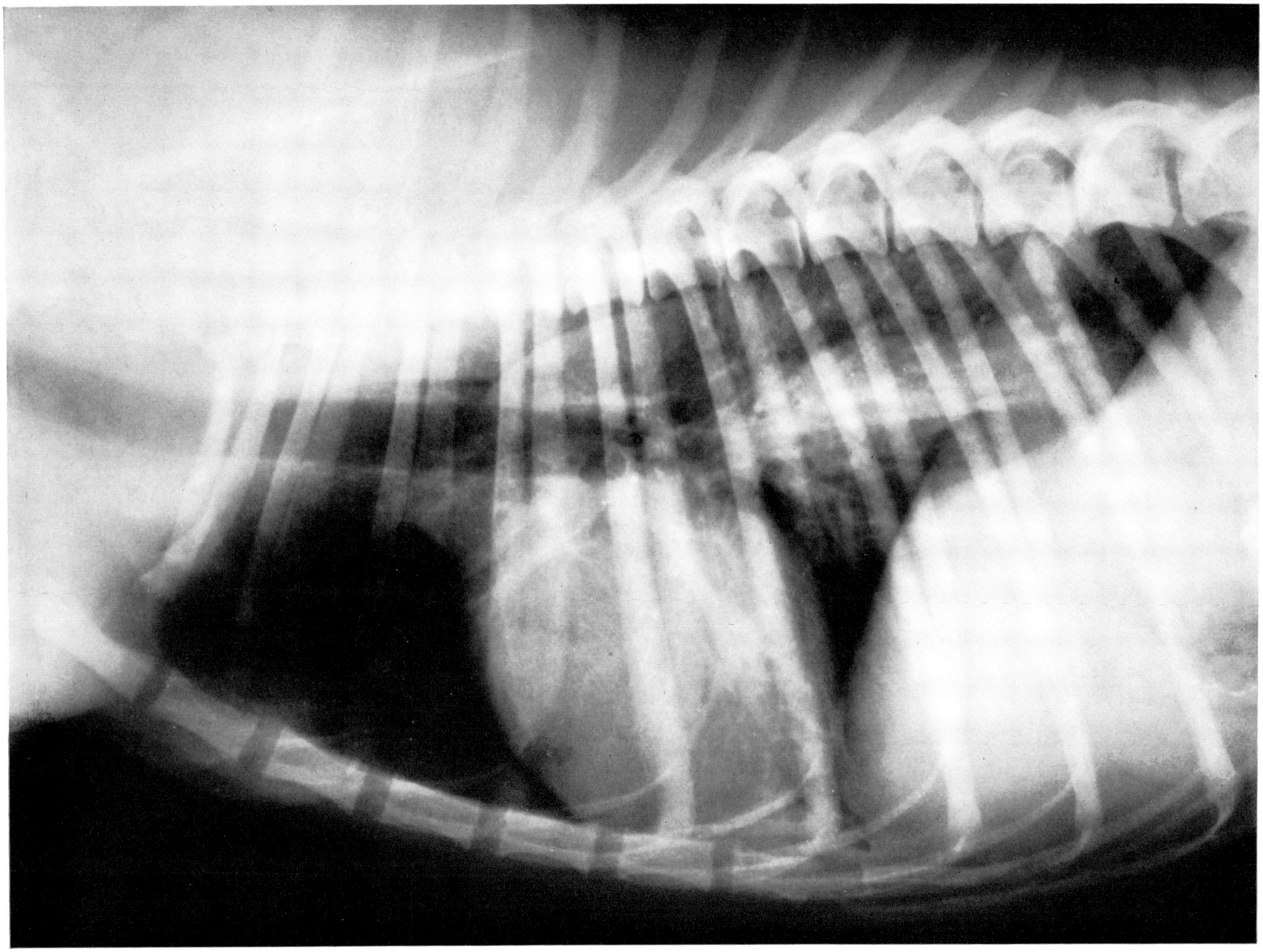

Case 8. **A,** There is a marked consolidation in the lung parenchyma caudal to the base of the heart and minor consolidations superimposed on the heart. The bronchial and vascular patterns of the entire lung field are somewhat more marked than normal.

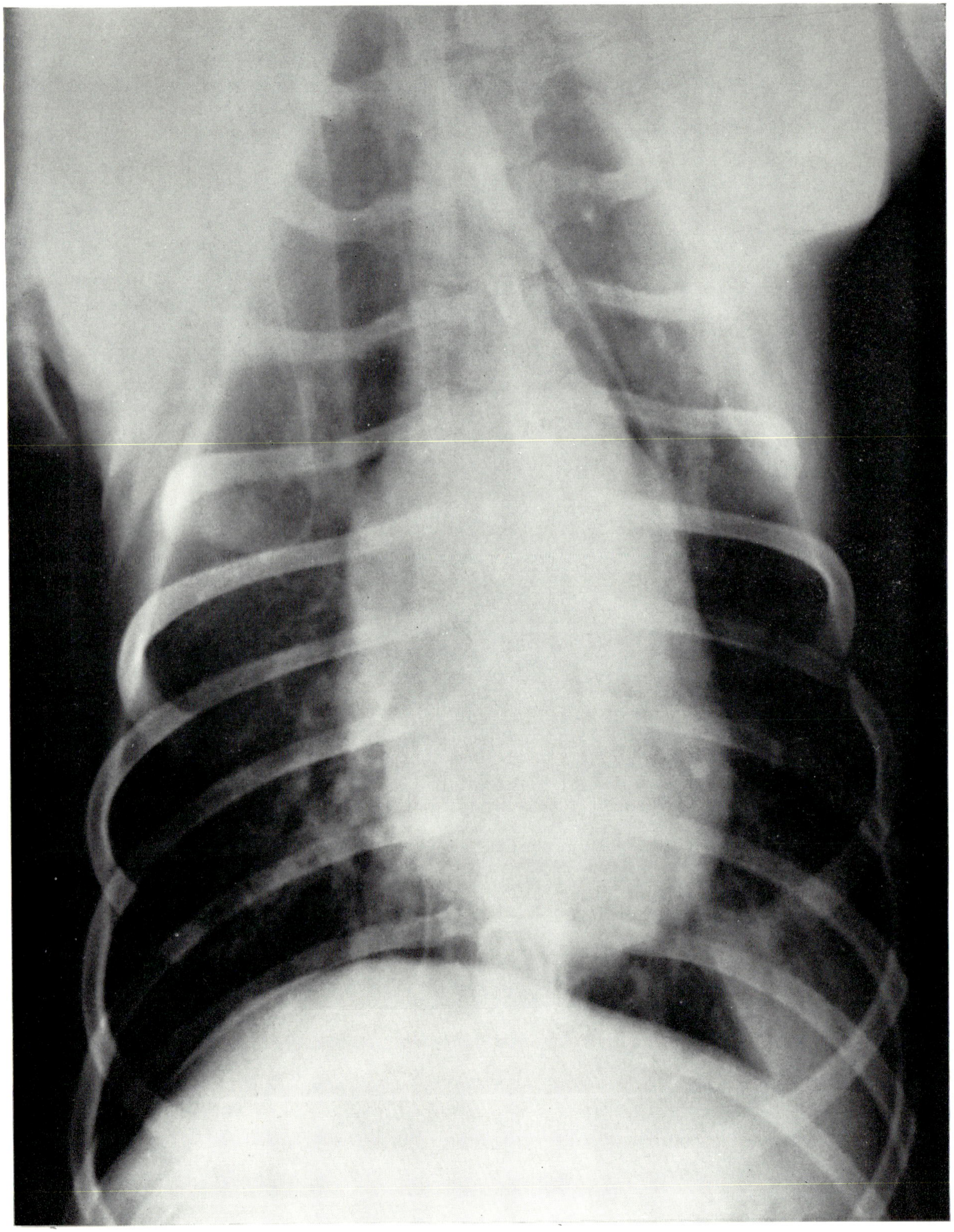

Case 8. **B,** In this ventrodorsal radiograph there is diffuse consolidation of part of the right cardiac lobe and a well-delineated consolidation in the left diaphragmatic lobe. There is a sharp demarcation line between the diseased part of the left diaphragmatic lobe and the normal intermediate lobe. There is an evident "air bronchogram" in the consolidated lung parenchyma.

Diagnosis: Pneumonia. The location and clinical history indicate aspiration as the cause.

Case 9

Miniature poodle, male, 4 months old. This dog was referred to the clinic because of severe dyspnea, which had begun while it was being clipped. On admission the animal suffered from respiratory distress, which was so severe that it refused to lie down. The respiratory sounds were very marked, but the heart sounds were weak. A diffuse radiographic density of both lungs was considered to be a sign of pulmonary edema. The dog was hospitalized and treated with lanatoside C and diuretics. Recovery was rapid and uneventful.

Differential Diagnosis: The main differential diagnostic concern in this case was pneumonia versus edema of the lungs. On the radiograph the diffuse bilateral density is very widespread and this speaks in favor of lung edema. Pneumonia involving the lungs to such a degree would hardly be compatible with life. The sudden onset of clinical signs also points towards lung edema as the most probable cause of the radiographic changes. In pneumonia the ventral parts of the lungs are usually more involved than the dorsal. In this case the base of the lungs was more dense than the periphery of the lungs, indicating a vascular origin of the density. The diagnosis of edema was, however, seriously questioned since the density is not completely symmetrical, the left lung being more dense than the right.

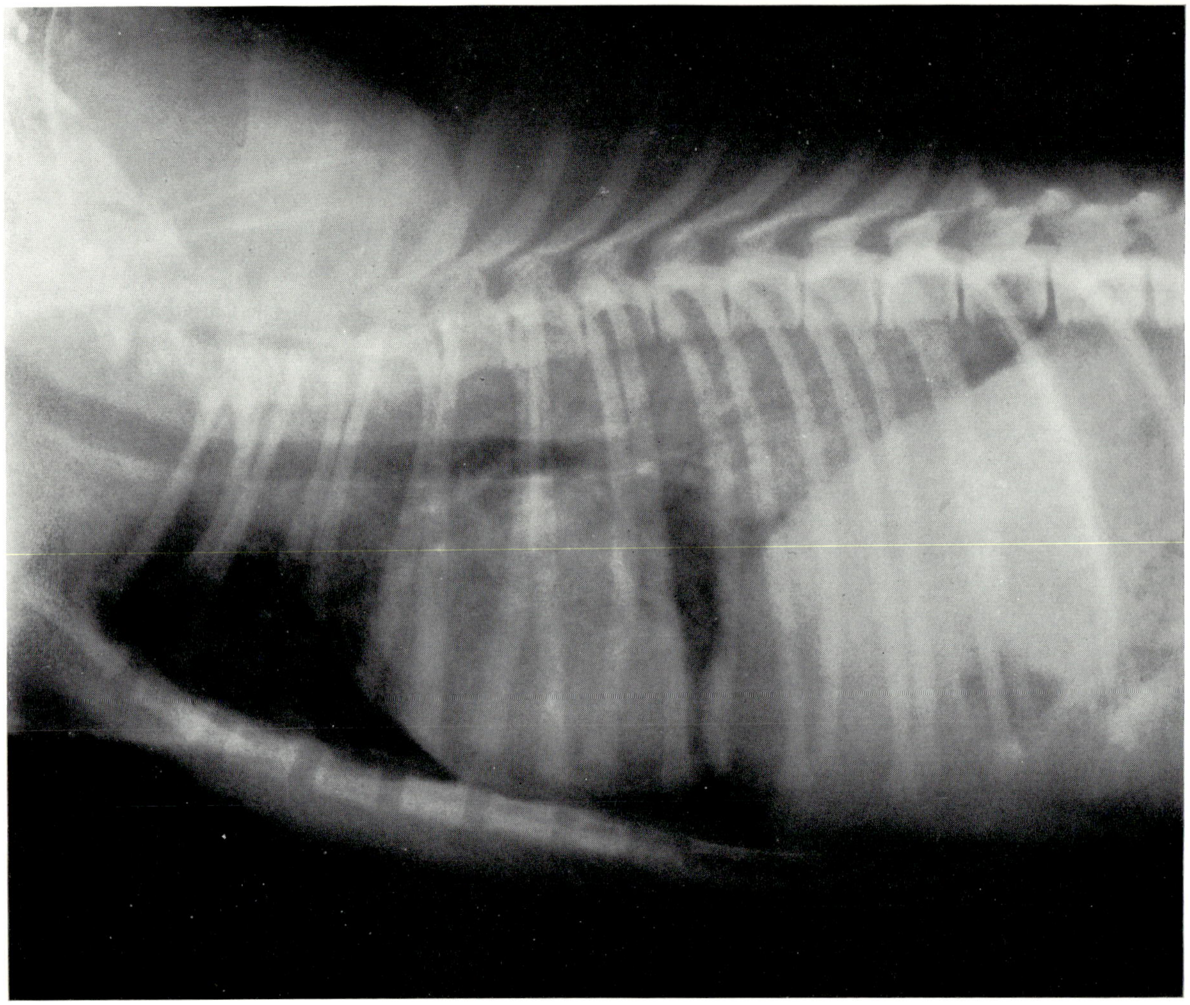

Case 9. **A,** There is a slightly enlarged heart shadow. The dorsal part of the lung field is very dense while the ventral appears only slightly denser than normal.

Case 9. **B,** There is a homogeneous density of the entire lung field on the left side. The density is less marked in the right lung.

Diagnosis: Pulmonary edema.

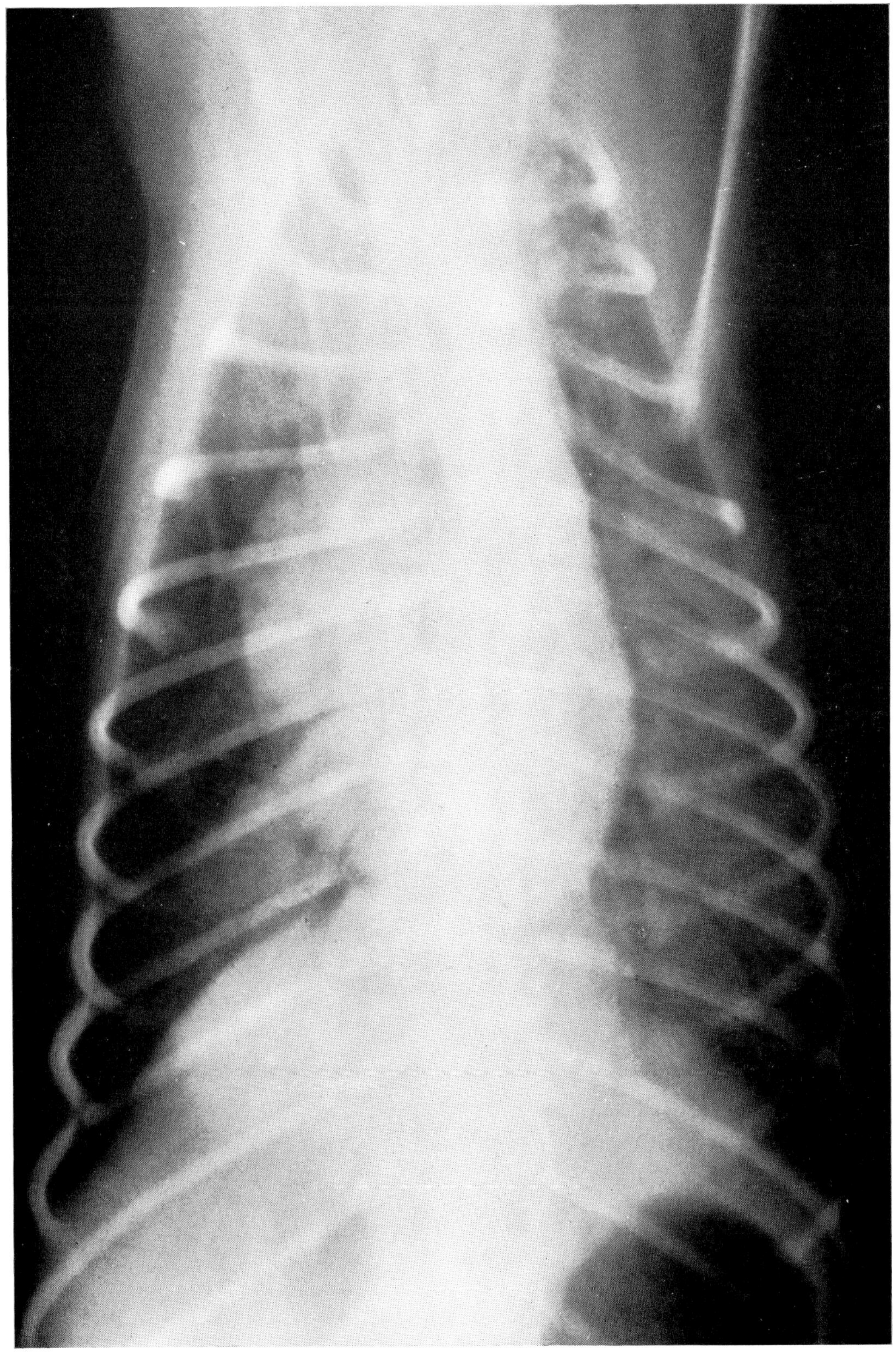

Case 10

Cairn terrier, female, 2 years old. A few hours prior to admission to the clinic this dog developed respiratory signs of "asthmatic type" and vomited several times. It was brought to a veterinarian, who prescribed streptomycin and penicillin. Since the animal did not improve it was referred to the clinic. A diaphragmatic hernia was suspected. At examination the predominant sign was expiratory dyspnea. Radiographs revealed a mediastinal emphysema and the dog was hospitalized. Its condition remained unchanged for several days, but suddenly signs of acute lung edema complicated the picture. During this attack the dog died.

Necropsy: Edema of the lungs, emphysema in the precardial mediastinum, and stasis in the liver were found. No underlying cause of the emphysema was revealed.

Differential Diagnosis: The air in the mediastinum along the trachea was easily found and the diagnosis was obvious.

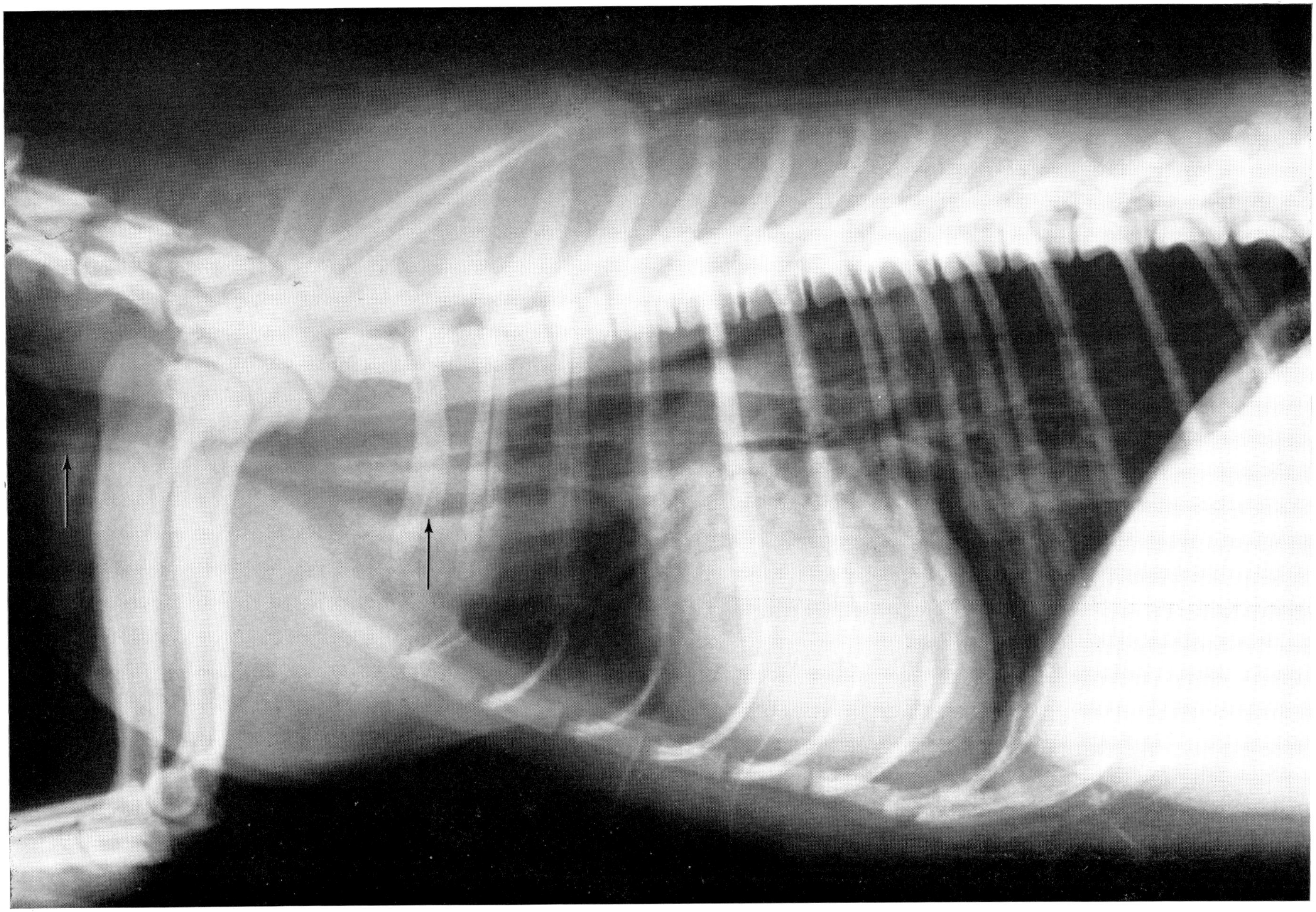

Case 10. The heart is of normal size and shape. There is a slightly increased vascularity of the lungs. There are also streaks of air in the precardial mediastinum extending into the neck (arrows). The diaphragm is flatter than normal.

Diagnosis: Mediastinal and intramuscular emphysema.

Case 11

Drever (Swedish driving dog), male, 1 year old. This dog was hit by a car. On admission to the clinic it had severe dyspnea. Radiographs revealed pneumothorax with marked atelectasis of both lungs. The thirteenth rib on the left side was fractured. The dog was hospitalized, put in an oxygen tent, and showed some improvement. After 2 days it began to vomit and GI series revealed a dilated stomach with no emptying of barium into the duodenum. Because of this finding, laparotomy was performed but the dog died during the operation. The duodenum was found to be strangulated in a tear in the mesentery.

Differential Diagnosis: No diagnostic problem as far as the thoracic cavity was concerned was presented. The characteristic features of pneumothorax, such as collapse of the lungs and elevation of the heart from the ventral wall of the thorax, were displayed.

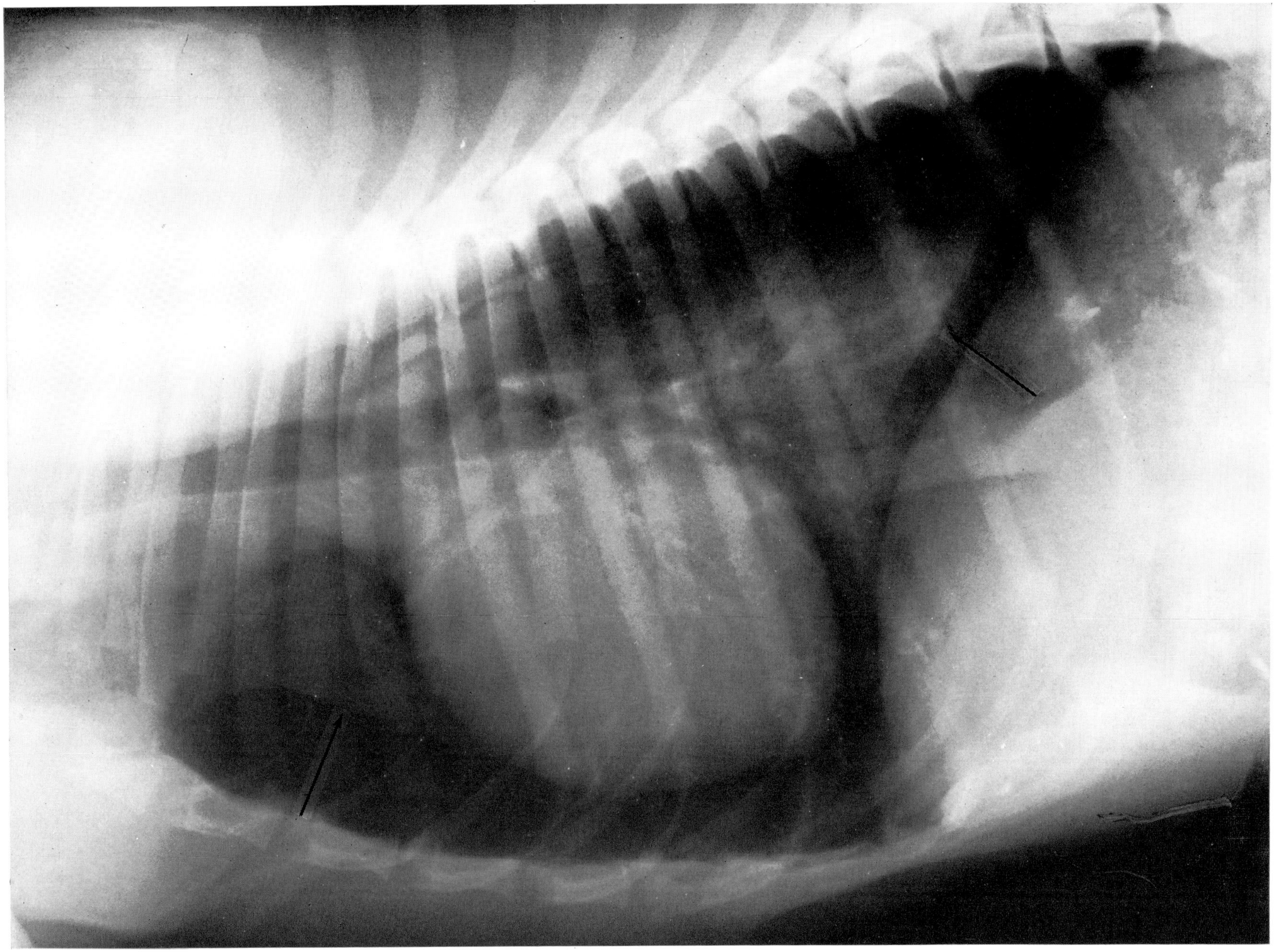

Case 11. **A,** The heart, which is of normal size and shape, is dislocated dorsally and the lungs have collapsed (arrows), leaving an "empty space" in the thoracic cavity. The aorta and the esophagus are seen more clearly than normal.

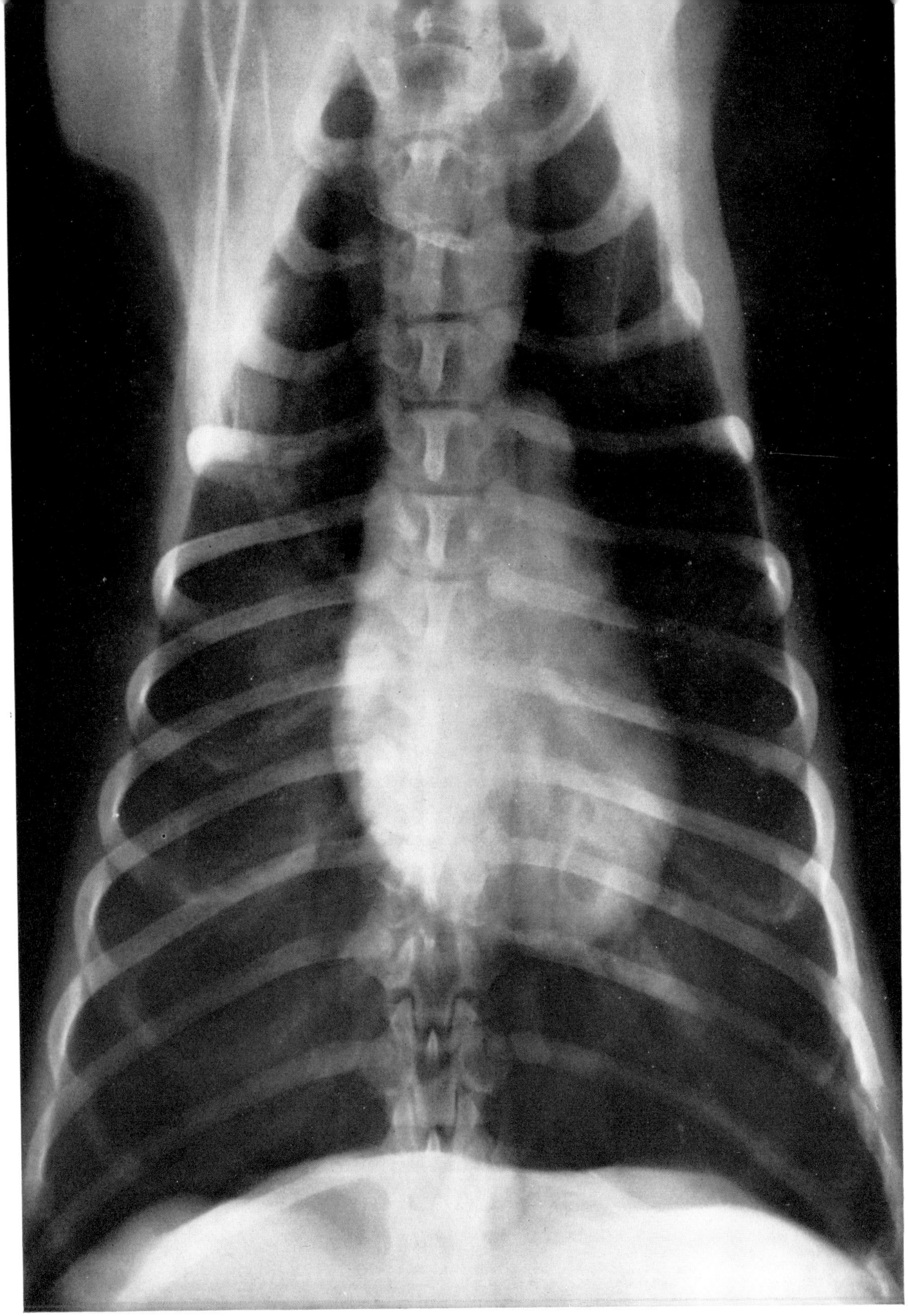

Case 11. **B,** The contour of the heart is more round than normal because of the apex of the heart being tipped in a cranial direction. The diaphragm is markedly flatter than normal. The lung lobes are collapsed.

Diagnosis: Pneumothorax.

Case 12

Mongrel, female, 12 weeks old. Four days prior to admission the puppy was given a bone meal. Since then it had difficulties in swallowing. On admission its general condition was good. Radiographs revealed a foreign body in the esophagus close to the cardia. A soft-tissue density surrounded the foreign body. The puppy was anesthetized, an endoscope was inserted, and the foreign body was pushed into the stomach. As soon as this was done the animal became dyspneic. Radiographic examination revealed a gas-filled esophagus and pneumothorax. The esophagus had apparenty been ruptured while the foreign body was manipulated. The puppy died during preparation for transthoracic surgery.

Necropsy: Necrosis of the esophagus at the site of the foreign body. Rupture of the esophageal wall. Pneumothorax.

Differential Diagnosis: The foreign body was easily detected. More attention should have been paid to the soft-tissue densities surrounding it. The foreign body had apparently been lodged in the esophagus for 4 days and had caused necrosis and inflammation of the wall. A direct transthoracic approach would probably have saved the puppy's life.

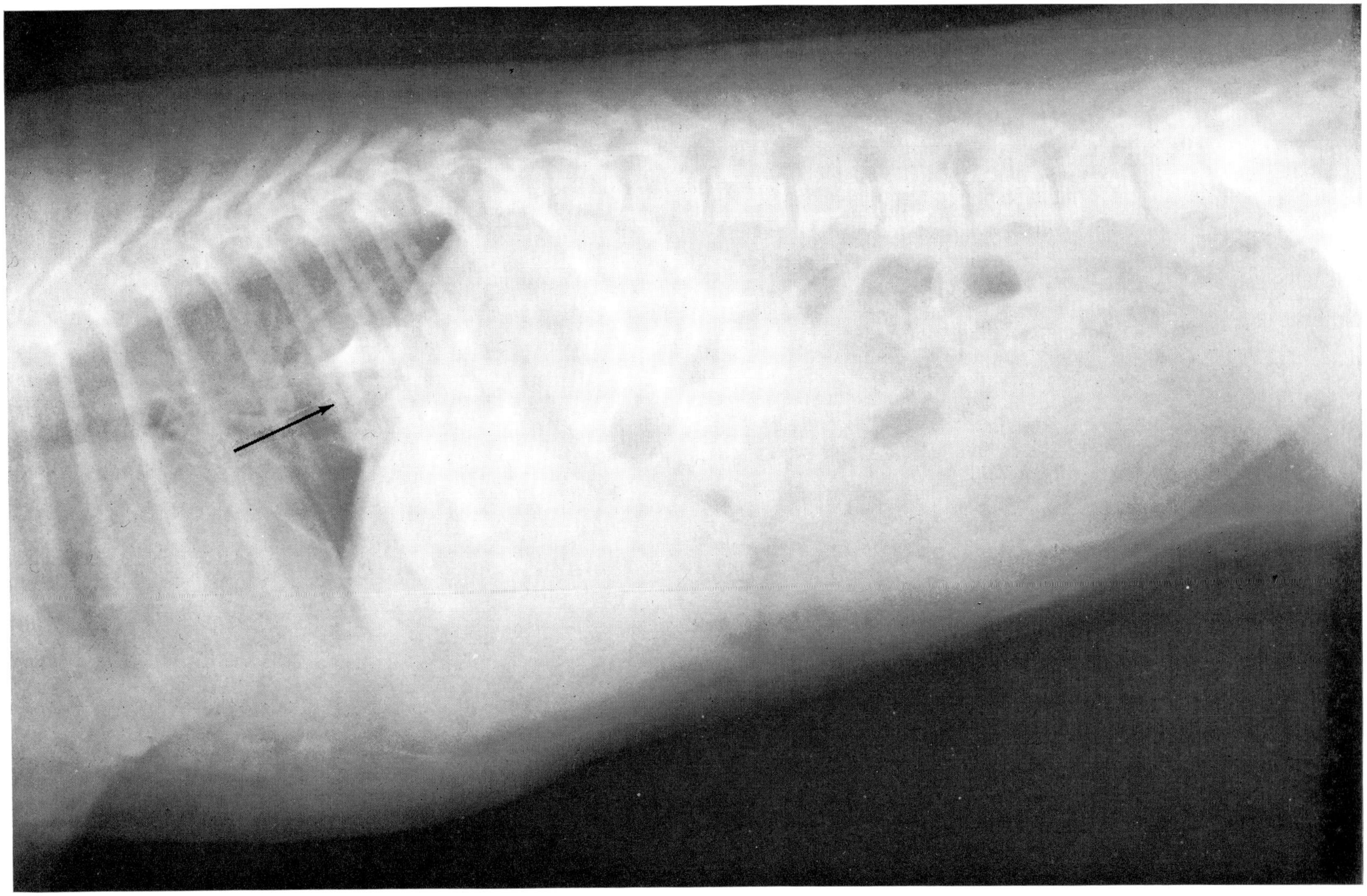

Case 12. **A,** There is a foreign body (apparently a piece of bone with sharp edges) in the esophagus close to the stomach. Around the foreign body there is a diffuse soft-tissue density (arrow).

Diagnosis: Esophageal foreign body causing inflammatory reaction in and around the esophagus.

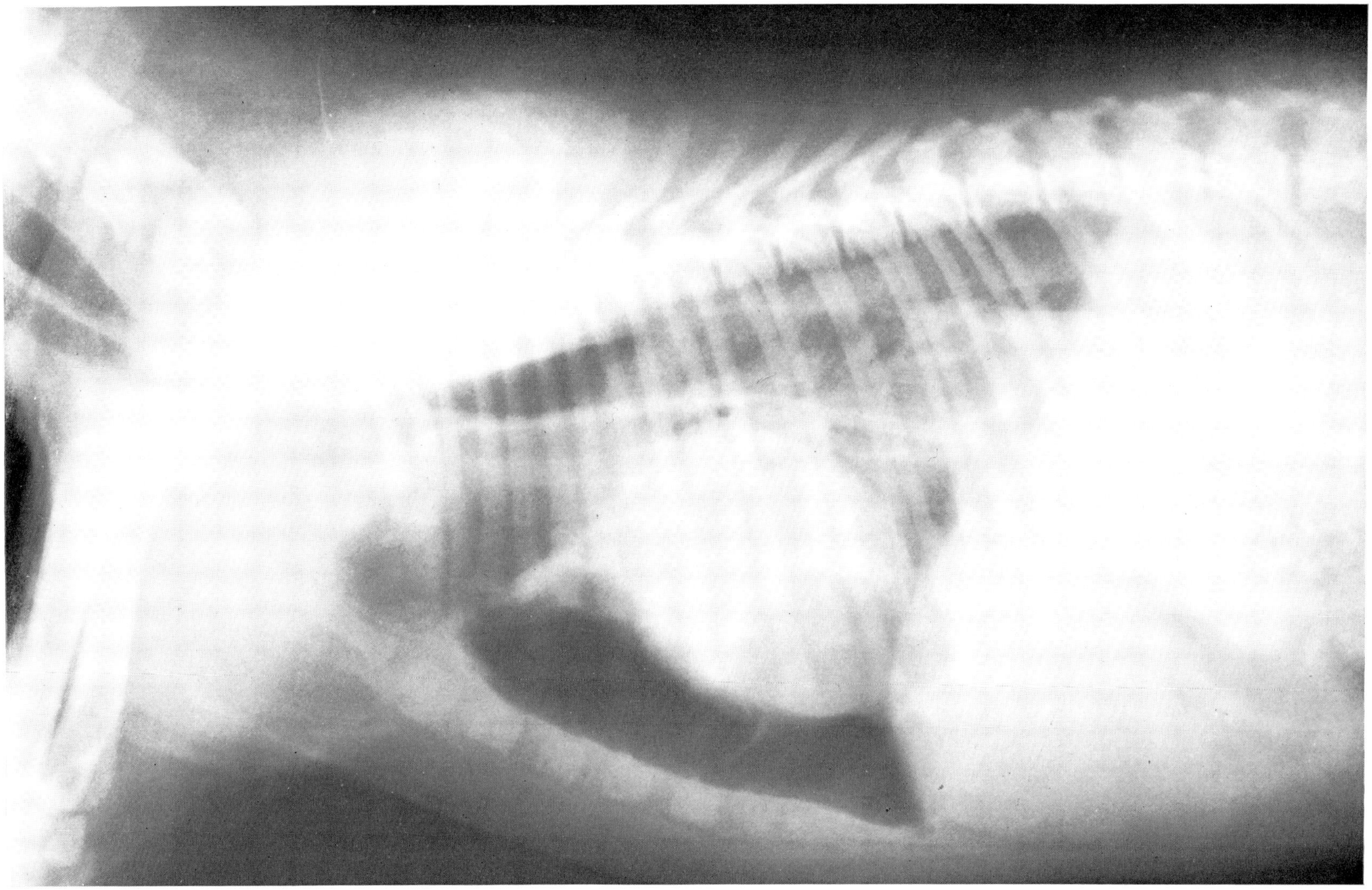

Case 12. **B,** After removal of the foreign body the esophagus is dilated and filled by air. This air has also leaked to the pleural cavity (pneumothorax).

Diagnosis: After removal of the foreign body there is rupture of the esophagus causing pneumothorax.

Case 13

Dachshund, male, 6 years old. This previously healthy dog had suddenly developed anorexia and started to cough. It was brought to the clinic after several days of illness and was hospitalized. Clinical examination revealed a soft systolic heart murmur. Changes on the ECG indicated myocarditis. The dog developed a gradually increasing dyspnea and had difficulties in lying down. For this reason only a lateral radiograph of the chest was made. This revealed a marked density dorsal to the heart. There was also a slight ventral curvature of the trachea cranial to the heart. A non-radiopaque esophageal foreign body was suspected. The dog's condition deteriorated and another radiographic examination was made the following day. Fluid was found in the thoracic cavity. The owner refused to have the dog operated upon. The animal was euthanatized at his request.

Necropsy: A foreign body (a piece of a tendon from a horse) was found in the esophagus. The esophageal wall was necrotic and had ruptured. There were about 300 ml of a grayish, slightly blood-tinged, thick fluid in the thoracic cavity. The pleura was hyperemic and had lost its normal glossiness.

Differential Diagnosis: The foreign body was overlooked when the "wet film" was viewed but the increased density was noticed and a tumor was suspected. Nothing in the clinical history pointed directly to a foreign body in the esophagus. The presence of a foreign body was noticed on the film which was reviewed the following morning, but when the radiographic examination was repeated the esophagus had already ruptured.

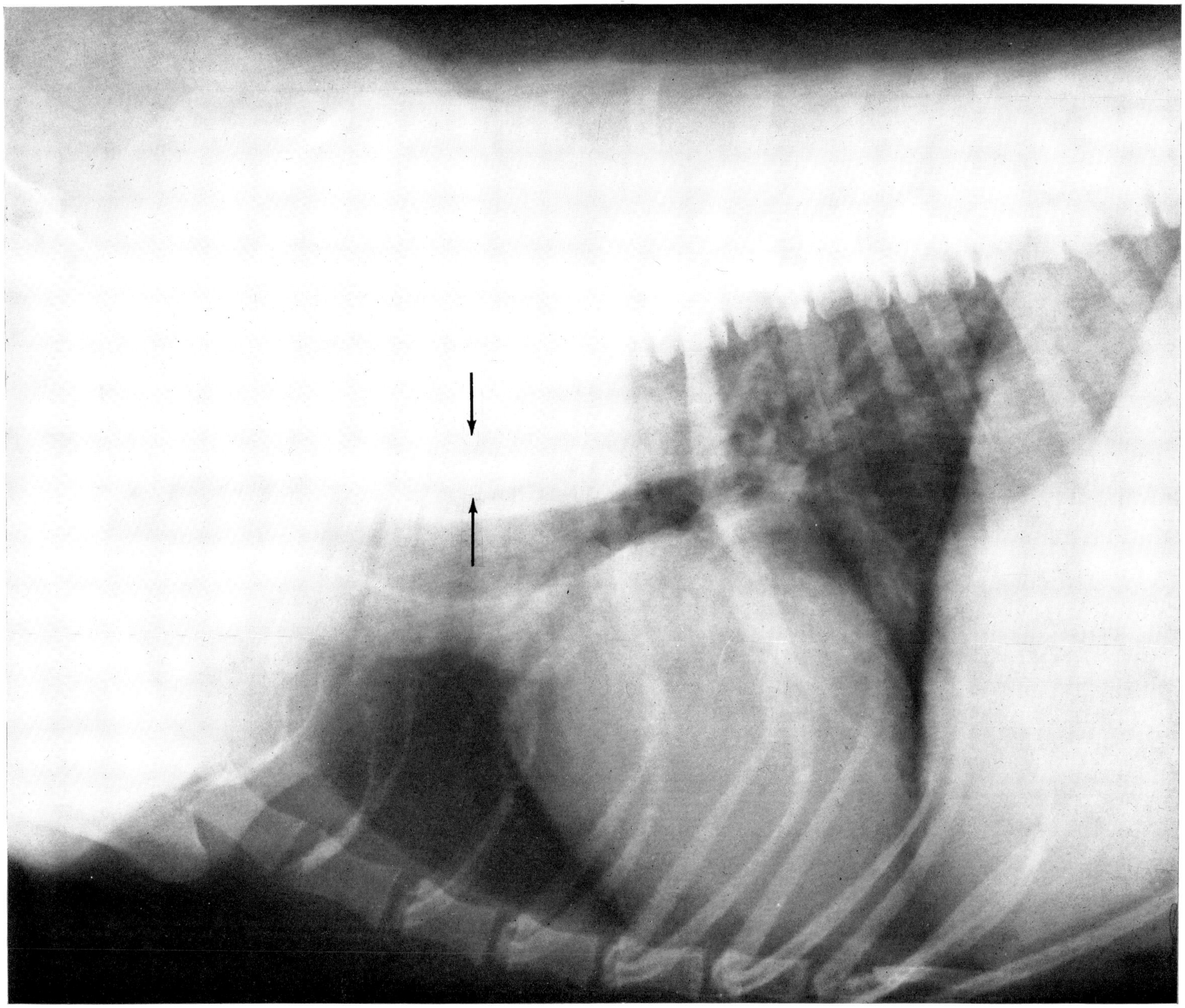

Case 13. **A,** The heart is of normal size and shape. There is a slightly increased vascularity of the lungs. Dorsal and cranial to the heart there is a diffuse density with two vaguely discernible, parallel air streaks (arrows). Cranial to the heart the trachea is pushed in a ventral direction.

Diagnosis: Non-radiopaque foreign body in the esophagus with surrounding increased soft-tissue density as a sign of esophagitis and mediastinitis.

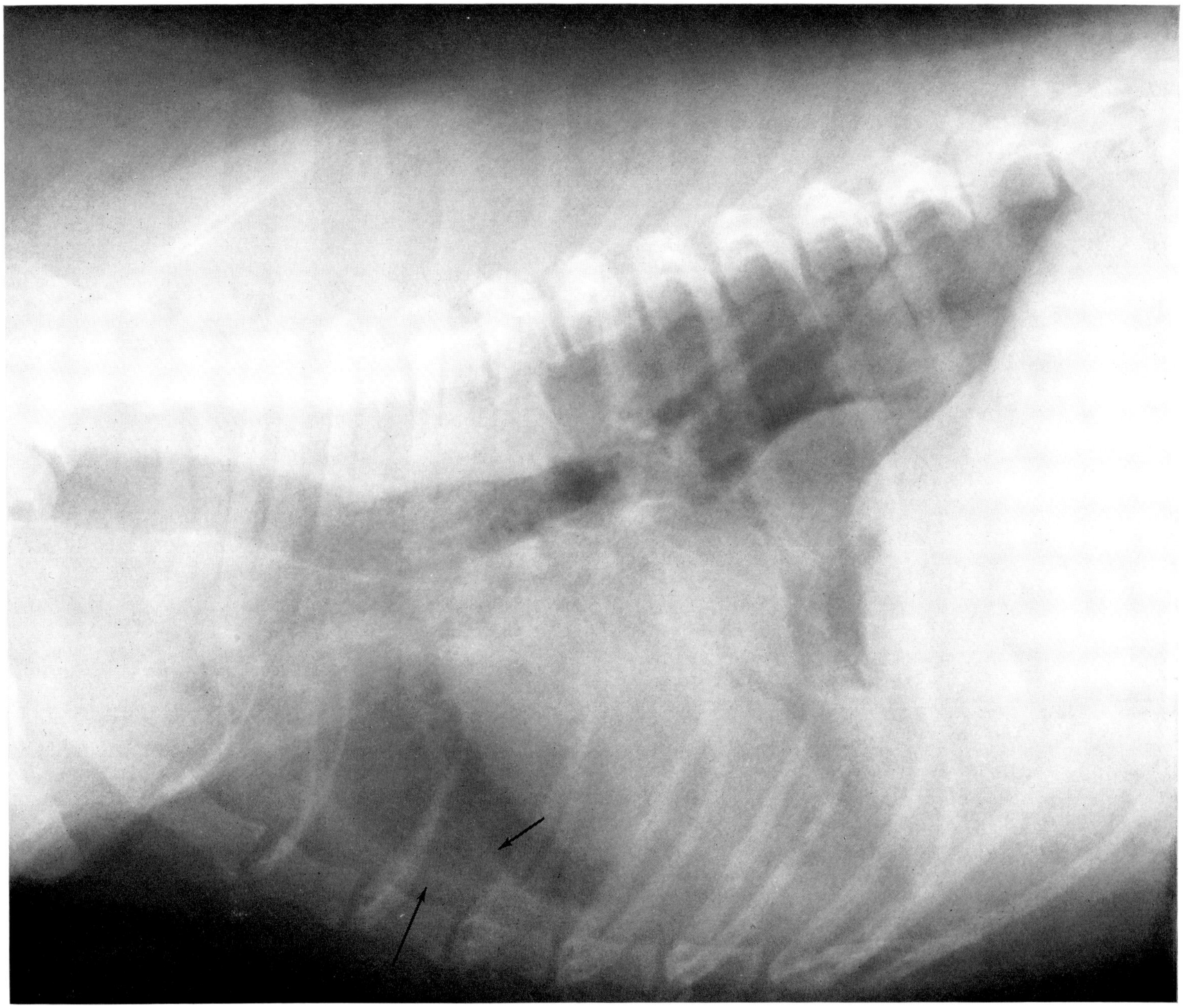

Case 13. **B,** Radiograph made 12 hours after the one shown in **A.** In addition to the changes described in the legend for **A** there is fluid between the lobes of the lung (short arrow) and also between the lobes of the lung and the thoracic wall (long arrow).

Diagnosis: Pleural effusion. Pleuritis caused by a perforating foreign body in the esophagus.

Case 14

Cat, male, 11 months old. After having been missing for 24 hours this cat was found in a miserable condition and unable to stand on its legs. It was immediately brought to the clinic, where it was found to have severe dyspnea and a large hernia of the abdominal wall. Radiographs revealed hemorrhage in the lungs and a slight pneumothorax. In the right lung the main location of the hemorrhage was in the apical lobe. In the left lung there were hemorrhages in the cardiac and diaphragmatic lobes as well. The cat was hospitalized. The respiratory signs subsided within 2 days. The hernia was then surgically repaired. Recovery was uneventful.

Differential Diagnosis: The combined clinical and radiographic picture was rather typical of pulmonary hemorrhage. The light pneumothorax could easily have been overlooked.

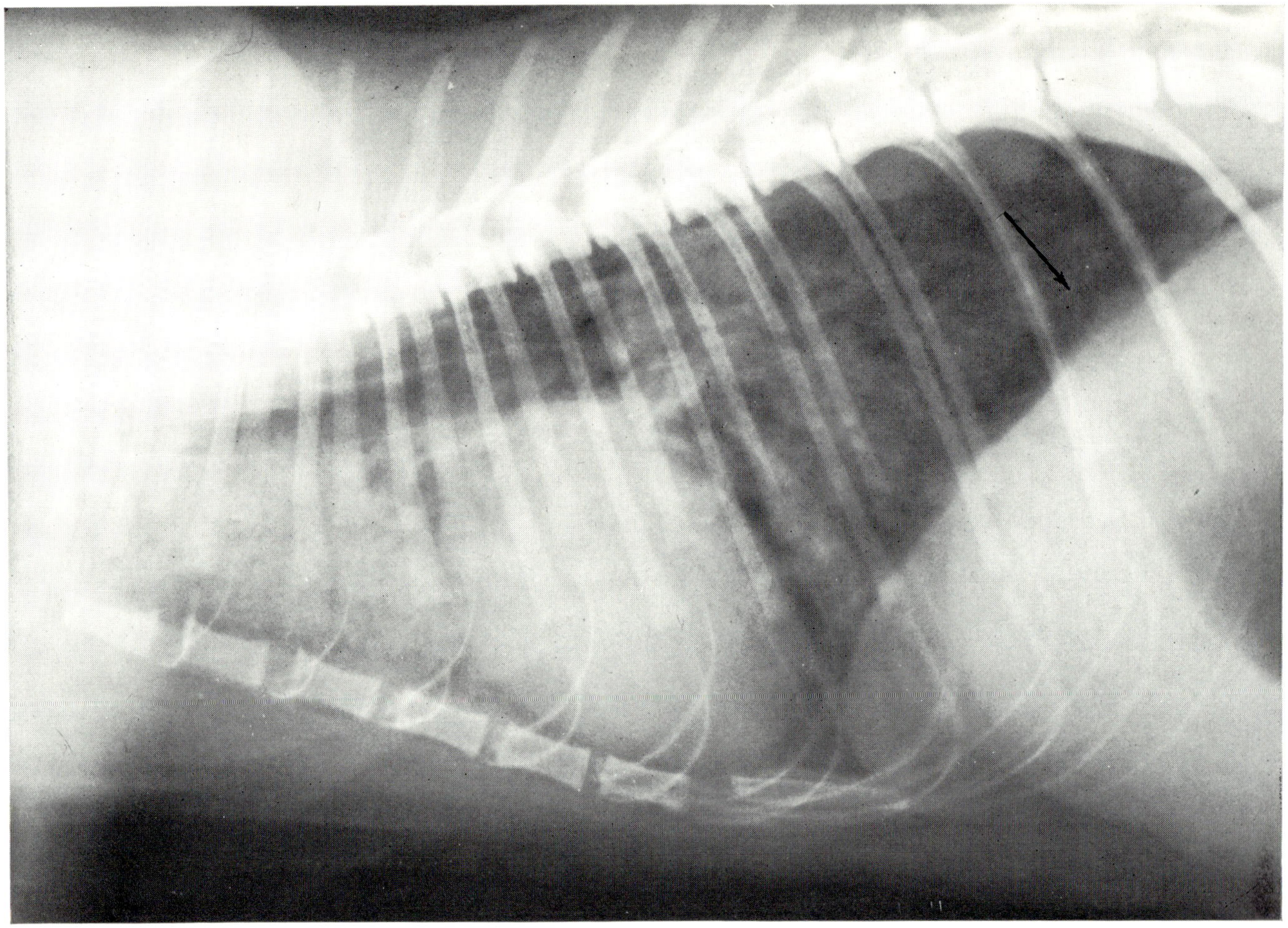

Case 14. **A,** The apical lobes are markedly consolidated and there are scattered densities also in the other portions of the lung field. Parallel to the diaphragm there is a vaguely discernible border of a lung lobe (arrow).

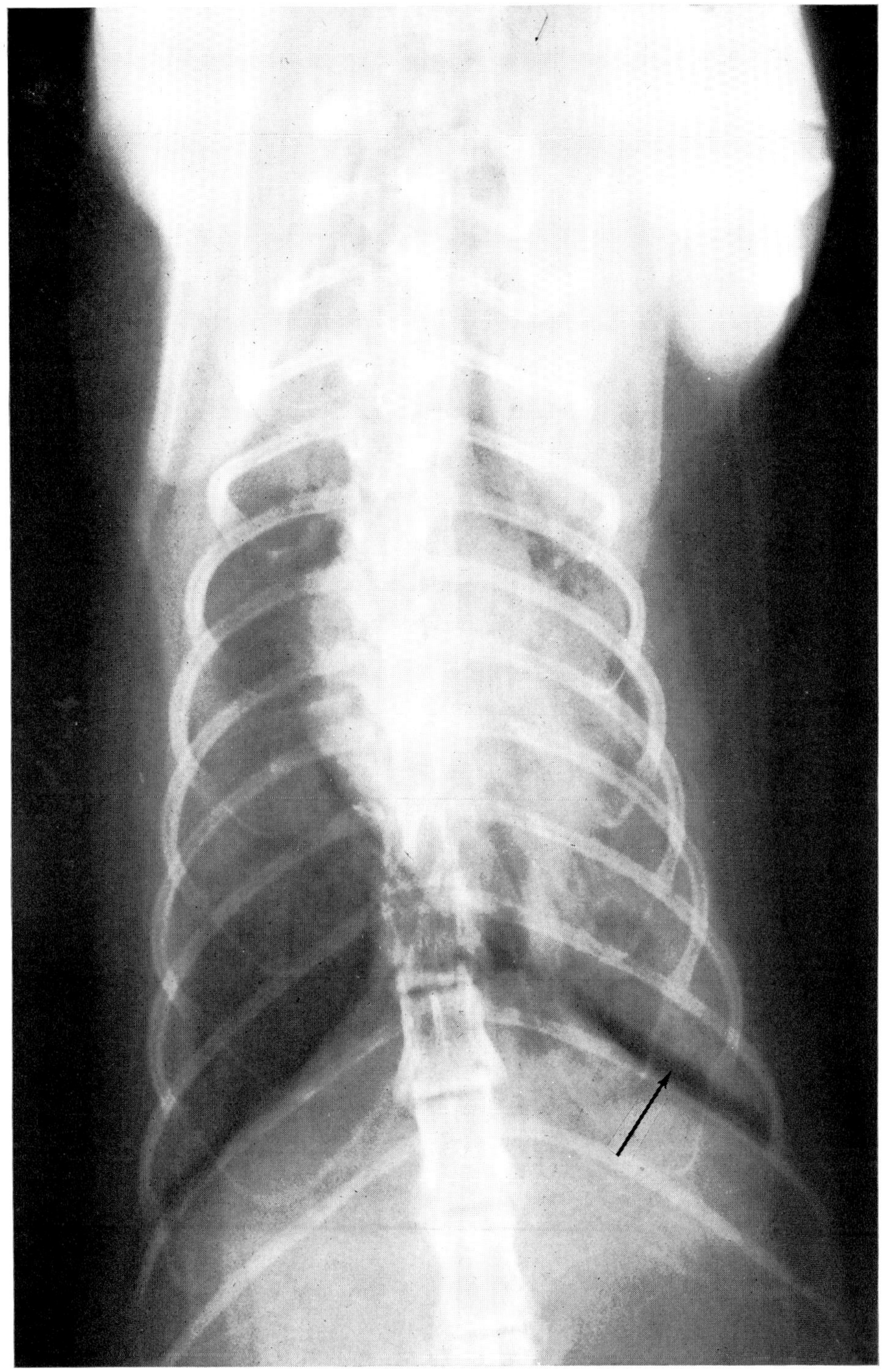

Case 14. **B,** Both apical lobes are denser than normal. There are irregular radiopaque areas in the left cardiac and left diaphragmatic lobe. There is pneumothorax seen as a streak of air between the left diaphragmatic lobe and the diaphragm (arrow).

Diagnosis: Bilateral pulmonary hemorrhage and pneumothorax.

Case 15

Drever (Swedish driving dog), female, 3 years old. Two hours prior to admission to the clinic the dog was hit by a car. On examination the animal was found to have pale mucous membranes and to be in severe respiratory distress. The right hind leg was lacerated. After blood transfusion the dog's condition improved and a radiographic examination of the chest was made. The radiographs revealed fluid in the left thoracic cavity and a partially collapsed left lung. In the right thoracic cavity there was only a minimal amount of fluid. Subcutaneous and intramuscular emphysema in the thoracic wall complicated the picture. The dog was hospitalized and recovered following cage rest.

Differential Diagnosis: This was a straight-forward case and no question was raised about the diagnosis.

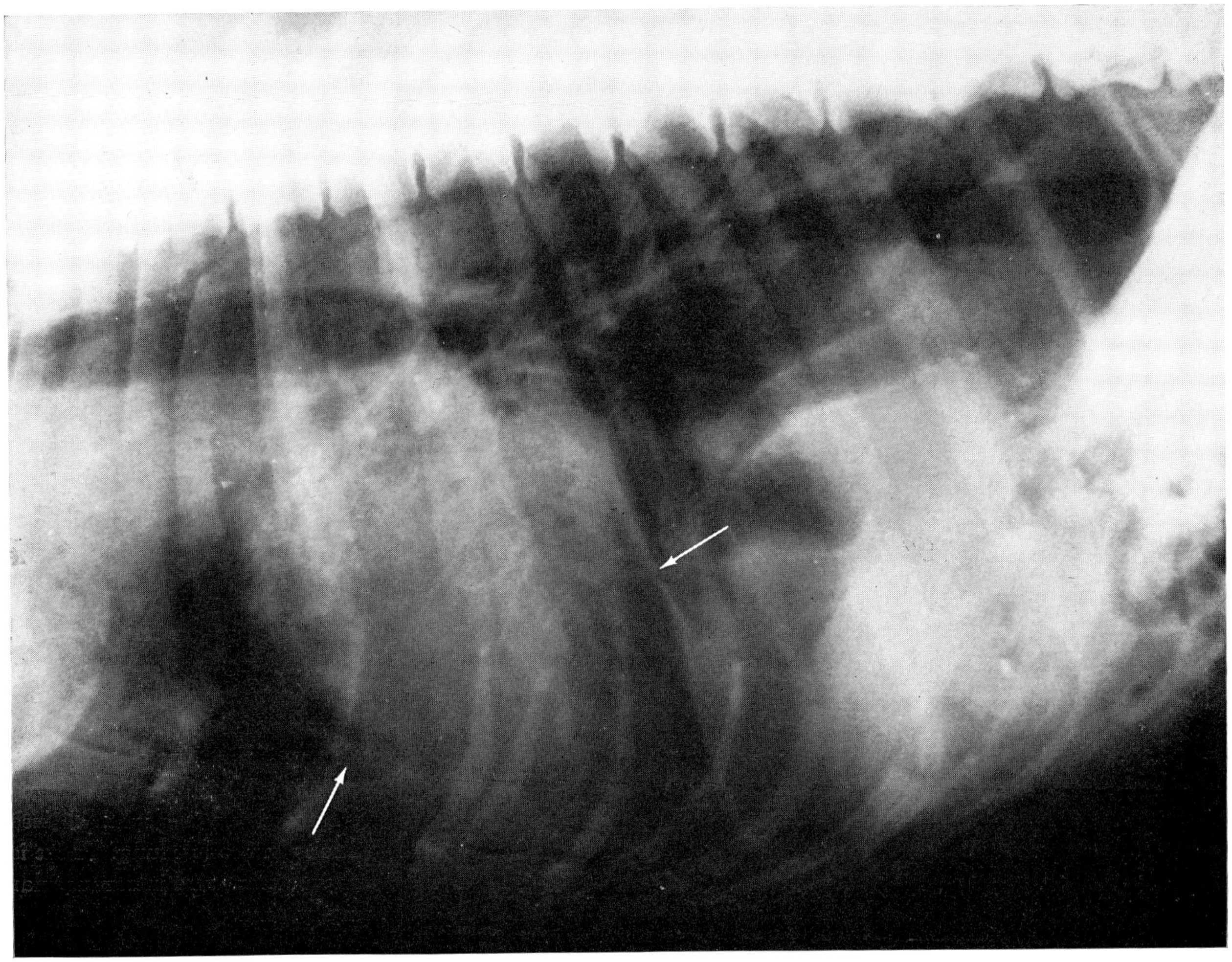

Case 15. **A,** The normal lung pattern is completely lost. A few inter-lobar borders (arrows) can be seen because of fluid in the pleural cavity. There is no distinct outline of the diaphragm. The precardial mediastinum is denser than is normal.

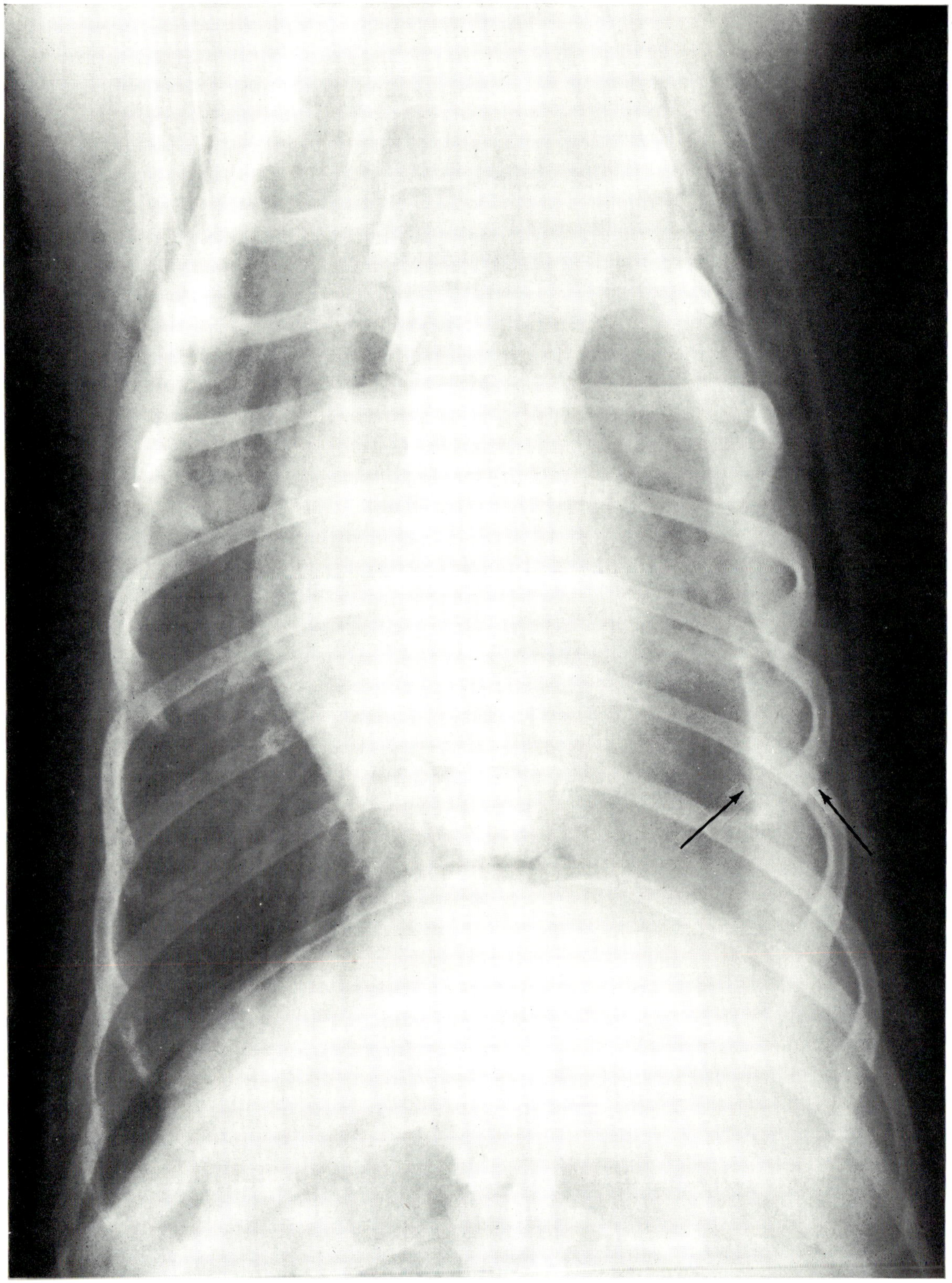

Case 15. **B,** On the ventrodorsal radiograph a homogeneous density is noted between the left lung and the thoracic wall (arrows), indicating the presence of fluid (blood) in the left portion of the pleural cavity. The left contour of the heart is blurred by a slight, diffuse density in the left lung. There is subcutaneous and intramuscular emphysema.

Diagnosis: Pulmonary, mediastinal, and intrapleural hemorrhage. Subcutaneous and intramuscular emphysema.

Case 16

Cat, male, 5 years old. This cat strayed away from its home for 2 days and returned in a very poor condition. On admission to the clinic it had severe inspiratory and expiratory dyspnea. On auscultation the normal respiratory sounds could not be heard. A diaphragmatic hernia was suspected; this diagnosis was confirmed radiographically. Abdominal organs were found in the thoracic cavity. The cat was euthanatized on the owner's request. The animal was not necropsied.

Differential Diagnosis: It is sometimes difficult to differentiate between pleural effusion and herniated abdominal organs. In this case no such problem arose because contours of organs such as the spleen and several lobes of the liver could be seen in the thoracic cavity.

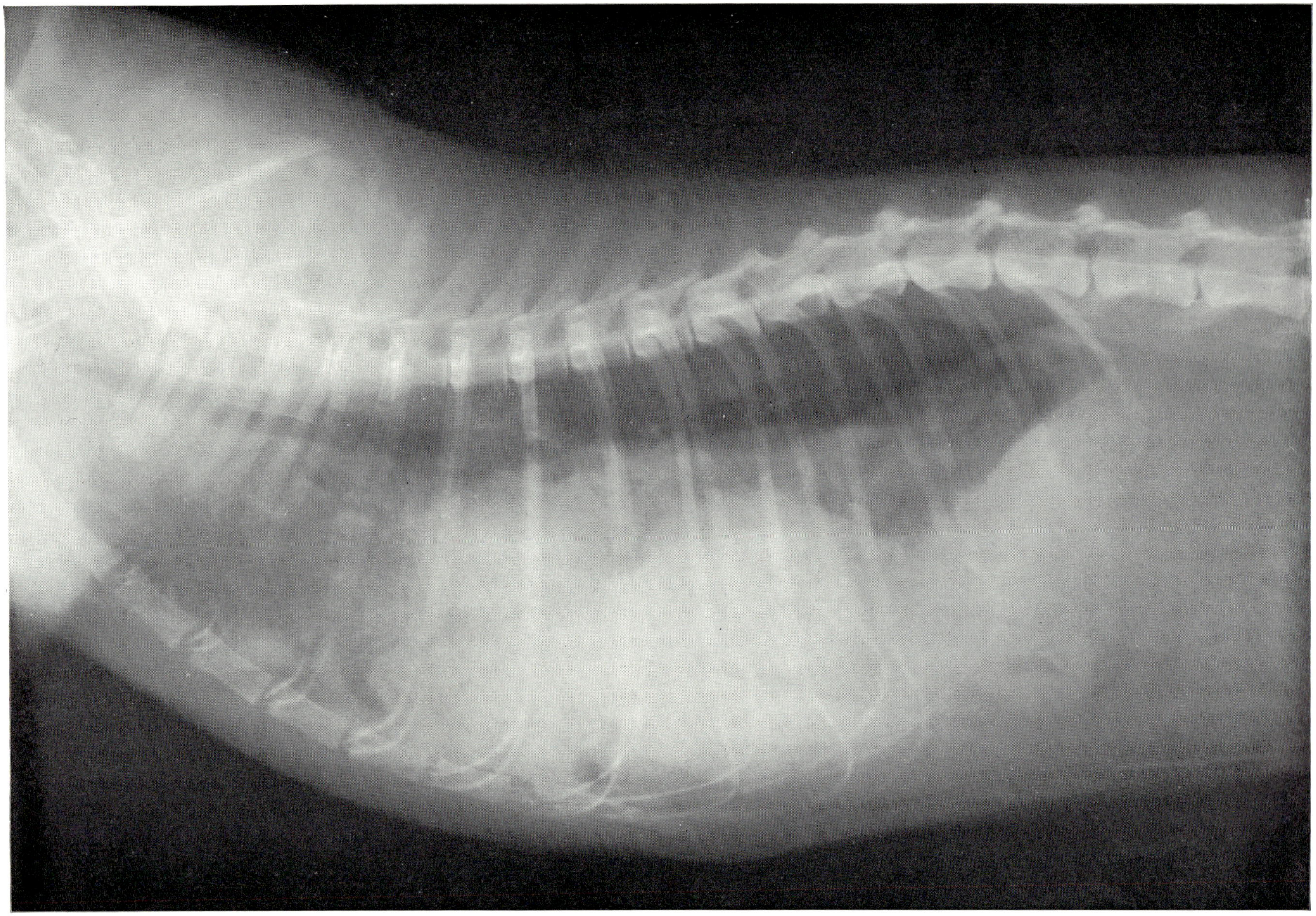

Case 16. **A,** The thoracic cavity is filled by a large irregular mass which obscures the contour of the heart. Only in the dorsal part of the thorax can normal lung tissue be seen.

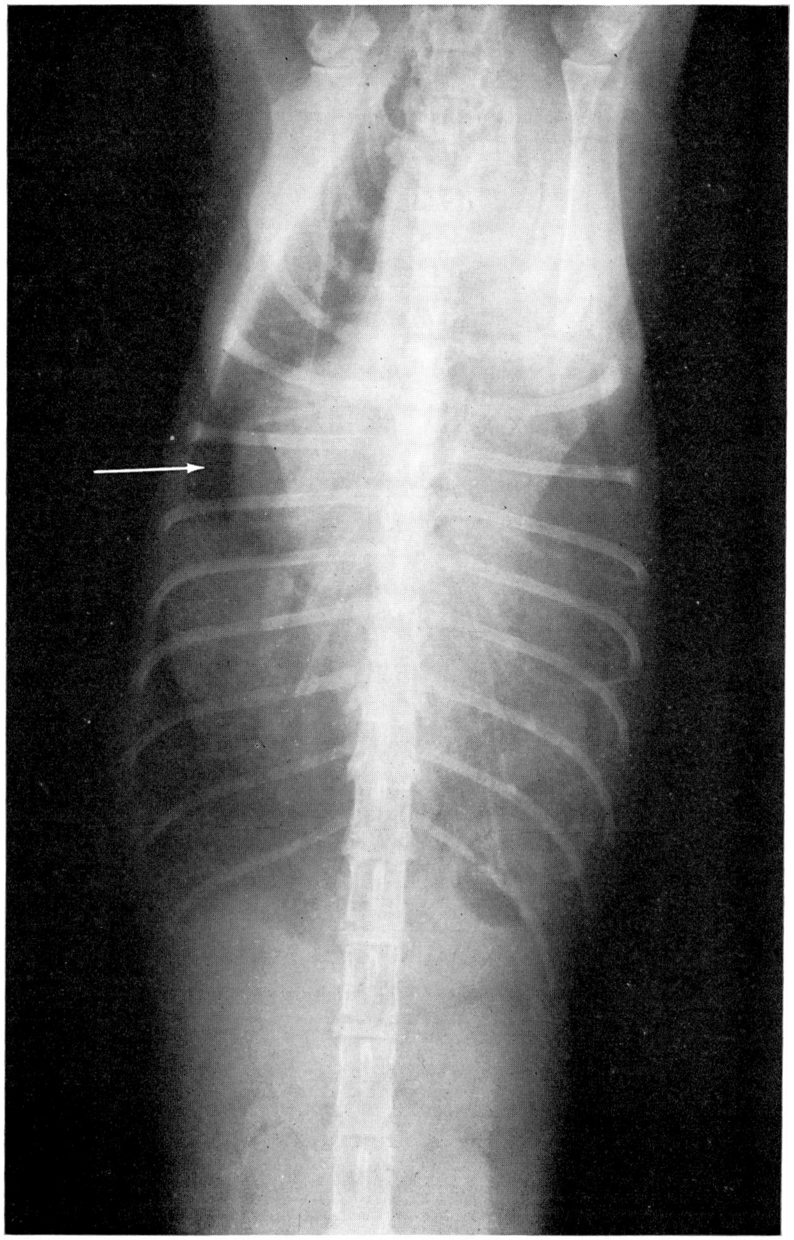

Case 16. **B,** There are large irregular densities in the thoracic cavity and the diaphragm cannot be seen. The heart (arrow) is pushed cranially and to the right. Several abdominal organs can be recognized in the herniated mass.

Diagnosis: Diaphragmatic hernia.

Case 17

Dachshund, female, 3 months old. Two days prior to admission to the clinic this dog started vomiting and became listless. The owner suspected that a foreign body was present in the intestines and brought the dog to the clinic late in the evening of the second day of illness. On admission the dog was alert. No immediate radiographic examination was made because of the late hour. About 25 ml of barium were given orally and the dog was hospitalized and left in a cage overnight. Radiographs of the abdomen were made the following morning. The contrast medium had all but completely passed out to the large bowel. On the lateral radiograph a speck of contrast medium was noted superimposed on the liver and there was also a diffuse density in the lung field caudal to the heart. On the ventrodorsal radiograph it could be demonstrated that the speck of contrast was localized in the left part of the thoracic cavity. There was a very conspicuous density in the caudal portion of the left pleural cavity. A second barium swallow, this time under fluoroscopic view, made clear that there was normal passage through the esophagus down to the abdominal cavity. Caudal to the diaphragm the esophagus made a dorsal loop and the contrast medium arrived in the stomach, which was lodged in the thoracic cavity. At operation it was found that the stomach and part of the omentum were herniated. The herniation was reduced and the opening in the diaphragm, which was apparently congenital, was closed by suture. Recovery was uneventful.

Differential Diagnosis: The herniated abdominal organs were less conspicuous on the radiographs than is usual in such cases. Because the empty stomach and the omentum were only slightly radiopaque and there was no flattening of the diaphragm, the diagnosis of diaphragmatic hernia was at first overlooked. Another reason for not making the right diagnosis in the first instance was the fact that the first barium swallow was not immediately followed by a radiographic examination. The second barium swallow under fluoroscopic view (also followed by radiographs) left no doubts concerning the correct diagnosis.

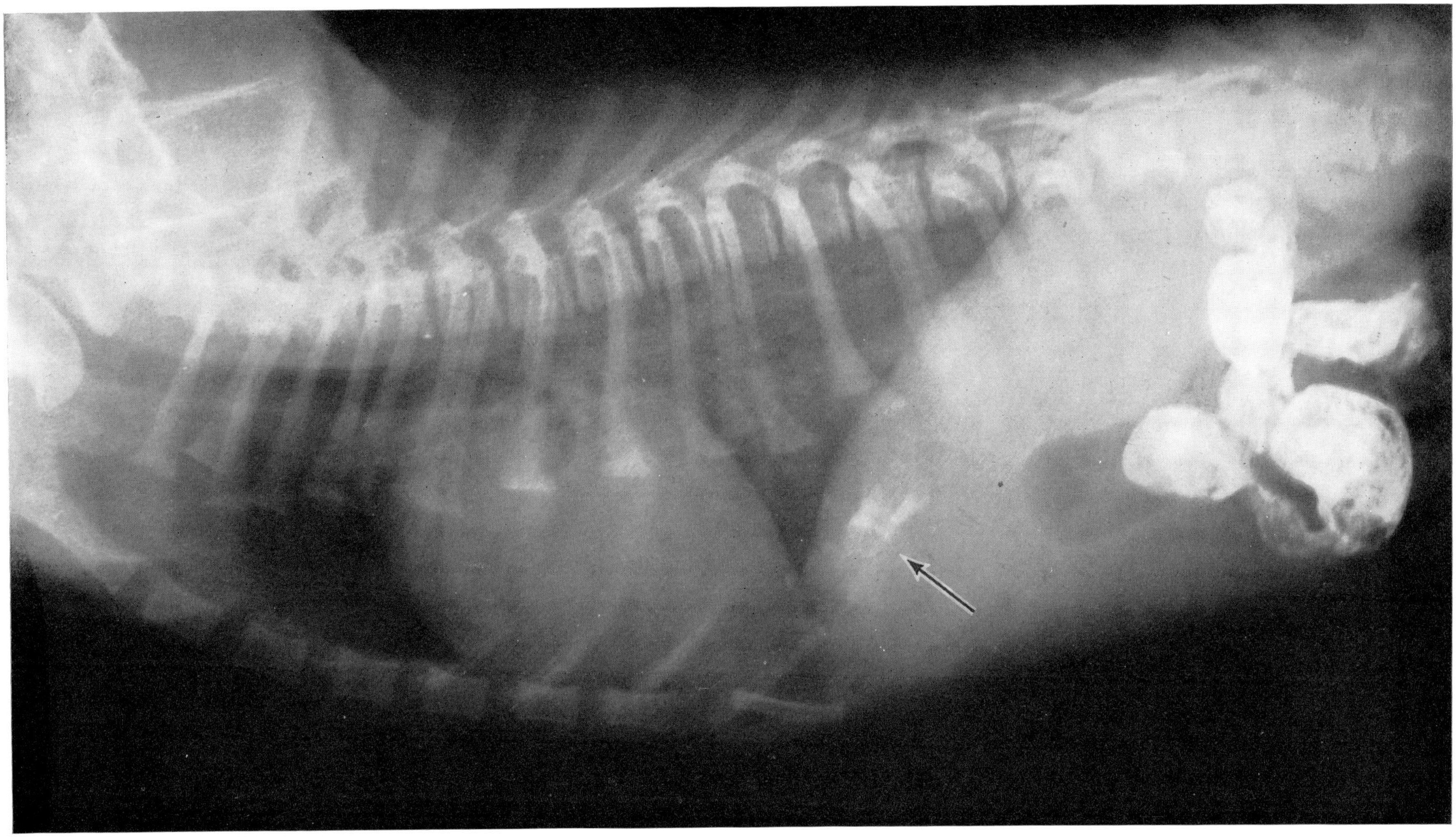

Case 17. **A,** Lateral radiograph. The heart is of normal size and shape and the diaphragm is normally curved. There is a diffuse density of the lung field, corresponding to the diaphragmatic lobes. There is a speck of contrast medium (arrow) superimposed on the shadow of the liver close to the diaphragm. The large bowel contains contrast medium.

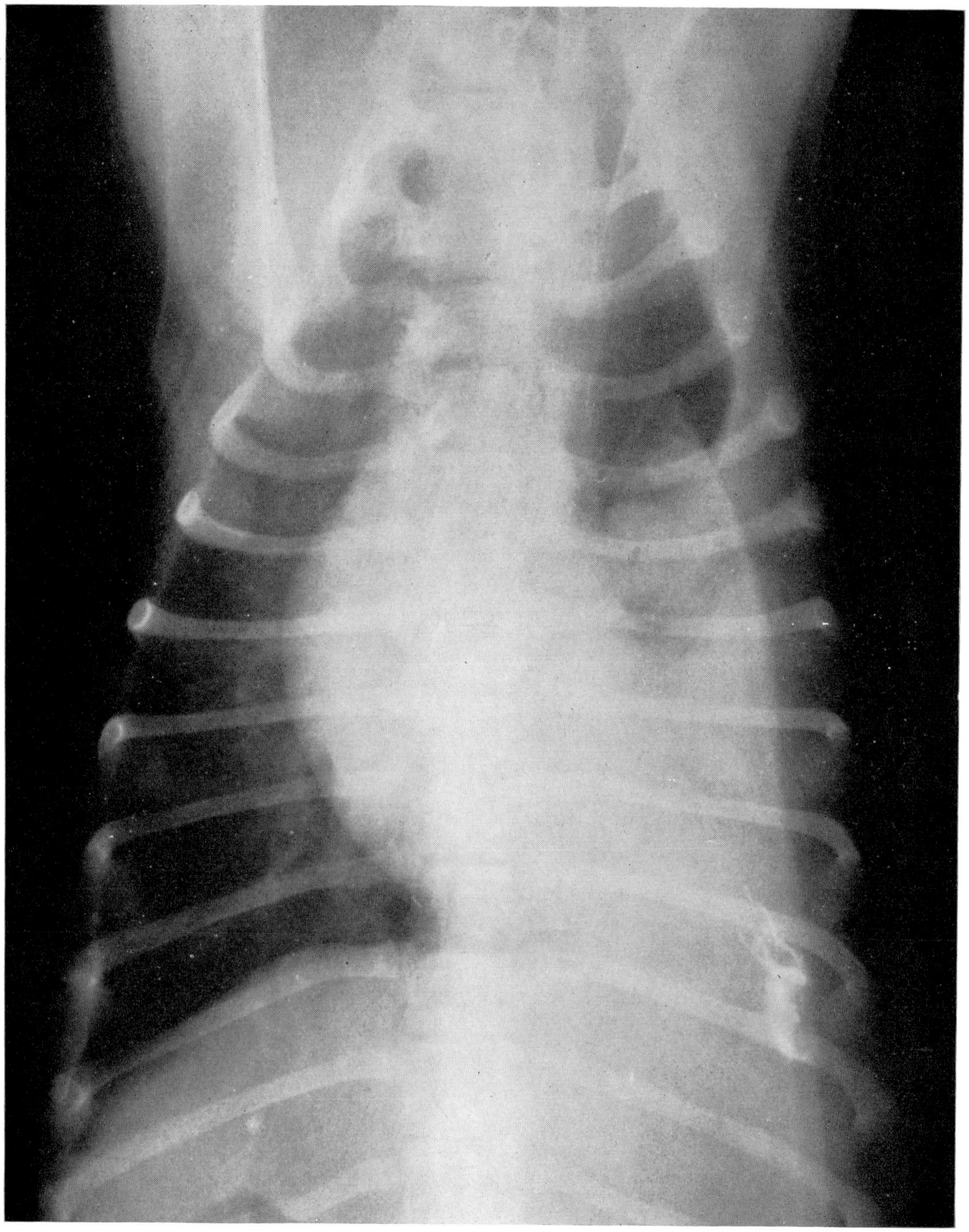

Case 17. **B,** In this ventrodorsal radiograph, there is a very marked, homogeneous consolidation in the caudal part of the left thoracic cavity. This consolidation has no lobar arrangement. The small speck of contrast medium is seen to be localized close to the thoracic wall within the left thoracic cavity.

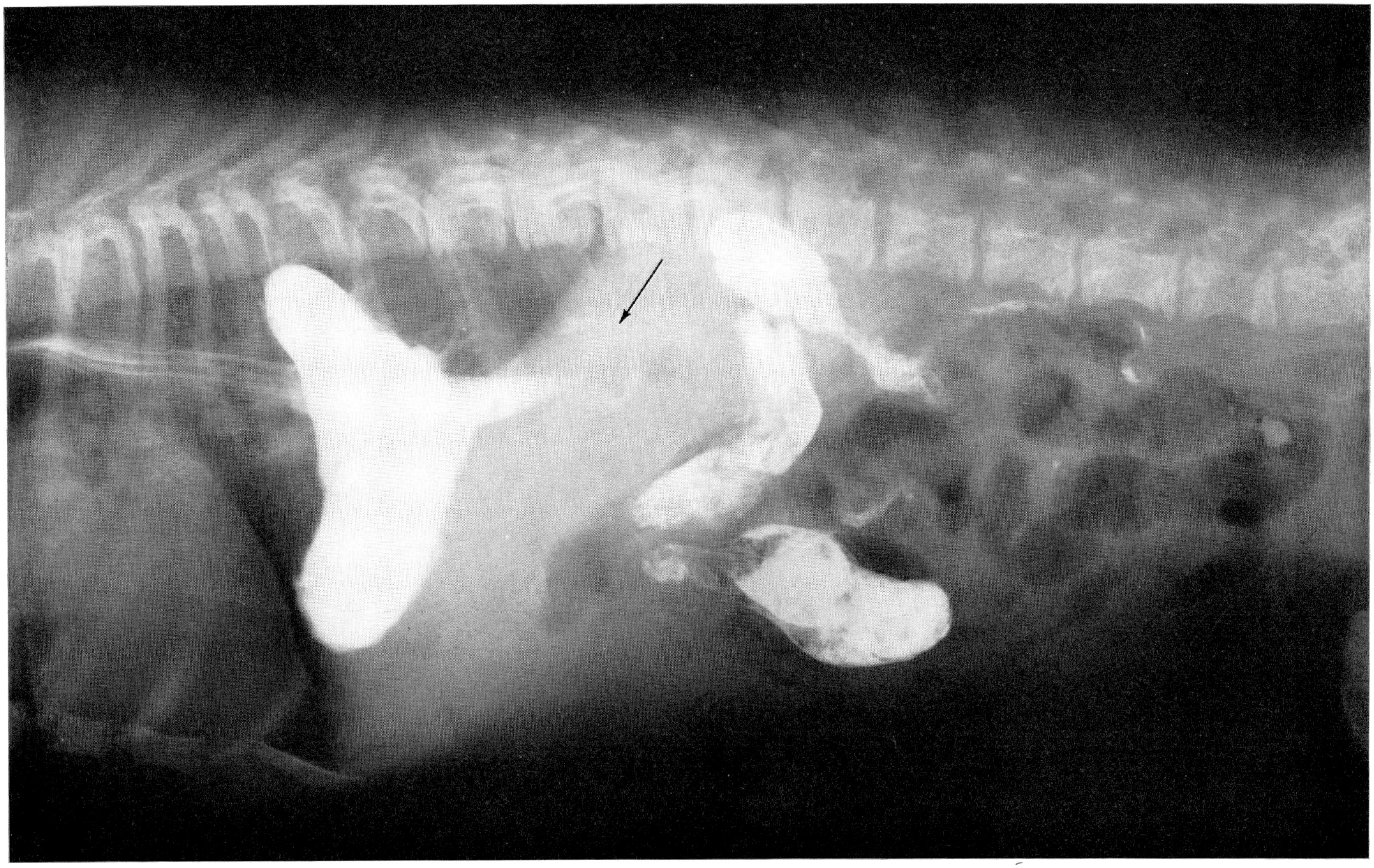

Case 17. **C,** Lateral radiograph made 5 minutes after a barium swallow. There is contrast material in the stomach, which is lodged in the thoracic cavity. After entering the abdominal cavity the esophagus makes a dorsal loop (arrow) into the stomach. The small bowel is gas-filled and partly distended.

Diagnosis: Diaphragmatic hernia. Herniation of the stomach and part of the omentum.

Part 2

The Abdomen

Chapter 3

The Digestive Tract

Changes seen in association with trauma and disease of the digestive tract are illustrated in this chapter. Included are pyloric stenosis; gastric torsion; mesenteric torsion; intestinal foreign bodies; intestinal stenosis; fecal impaction; intussusception; splenic, hepatic, and tumor hemorrhages; intestinal perforation; intestinal rupture; rupture of the mesentery; pancreatitis; peritonitis; traumatic abdominal hernia; and rupture of the gallbladder.

Many of these lesions and diseases present considerable differential diagnostic problems; others, such as gastric and mesenteric torsions, have a characteristic radiographic appearance.

A common radiographic manifestation of many abdominal disorders is a mottled, flaky density due to either blood or inflammatory reaction of the peritoneum. This density blurs the abdominal organs.

There are other features which do not make the differential diagnosis of abdominal disorders easy. The initial signs of a traumatic lesion in the abdomen may easily be overlooked because of more obvious other signs of trauma such as fractures, bruises, laceration, and hemothorax. The abdominal signs may only gradually become evident and, if this possibility is not kept in mind and repeated radiographs are not made, necessary surgical treatment may be given too late to save the animal's life. It is imperative that the animal be kept under close observation for several days.

Plain radiographs of the entire abdomen in two projections, one lateral and one ventrodorsal, should always be made as the first step in a radiographic examination of the digestive tract. Only after careful examination of such radiographs should a decision be made concerning the use of special procedures such as GI series, barium enemas, or fluoroscopy.

If there are radiographic signs of an obstructive, traumatic or inflammatory lesion without sufficient indication for an immediate operation, the animal should be kept under close clinical observation and the radiographic examination repeated one or several times.

A foreign body in the digestive tract, intestinal stenosis (inflammatory or neoplastic), or intussusception gives rise to partial or complete obstruction. Partial obstruction may cause only mild clinical signs and small radiographic changes. Nevertheless, necrosis and perforation of the intestinal wall leading to fatal peritonitis may occur. It is therefore safer to perform laparotomy immediately following the radiographic examination (if the condition of the animal permits) rather than wait, hoping for a normal passage. Location of a foreign body should be carefully checked before operation is undertaken. The foreign body may have passed to the large bowel during the period between the radiographic examination and the operation, thus making the operation unnecessary. Signs of obstruction such as distended gas- and fluid-filled loops of small bowel may be seen on the radiographs for a time after the foreign body has disappeared.

The location of a foreign body can be established in three ways. Inflation of air through a tube immediately followed by radiographs in two projections is often a good way to demonstrate the presence of a foreign body in the stomach. If there is reason to believe that there is a foreign body in the small bowel, a barium swallow (10 ml per kilogram of body weight) and subsequent radiographs after 1, 3, 6, and 12 hours will reveal its location. Meglumine diatrizoate (1 ml per kilogram of body weight) can also be used. Under normal conditions this contrast medium reaches the large bowel 1 to 2 hours following its administration. If the intestinal mucosa is damaged or is the site of an inflammation, the meglumine diatrizoate can be resorbed, excreted by the kidneys, and collected in the bladder. Unfortunately, this sometimes occurs in clinically normal animals.

If there is reason to believe that the foreign body is in the large bowel, a barium enema given under fluoroscopic observance or followed by one or more radiographs is the best means of determining the exact position of the foreign body.

Case 18

Boxer, male, 13 years old. For several months this dog had vomited occasionally. On the day prior to admission to the clinic the animal became listless and vomited several times. It continued to vomit after each meal and also after intake of water. On admission it was listless and dehydrated. Following hospitalization a radiographic examination, including a GI series with meglumine diatrizoate as contrast medium, was made. On all radiographs the pyloric antrum was seen to be gas-filled and distended. The contrast medium passed slowly from the stomach. As long as 6 hours after its administration most of it remained in the stomach. The stomach continued to show a distended pyloric antrum. Fluoroscopic examination revealed good peristaltic movements in the stomach with little effect in terms of emptying. The dog improved on fluid and electrolyte therapy. Food and water given in small quantities were retained. The owner requested the dog's release but was told to return with the dog to the clinic after 3 weeks. He did not follow this advice and the dog did not become available for repeated examination. On the basis of the clinical and radiologic findings the diagnosis of pyloric stenosis of unknown cause was made.

Differential Diagnosis: No foreign body or other obstruction could be found. A functional stenosis was the only explanation for the clinical and radiographic findings.

A large, round, gas-filled pyloric antrum, which is consistently found on repeated radiographs of the stomach, could indicate the presence of a functional or mechanical obstruction of the pylorus, duodenum, or first portion of the jejunum.

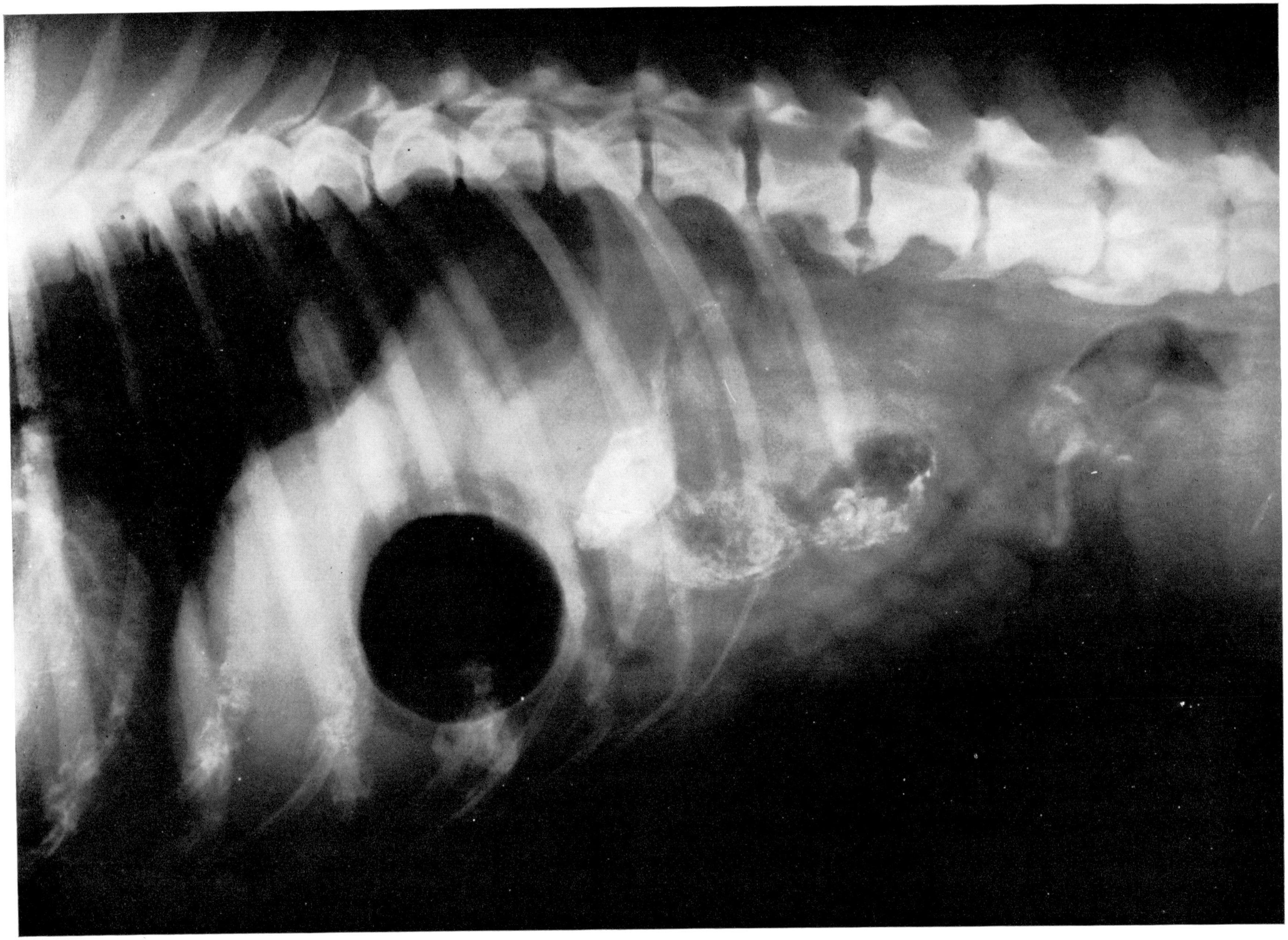

Case 18. **A,** There is a normal outline of the organs of the abdominal cavity. The stomach is slightly distended and filled with gas lodged in the cardia, part of the fundus, and in the pyloric antrum. There is dense ingesta in the large bowel.

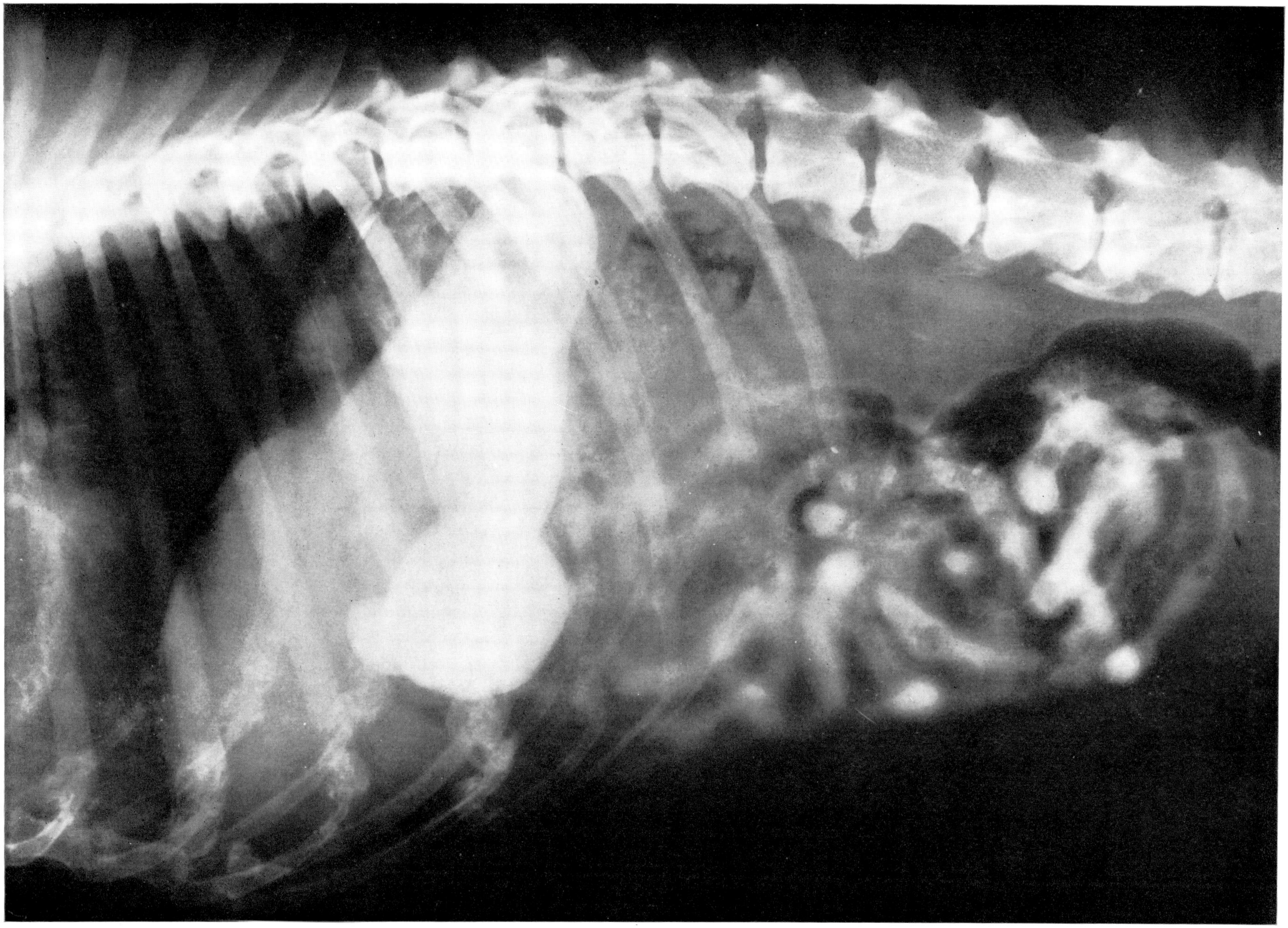

Case 18. **B,** Lateral radiograph made 6 hours after the oral administration of meglumine diatrizoate. Most of the contrast medium is still in the stomach. The pyloric antrum remains round and distended. There is no indication of an obstructive lesion of the bowel.

Diagnosis: Functional pyloric stenosis.

Case 19

Boxer, female, 10 years old. Three weeks prior to admission to the clinic this dog showed transient signs of meteorism. On the day of admission it "suddenly blew up." It was brought to a veterinarian, who emptied the stomach with the aid of a gastric tube. The dog's condition improved somewhat, but it continued its efforts to vomit and seemed to be in great pain. On admission it was in a state of shock. The diagnosis of gastric torsion was obvious both clinically and radiographically. The dog died during preparation for surgical treatment.

Necropsy: The diagnosis of gastric torsion was confirmed.

Differential Diagnosis: In this case the diagnosis of gastric torsion was easily made. Overeating and acute gastric distention may occasionally simulate gastric torsion, but in these conditions the clinical signs of acute gastric distention are usually less severe than in gastric torsion and the stomach remains in normal position even though it is greatly distended and partly gas-filled. In gastric torsion the pylorus is dorsal to the fundus and to the right in the abdomen.

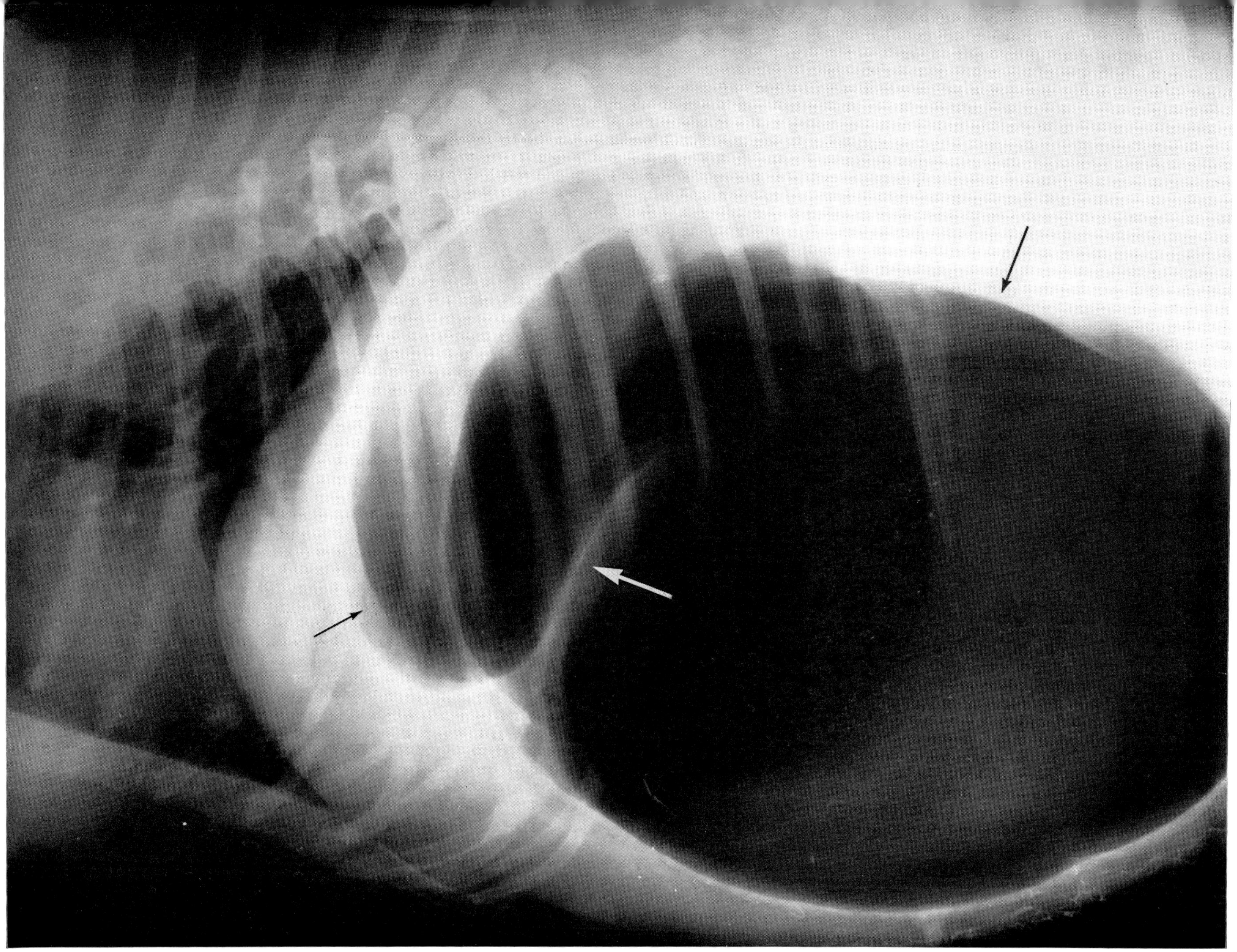

Case 19. The markedly distended and gas-filled stomach is abnormally positioned. The pyloric antrum (small black arrow) is located dorsal and cranial to the fundus. The wall of the fundus and the wall of the antrum are combined to form a fold (white arrow). The greater curvature of the stomach (large black arrow) lies in a dorsal instead of ventral position.

Diagnosis: Gastric torsion.

Case 20

Doberman, male, 4 years old. This dog had always been a poor eater and had remained very thin. One day prior to admission to the clinic it started to vomit after excessive intake of water. On examination it was found to be in poor condition, very dehydrated, and its abdomen was distended. Radiographs revealed the typical picture of gastric torsion.

A large amount of gas was evacuated through a stomach tube, followed by a radiographic examination which showed that the stomach was still rotated 180 degrees. Transesophageal reposition under fluoroscopic view was then tried and proved to be successful. The dog's condition remained serious however. Repeated transfusions of blood and electrolytes did not result in improvement of any appreciable degree. Twelve days later the dog suffered a relapse of gastric torsion. After surgical reduction, gastropexia was performed, but the animal refused to eat, did not regain strength, and died 6 days later.

Necropsy: The stomach was in normal position but dilated.

Differential Diagnosis: In this case, the clinical as well as the radiographic picture gives little room for a diagnosis other than that of gastric torsion.

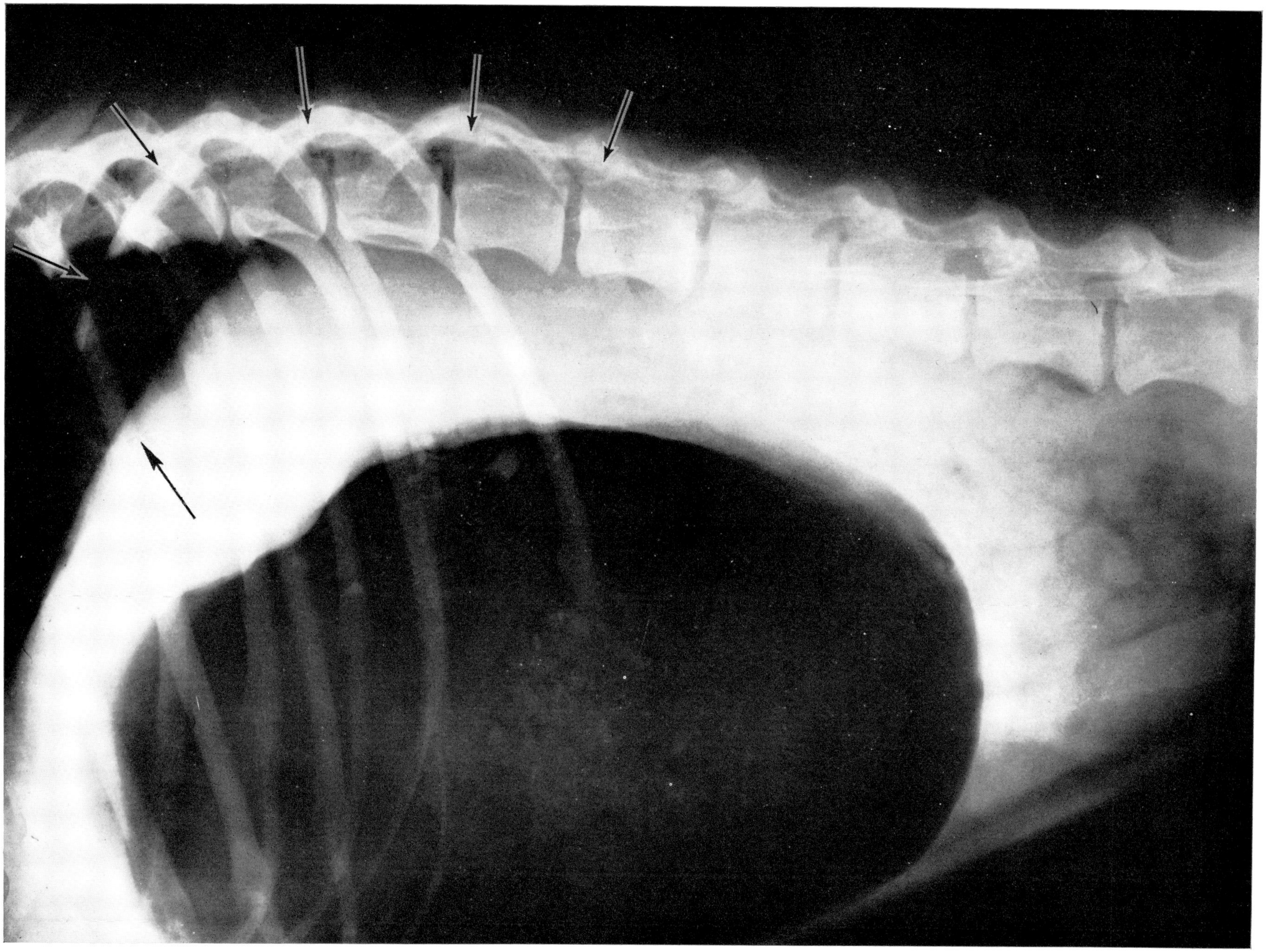

Case 20. **A,** Lateral radiograph made before removal of gas from the stomach. The greater part of the abdomen is filled by the distended stomach. The fundus constitutes the greatest part and is seen in a position ventral to the pyloric antrum (black and white arrows) which is pressed dorsally against the ribs. The pylorus (black arrow) is cranial and dorsal to the fundus.

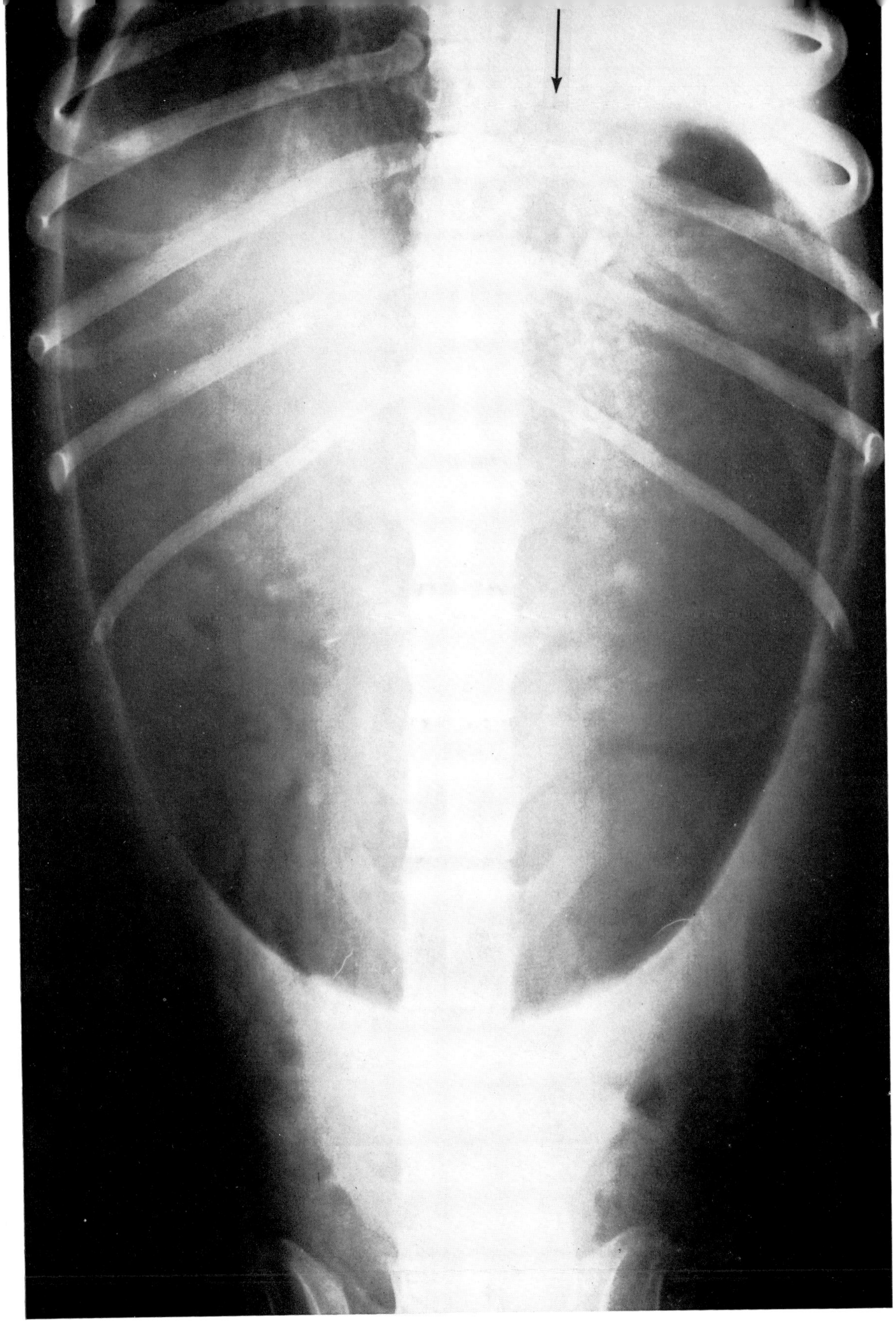

Case 20. **B,** Ventrodorsal radiograph made immediately after the radiograph shown in **A.** There is no difficulty in recognizing that the stomach is rotated 180 degrees. The cardia and the fundus are to the right, while the pyloric antrum and the pylorus (arrow) are positioned to the left.

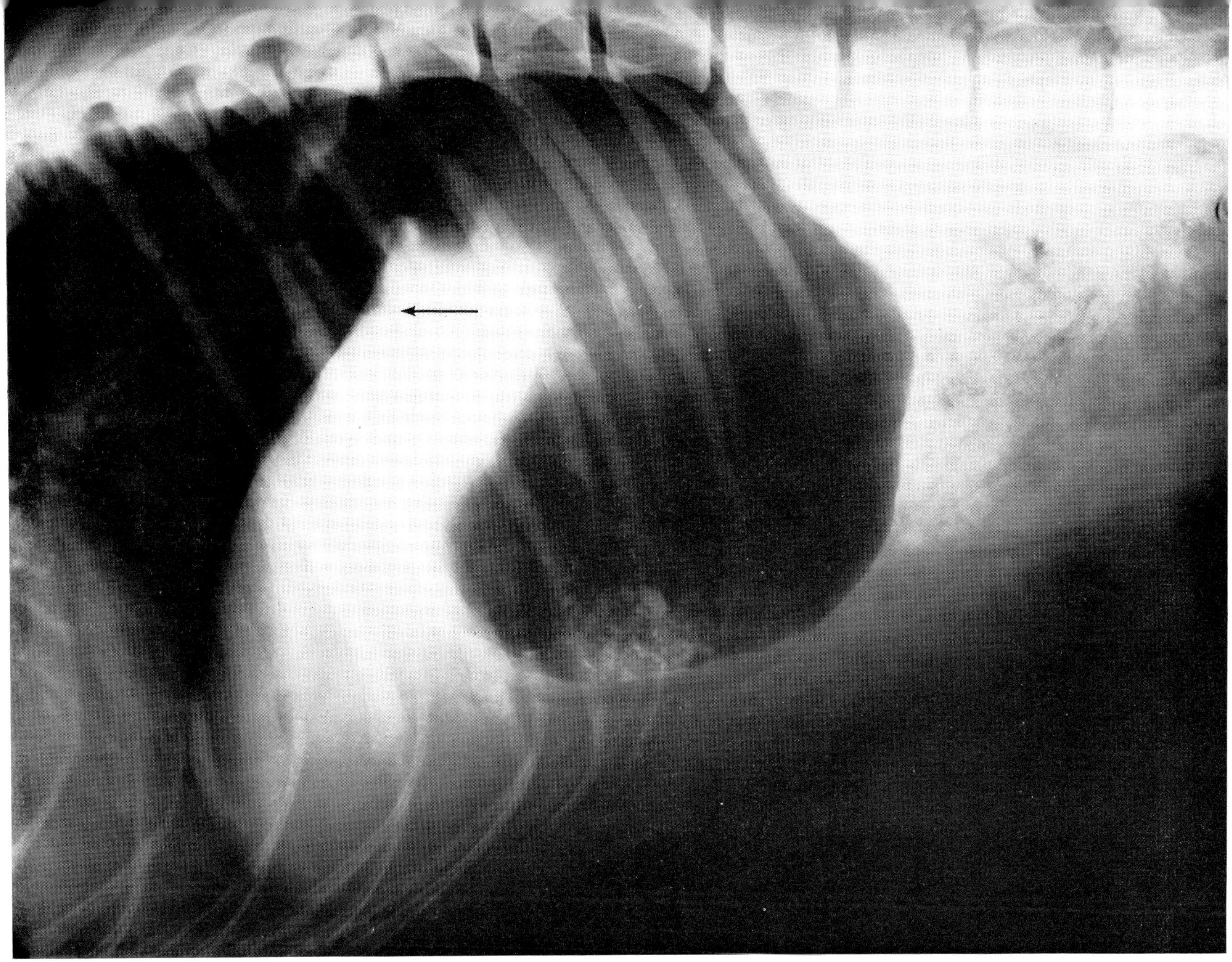

Case 20. **C,** Lateral radiograph made after removal of gas from the stomach. The 180-degree rotation of the stomach is well demonstrated on this radiograph, as the pyloric antrum and the pylorus (arrow) are positioned dorsal to the fundus.

Diagnosis: Gastric torsion.

Case 21

Rottweiler, male, 10 years old. This dog was admitted to the clinic because of difficulty in urinating. The urinary bladder was found to be retroflexed and lodged in a perineal hernia. It was emptied through a catheter. At operation on the following day, it was sutured to the rectum. Recovery was uneventful, but ten days later the dog's condition suddenly deteriorated. Radiographic examination revealed a gastric torsion. After removal of gas through a stomach tube the dog's condition improved and the stomach regained normal position. However, after 14 days the gastric torsion recurred. Removal of gas through a stomach tube improved the dog's condition, but the owner refused further treatment of the animal and it was euthanatized at his request.

Necropsy: The stomach was in normal position but dilated.

Differential Diagnosis: At both instances of gastric torsion the radiographic and clinical signs were such that the diagnosis was made with relative ease.

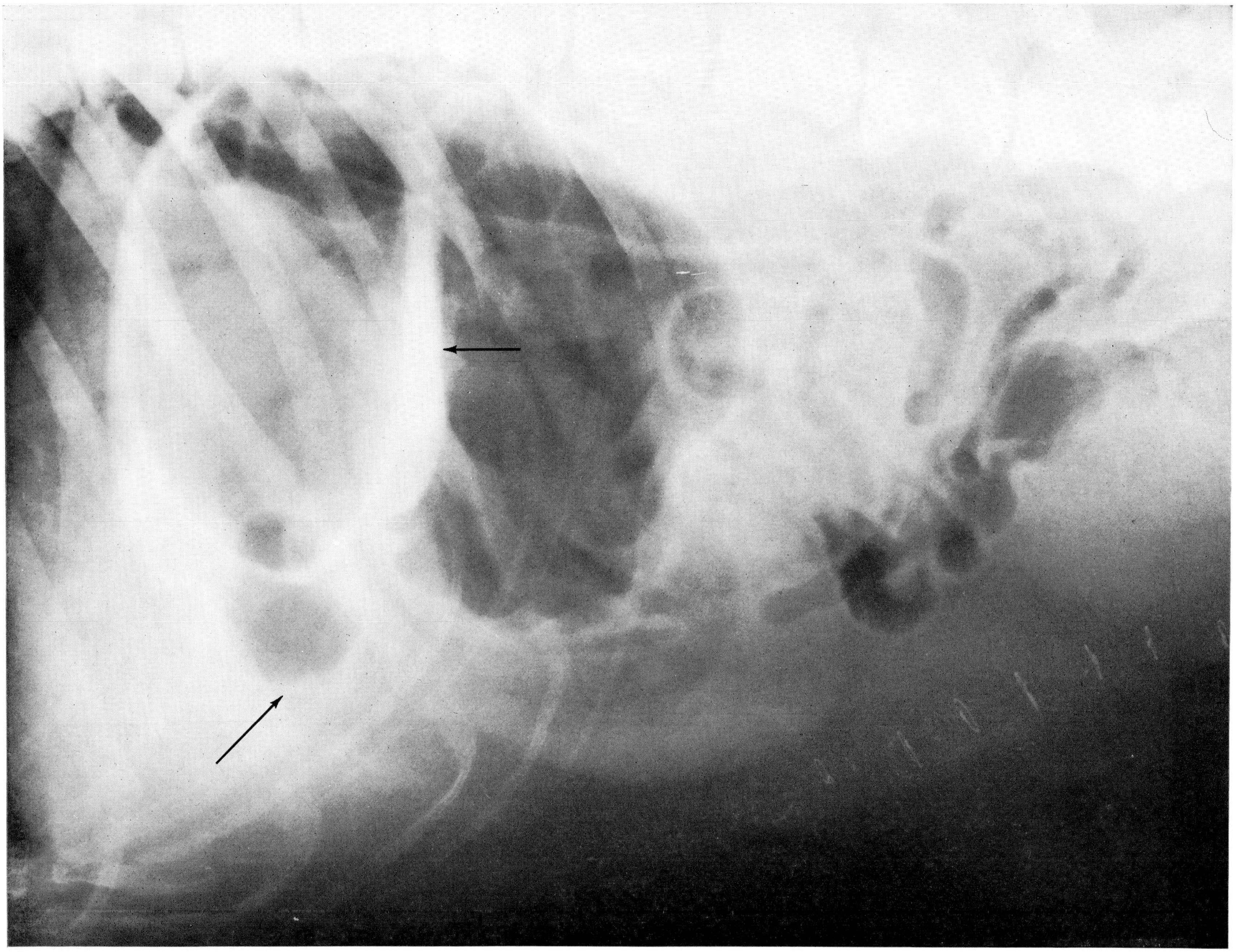

Case 21. **A,** Lateral radiograph made after recurrence of gastric torsion Gas was removed prior to the radiographic examination. The pylorus (lower arrow) is situated cranial and somewhat ventral to the fundus. The stomach is folded. The fold (upper arrow) consists of the walls of the antrum and the fundus.

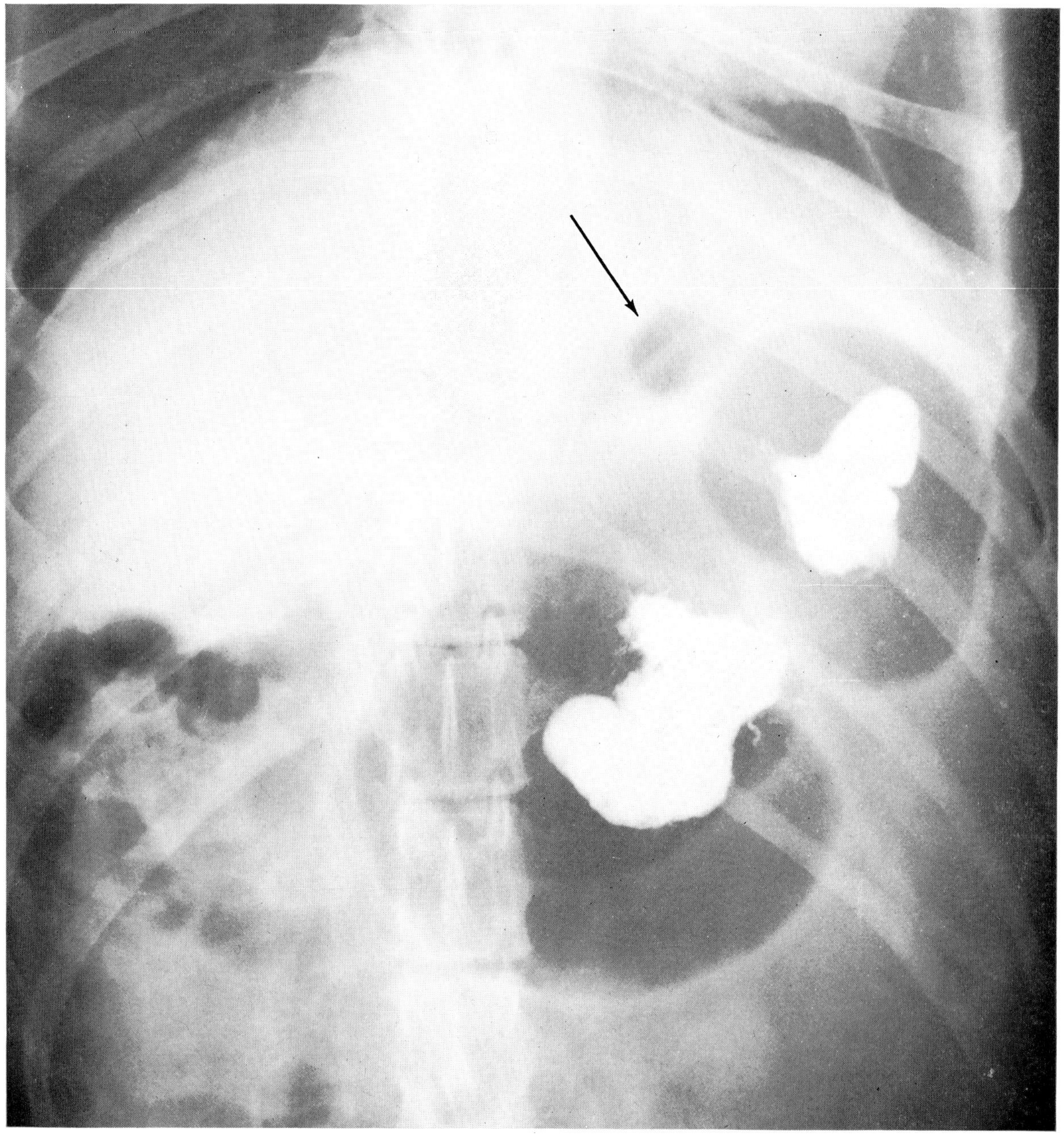

Case 21. **B,** Ventrodorsal radiograph made after a barium swallow. The two "compartments" of the stomach are well demonstrable. The pyloric antrum is to the left and cranial to the fundus. The pylorus (arrow) is well over on the left side.

Diagnosis: Gastric torsion with little distention of the stomach after removal of gas.

Case 22

Boxer, female, 8 years old. This dog became ill suddenly. It unsuccessfully tried to vomit and after a while could not stand on its legs. Its abdomen became very distended. It was brought to the clinic and, because of the distended abdomen, the diagnosis of gastric torsion was made. The stomach was intubated but little gas could be removed and the abdomen continued to be distended. A needle was inserted through the abdominal wall at the costal arch on the right side, but no gas or fluid could be withdrawn. Radiographs made at this time revealed the entire bowel to be distended and gas-filled. Laparotomy was performed. The entire small bowel was found to be gas-filled and very distended. Because of the bowel loops "ballooning" through the abdominal incision, the surgeon could not determine the cause of the problem. Most probably a complete torsion of the mesentery was responsible for the severe changes seen in the entire small bowel and the ensuing paralytic ileus. The prognosis was considered to be poor and the dog was put to sleep.

Necropsy: There were signs of strangulation of the mesentery, but because of the surgical procedure, which apparently had reduced the mesenteric torsion, this diagnosis could not be definitely confirmed on the postmortem table.

Differential Diagnosis: No other condition than mesenteric torsion would cause the enormous "ballooning" of the entire bowel.

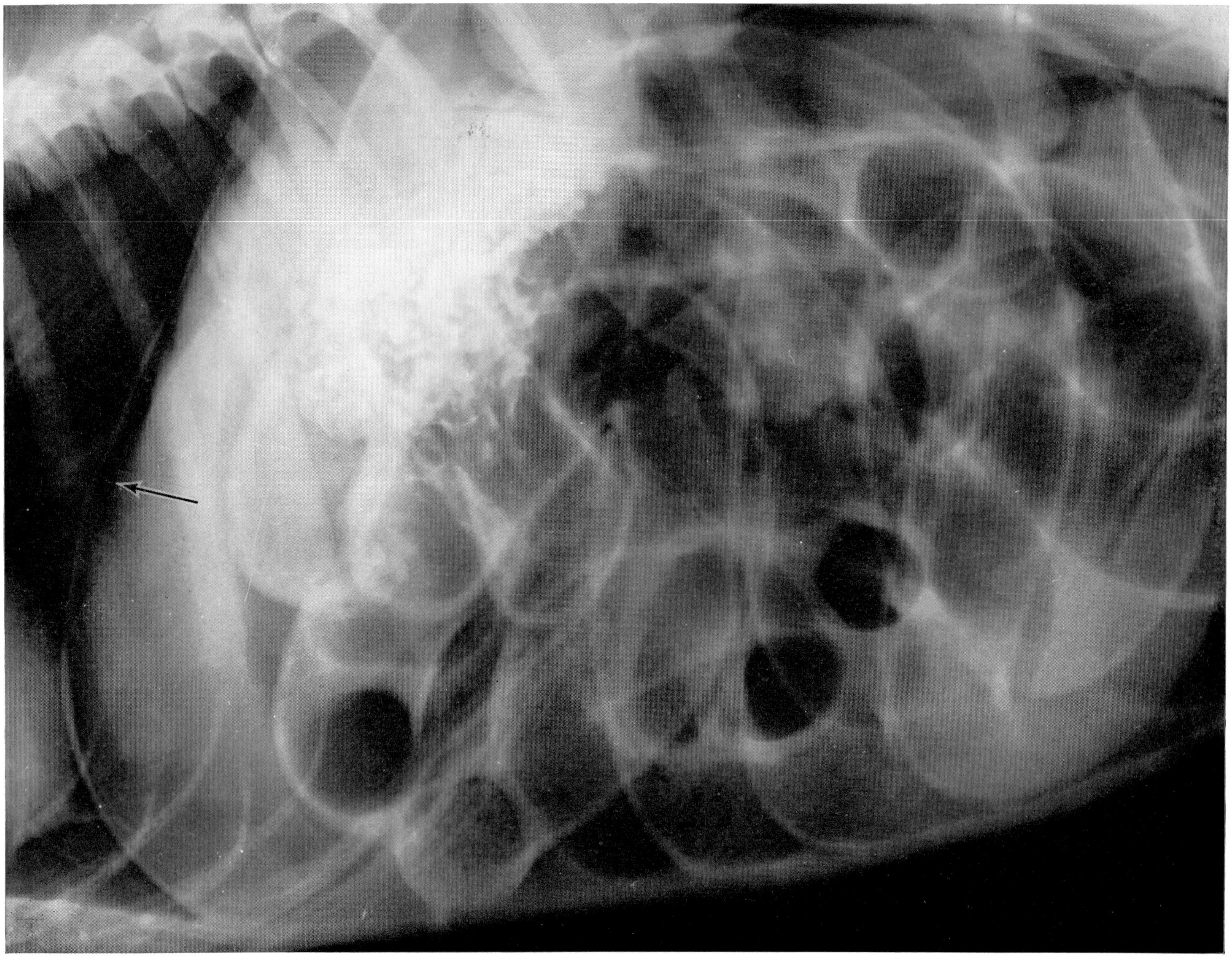

Case 22. Lateral radiograph of cranial and mid portion of the abdomen. The picture is dominated by the distended and gas-filled bowel loops. There is free gas in the abdomen as demonstrated by the presence of gas between the diaphragm and the liver (arrow).

Diagnosis: Paralytic ileus most likely caused by torsion of the mesentery.

Case 23

Dachshund, female, 3 years old. Three days prior to this dog's admission to the clinic, its owner had seen the dog swallow a piece of a pacifier. The animal became anorectic and started to vomit two days later.

On admission the dog was dehydrated and very listless. Palpation of the abdomen produced pain. A small mass as well as gas- and fluid-filled bowel loops was felt in the mid abdomen. Radiographic examination revealed a few somewhat distended fluid- and gas-filled bowel loops close to a barely visible foreign object. This made the diagnosis of an obstructive ileus almost certain. Meglumine diatrizoate was given, but the dog vomited and after 1 hour no contrast medium was seen in the stomach or the bowel. Laparotomy was performed. The tip of a pacifier was found to be obstructing the jejunum. There were rather severe changes in the wall of the bowel about 15 cm cranial to the foreign body. The foreign body was removed, but the surgeon did not consider resection of this part of the bowel necessary. The dog died two days after the operation.

Necropsy: Necrosis of the wall of the intestine at the site of the sutures had caused peritonitis.

Differential Diagnosis: The radiographs were characteristic of those seen in animals with relatively small foreign bodies lodged in the small intestine. A hazelnut in the bowel of a dachshund, would, for example, produce such a picture. Such a foreign body seems to move slowly through the intestine for a time before becoming firmly stuck in one bowel loop. The clinical signs are usually more severe than the radiographic signs would indicate.

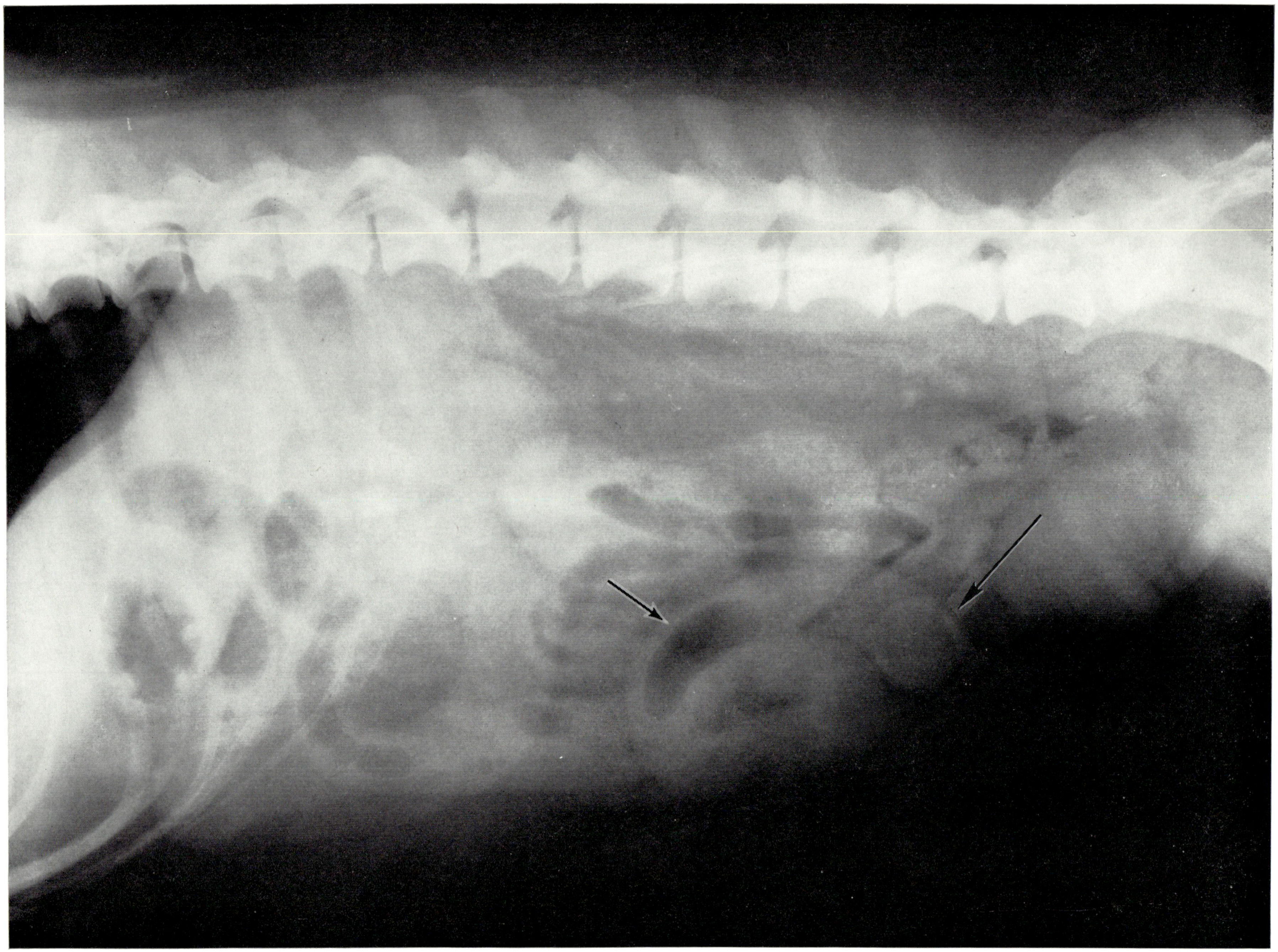

Case 23. Lateral radiograph on which a barely visible foreign body (large arrow) is noted in the small bowel. The foreign body is lodged in a bowel loop just cranial to the urinary bladder. Cranial to the foreign body, there is a bowel loop which is distended by fluid and some gas (small arrow). Other bowel loops containing only small amounts of gas are slightly distended by fluid.

Diagnosis: Ileus caused by an obstructing radiolucent foreign body.

Case 24

Stövare (Swedish driving dog), female, 2 years old. Previously this dog had had surgical treatment because of obstructive ileus. Recovery from the operation was uneventful. Eighteen hours prior to admission to the clinic the owner had seen the dog playing with two glass balls. Twelve hours later the dog vomited one of the balls. Because it continued to vomit and became anorectic and listless it was brought to the clinic. On examination a foreign object could be palpated in the abdomen. Radiographic examination revealed a radiopaque ball in the small intestine. Cranial to the foreign object was a gas and fluid-filled distended loop of the small bowel. The pyloric antrum was gas-filled and distended. This was indicative of complete obstruction. At operation a glass ball was removed from the cranial portion of the jejunum. The animal's recovery was uneventful. One month later it was again referred to the clinic because of signs of intestinal obstruction. Radiographs at this time revealed a foreign object, probably a piece of a rock, lodged in the small bowel. Several bowel loops were dilated and gas-filled. The dog was scheduled for operation the following day. When it was brought from its cage to the operating room, it was apparently in a much better condition than it had been on the previous day. A radiographic examination at this time showed that the foreign body was lodged in the rectum.

Differential Diagnosis: In both instances there was little question that the dog suffered from an ileus.

The radiographs illustrating this case are of interest mainly because they demonstrate the difference between a complete (radiograph **A**) and an incomplete (radiograph **B**) obstruction. The appearance of the stomach and the bowel in **A** indicates that there is little chance that the foreign body will move on further. In **B,** no retention of gas in the pyloric antrum can be seen and the moderate, uneven distention of the bowel (gas-filled but not fluid-filled) is more promising for a natural "removal" of the foreign object.

The foreign body seen in radiograph **B** was a piece of rock, flat in shape allowing some ingesta to pass by it. In contrast, the foreign body in **A** was a glass ball which completely obstructed the small bowel.

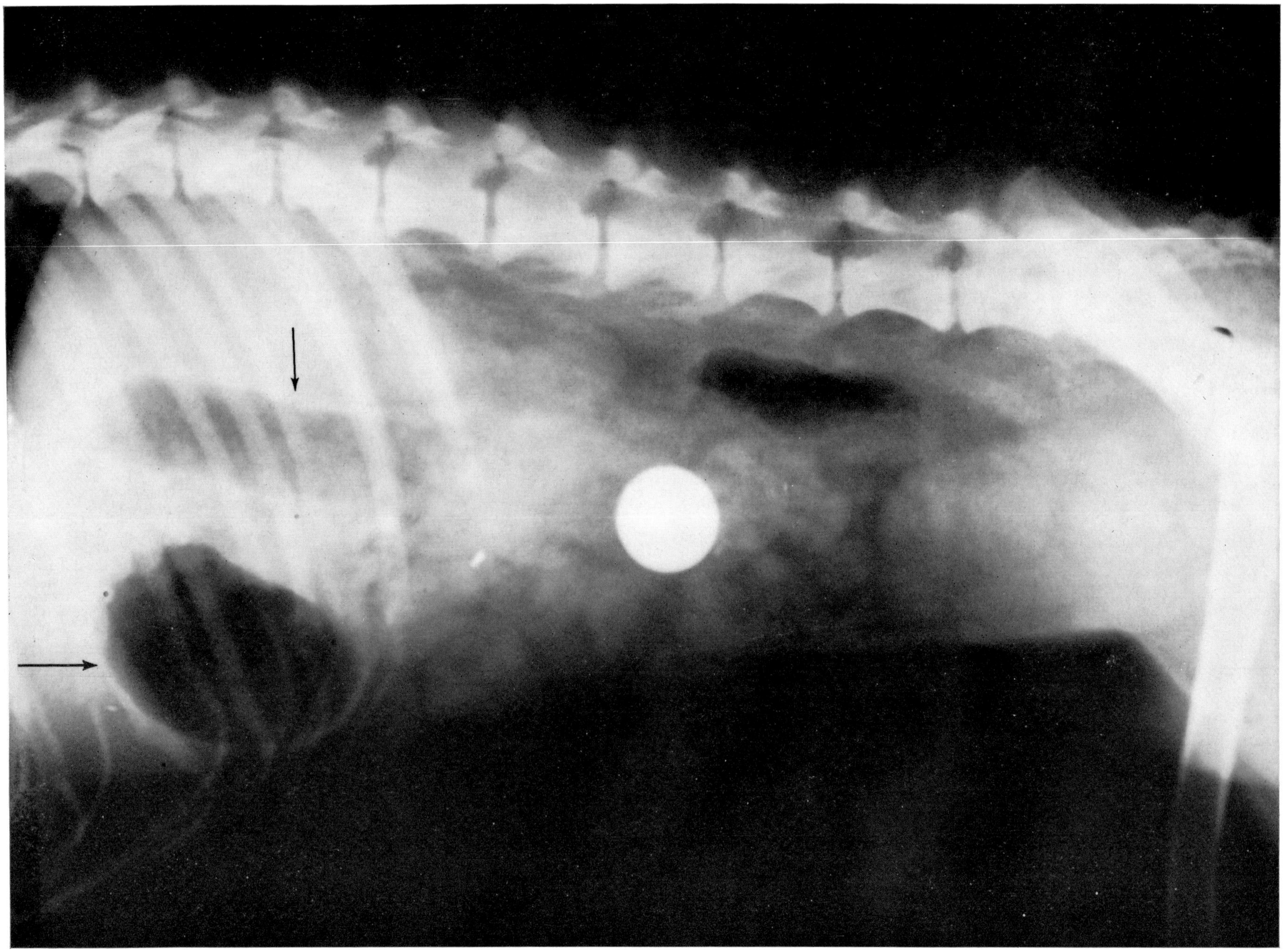

Case 24. **A,** Lateral radiograph made on the second hospital admission. A round, radiopaque foreign object is seen in the mid abdomen. The bowel loop cranial to the foreign body (probably the duodenum or the first part of the jejunum) is distended by gas and fluid (vertical arrow). The pyloric antrum is gas-filled and distended (horizontal arrow). The larger part of the small bowel and the large bowel are not distended and there is only one other pocket of gas. This gas is apparently lodged in the descending colon.

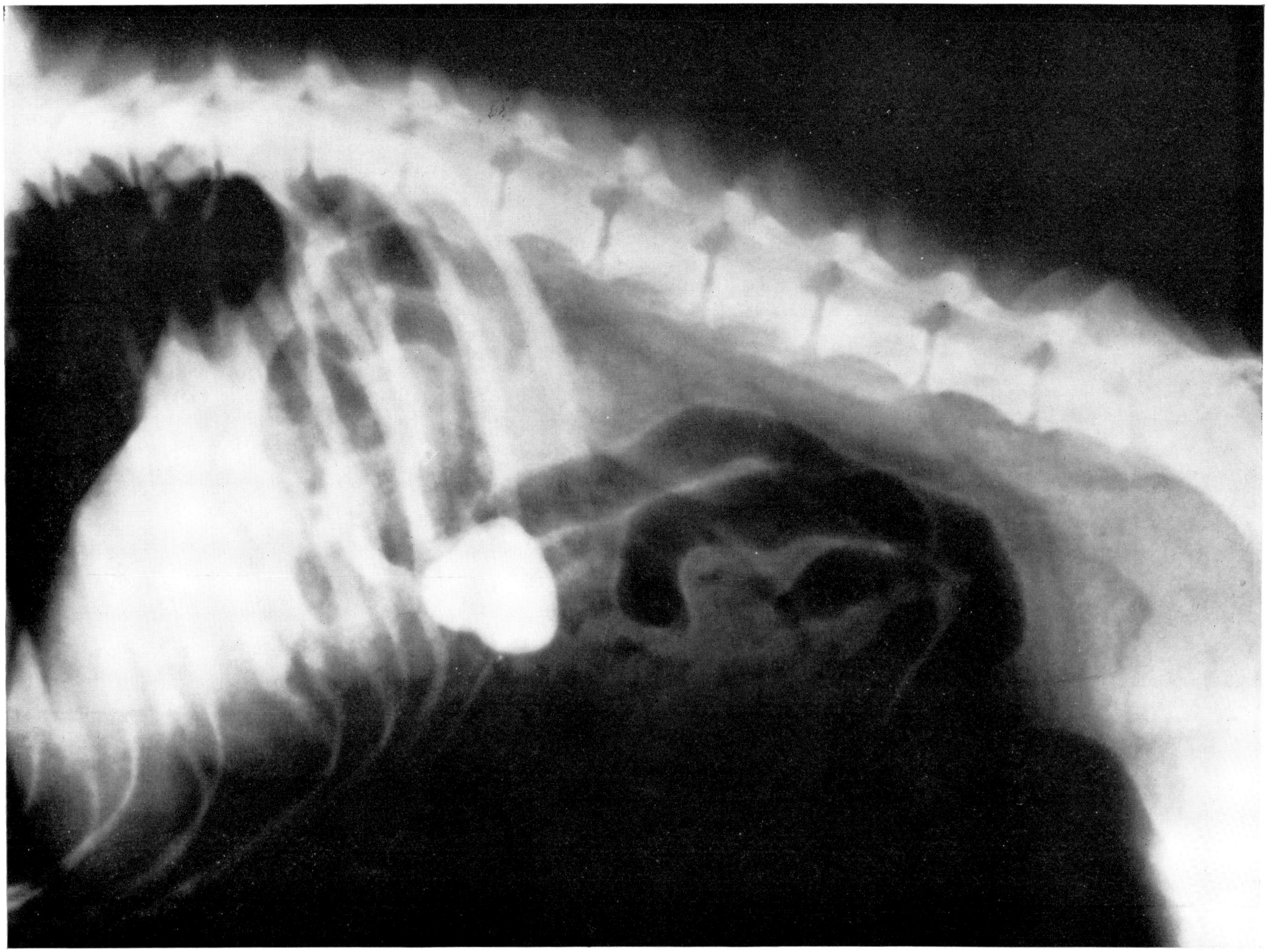

Case 24. **B,** Lateral radiograph made on the third hospital admission. A foreign body of irregular shape (a piece of a rock) is seen in the small bowel. The greater part of the small bowel is distended and gas-filled, but contains only traces of fluid. No part of the stomach is abnormally distended by gas.

Diagnosis: Recurrence of obstructive ileus.

Case 25

Dachshund, female, 11 years old. This dog had been anorectic and had vomited for three days before it was brought to the clinic. On admission it was dehydrated and in poor general condition. Radiographs revealed that several bowel loops were distended and gas-filled. Other loops were filled with fluid. A lump of ingesta with two metal objects was noted in the mid abdomen. Barium was given and a radiographic examination made 6 hours later showed that barium was still left in the stomach. Only about half of the small bowel was filled by contrast medium. Barium had not reached the gas-filled bowel loops.

The diagnosis of an obstructive ileus was made and the dog was operated upon. Tissue of a sausage with adhering metal clamps was found to be the cause of obstruction. The mesentery adhered to the bowel loop in which the foreign body was lodged. Recovery was uneventful following removal of the foreign body.

Differential Diagnosis: The clinical and radiographic diagnosis of ileus was obvious in this case. The slow passage of barium was the final evidence of an obstructive lesion.

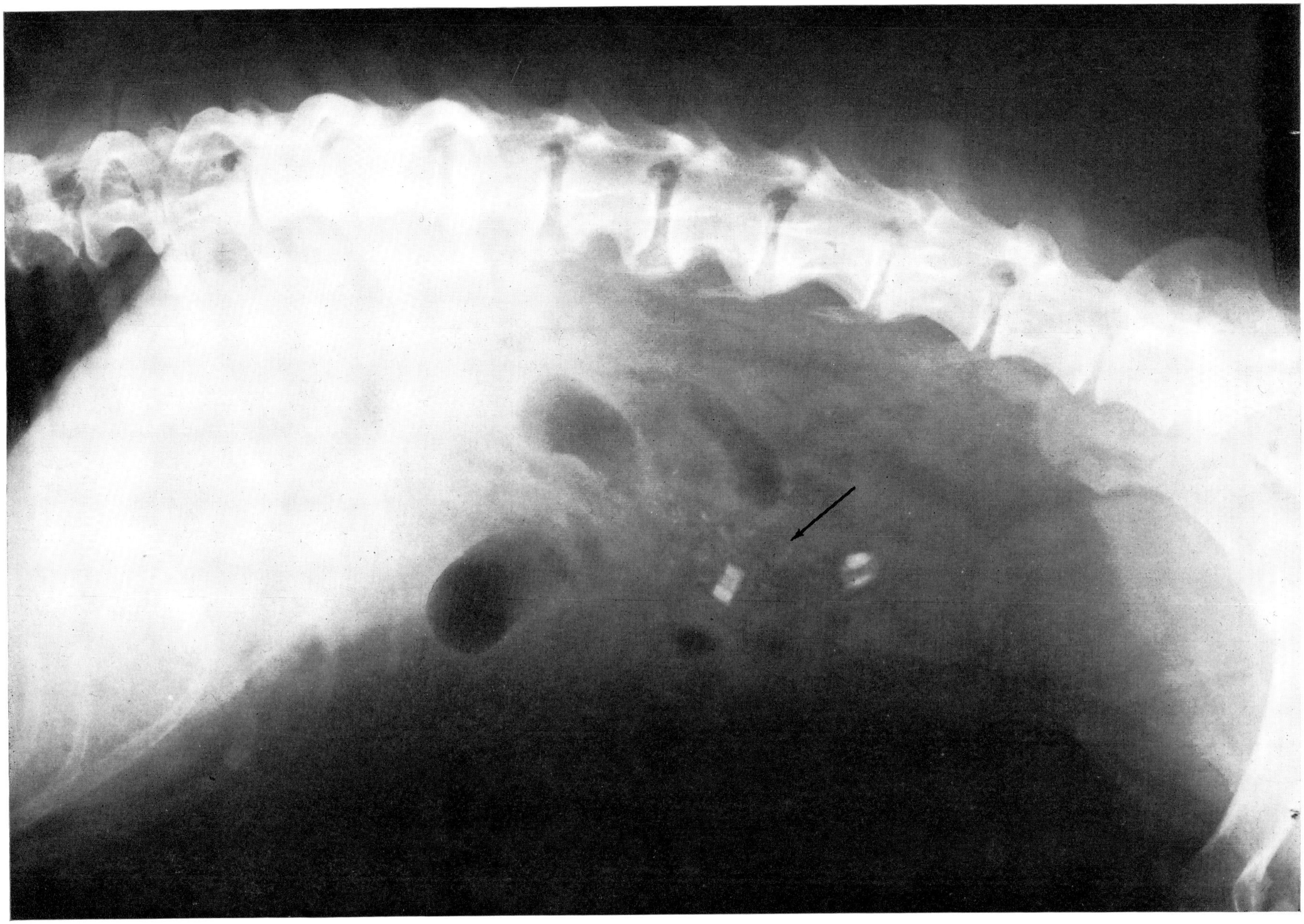

Case 25. **A,** Lateral radiograph. In the mid abdomen there is a lump of ingesta (arrow) with two metal objects. Gas-filled, distended bowel loops encircle the lump of ingesta. Incidental findings are: intervertebral disc degeneration (calcification), disc protrusions, and spondylosis deformans.

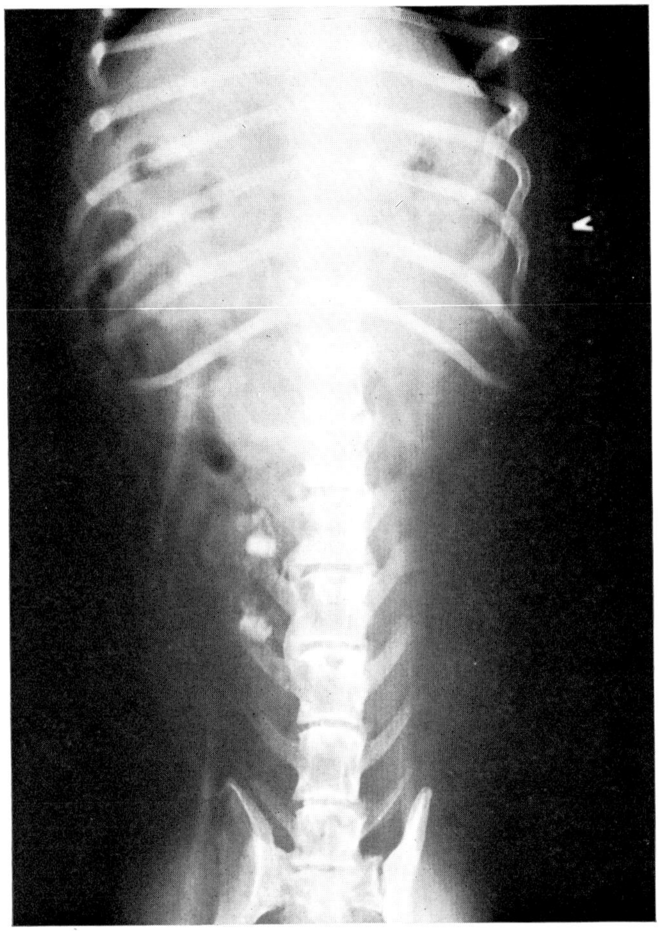

Case 25. **B,** In this ventrodorsal radiograph the two metal objects and the lump of ingesta are easily seen. Also several gas-filled bowel loops are visible cranial and to the right of the foreign object.

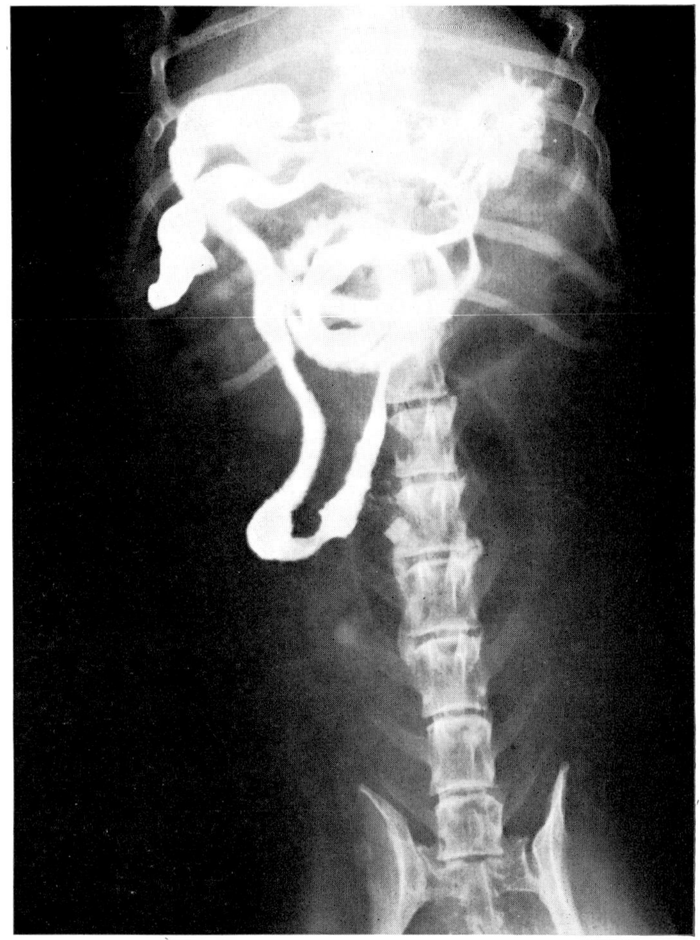

Case 25. **C,** Radiograph made 6 hours after a barium swallow. A considerable amount of contrast medium remains in the stomach. Barium does not reach the distended, gas-filled loops of the bowel close to the foreign object. The passage of barium is markedly delayed.

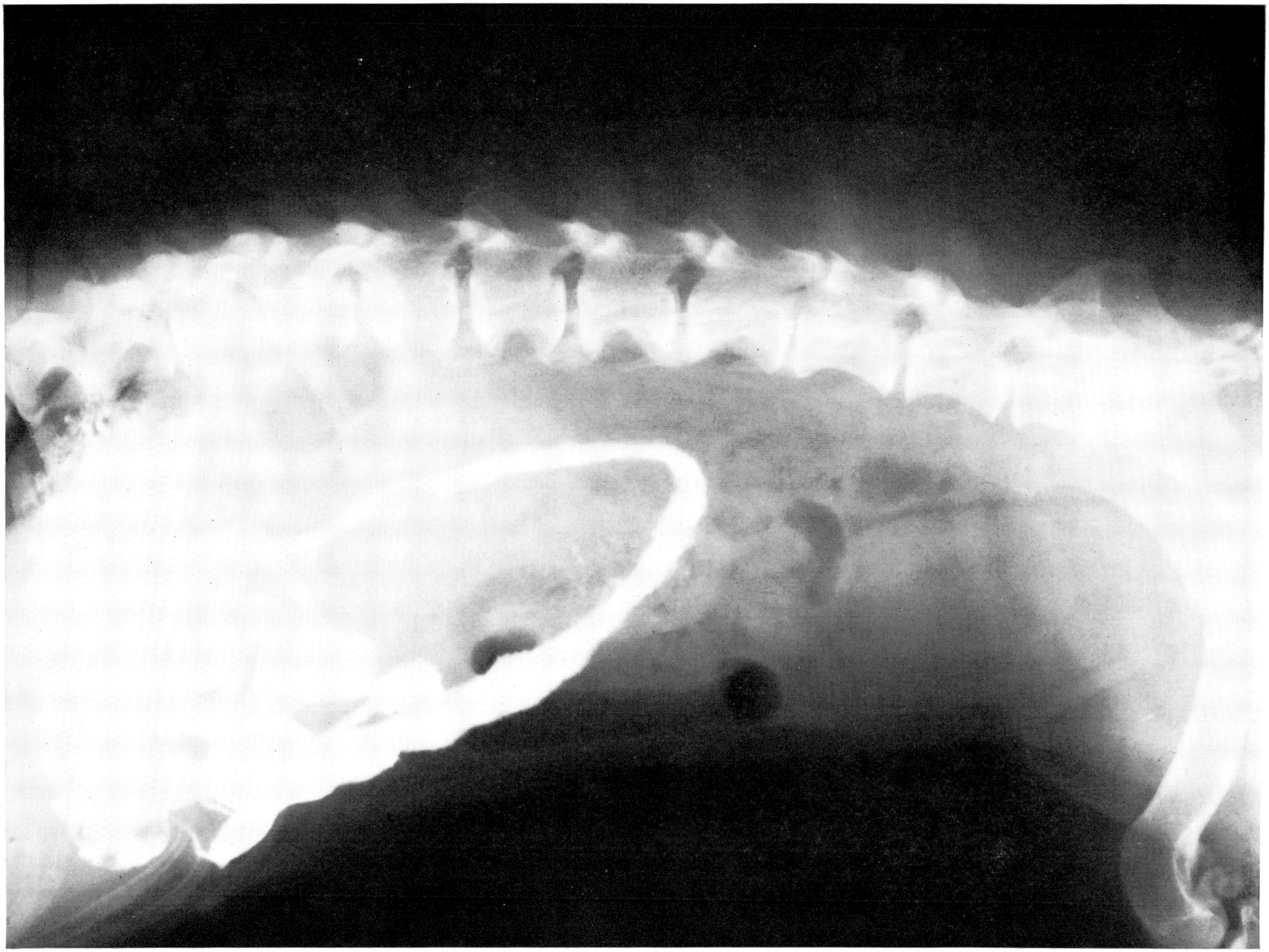

Case 25. **D,** Lateral radiograph made at the same time as the ventrodorsal radiograph shown in **C.**

Diagnosis: Obstruction of the small bowel by a soft foreign body.

Case 26

Spitz, female, 6 years old. This dog became listless after a large bone meal. Two days later it began to vomit. The following day the owner brought the dog to the clinic. On admission the dog vomited repeatedly and its abdomen was extremely painful on palpation. Radiographic examination revealed several distended, gas-filled bowel loops. There was also a small, partly radiopaque object in one of the loops. Intensive electrolyte and fluid therapy was instituted. Surgical exploration was postponed in order for the dog's condition to improve. Six hours following barium administration the radiographic examination was repeated. Several loops of the small bowel were seen to be distended and filled with barium. The contrast medium reached and, to a certain extent, bypassed the foreign body. After another 6 hours, most of the barium had passed out of the large bowel, but some still adhered to the foreign body.

At operation a sharp piece of bone was removed from the jejunum. At one point the wall of the bowel was found to be perforated to the serosa and much of the intestinal wall around the foreign body was necrotic. The foreign body and about 7 cm of the bowel were removed. Recovery was uneventful.

Differential Diagnosis: The diagnosis of ileus (in this case, rather, sub-ileus) was obvious. The foreign body was radiopaque and the passage of barium was delayed. There was, however, some discrepancy between the fact that the foreign body was not completely obstructing the intestine and the dog's poor general condition. Severe damage to the bowel wall was suspected because the foreign body was sharp and at one point nearly perforating the wall. A complete perforation was unlikely since there were no signs of peritonitis.

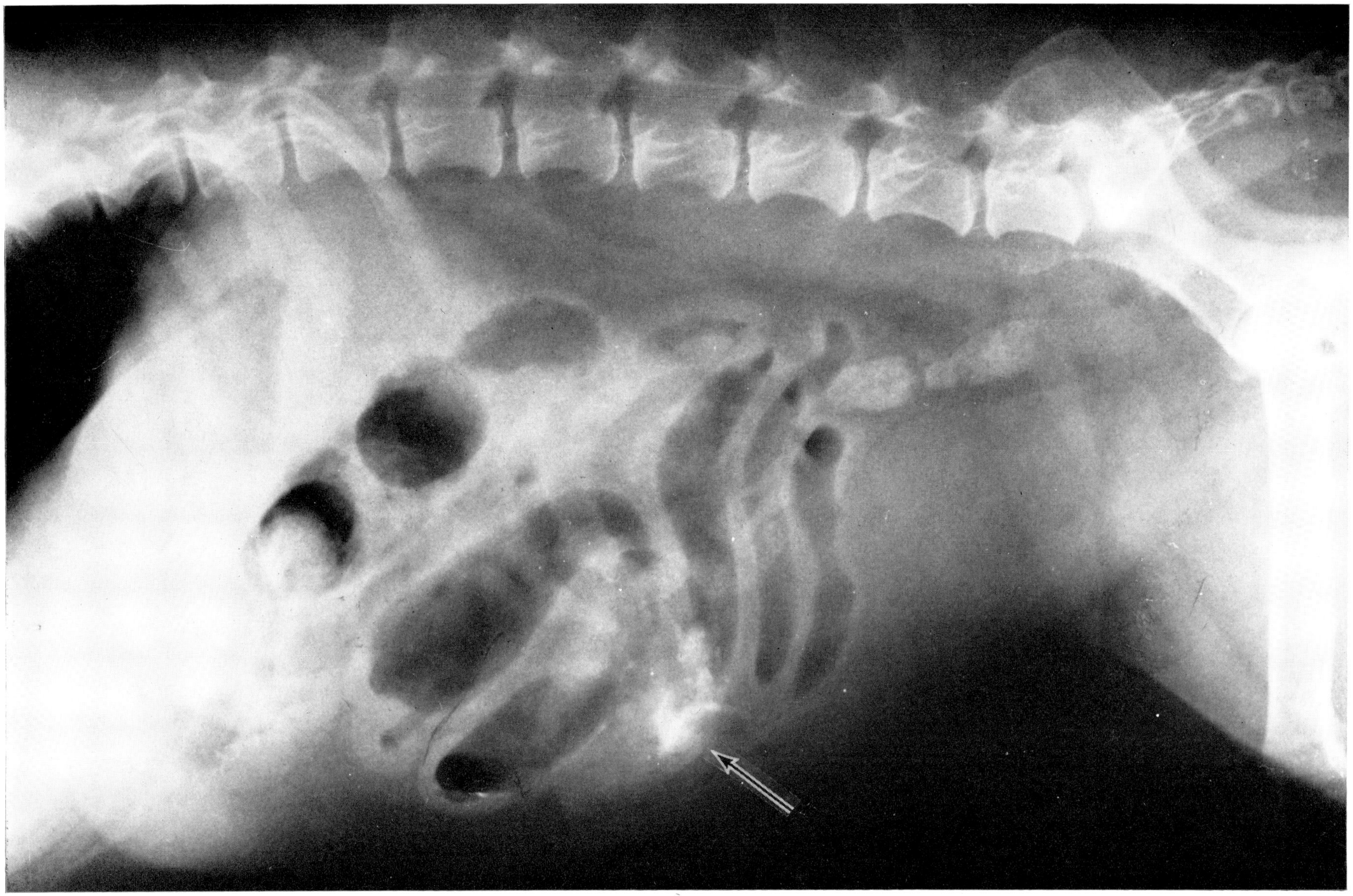

Case 26. **A,** A small foreign object with sharp edges is seen in the mid abdomen (arrow). The bowel loops surrounding it are gas-filled and somewhat distended.

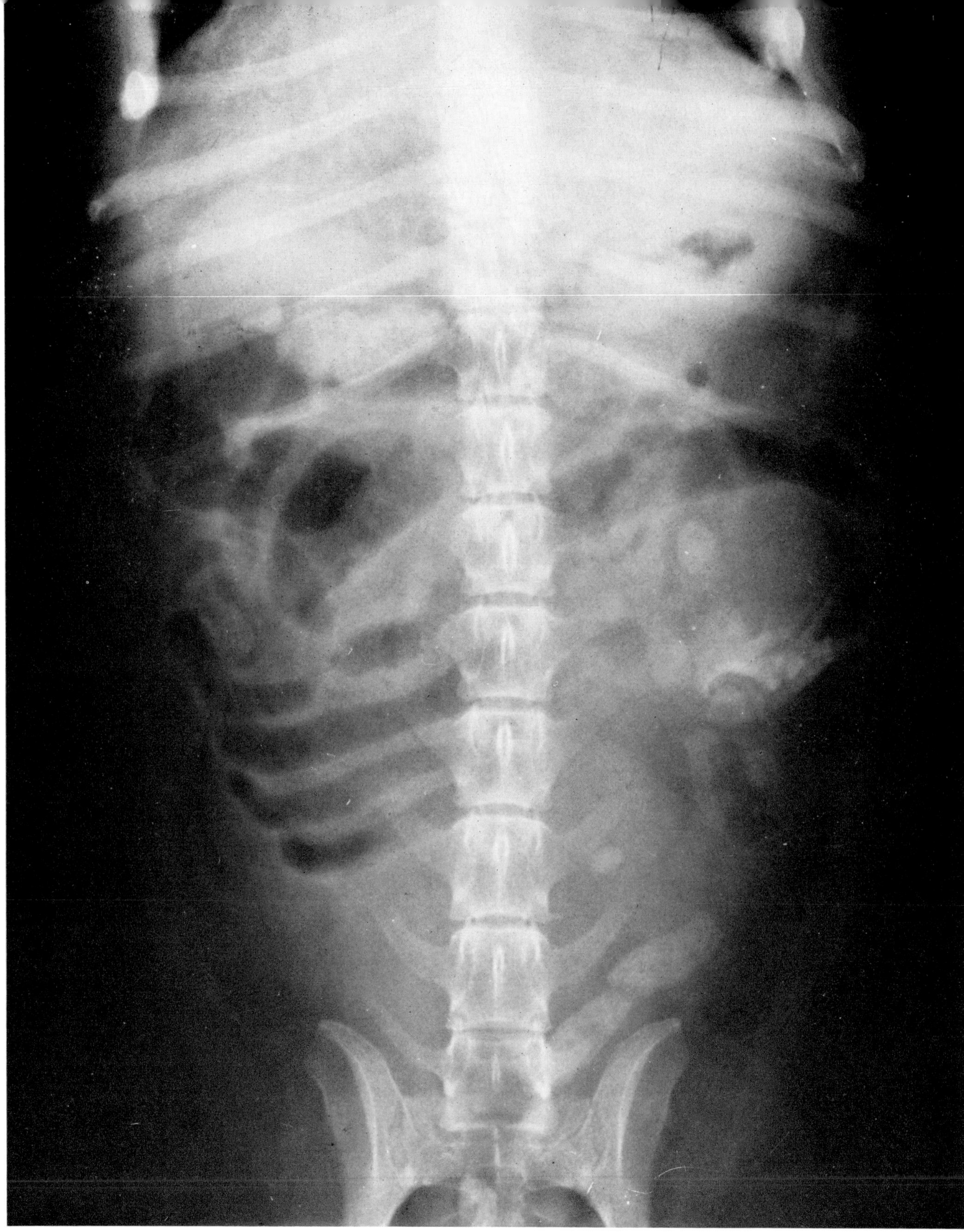

Case 26. **B,** On this ventrodorsal radiograph the bowel loop leading to the foreign body is noted to be distended and gas filled. The foreign object seems to be surrounded by ingesta.

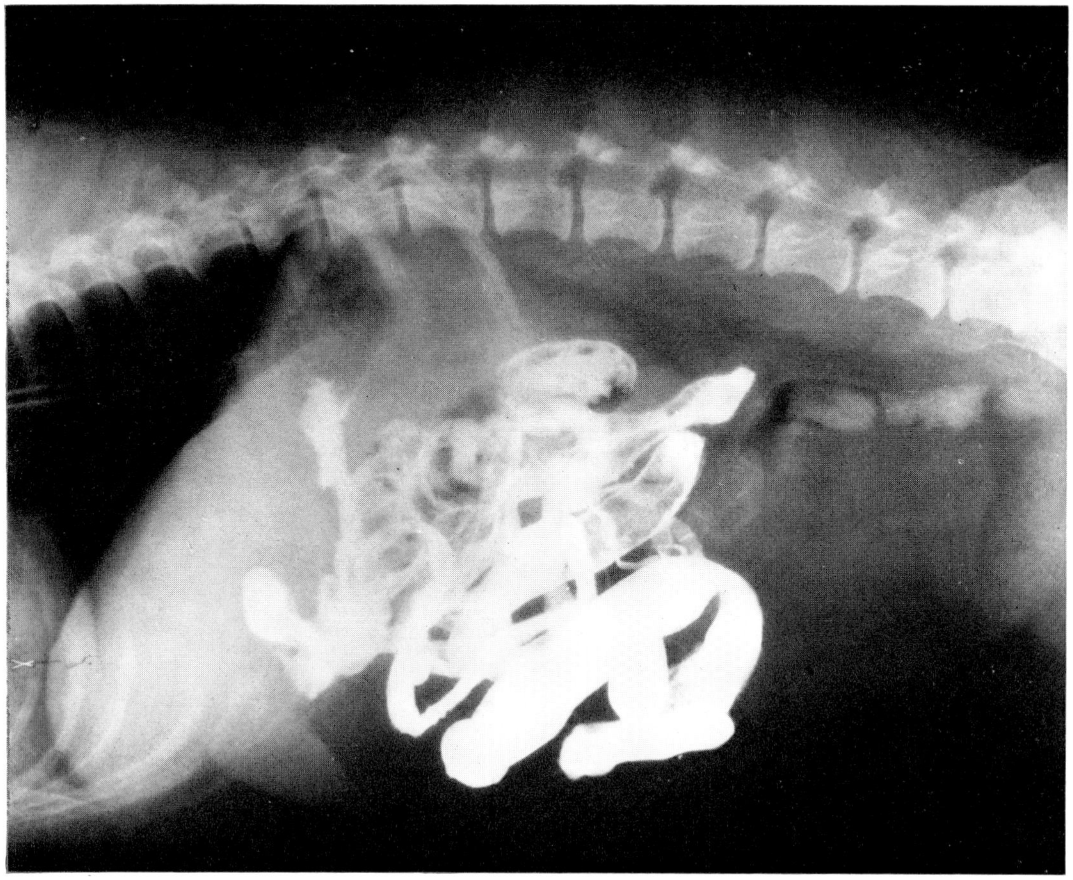

C

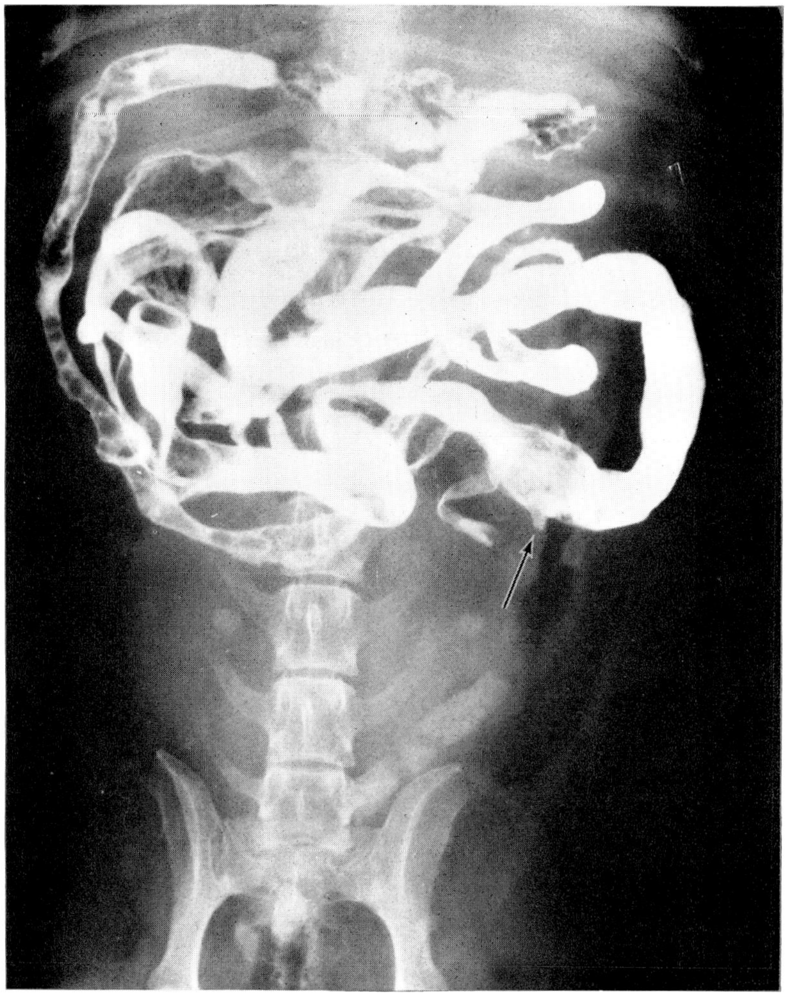

D

Case 26. **C** and **D,** Six hours after a barium swallow. Most of the contrast medium has left the stomach. The bowel loop close to the foreign body which on the previous radiographs was distended and gas-filled is now packed with contrast medium. The foreign body is outlined by the contrast material which passes by it. The two opposing indentations in the abdominal wall are apparently caused by the sharp edges of the foreign body (arrow).

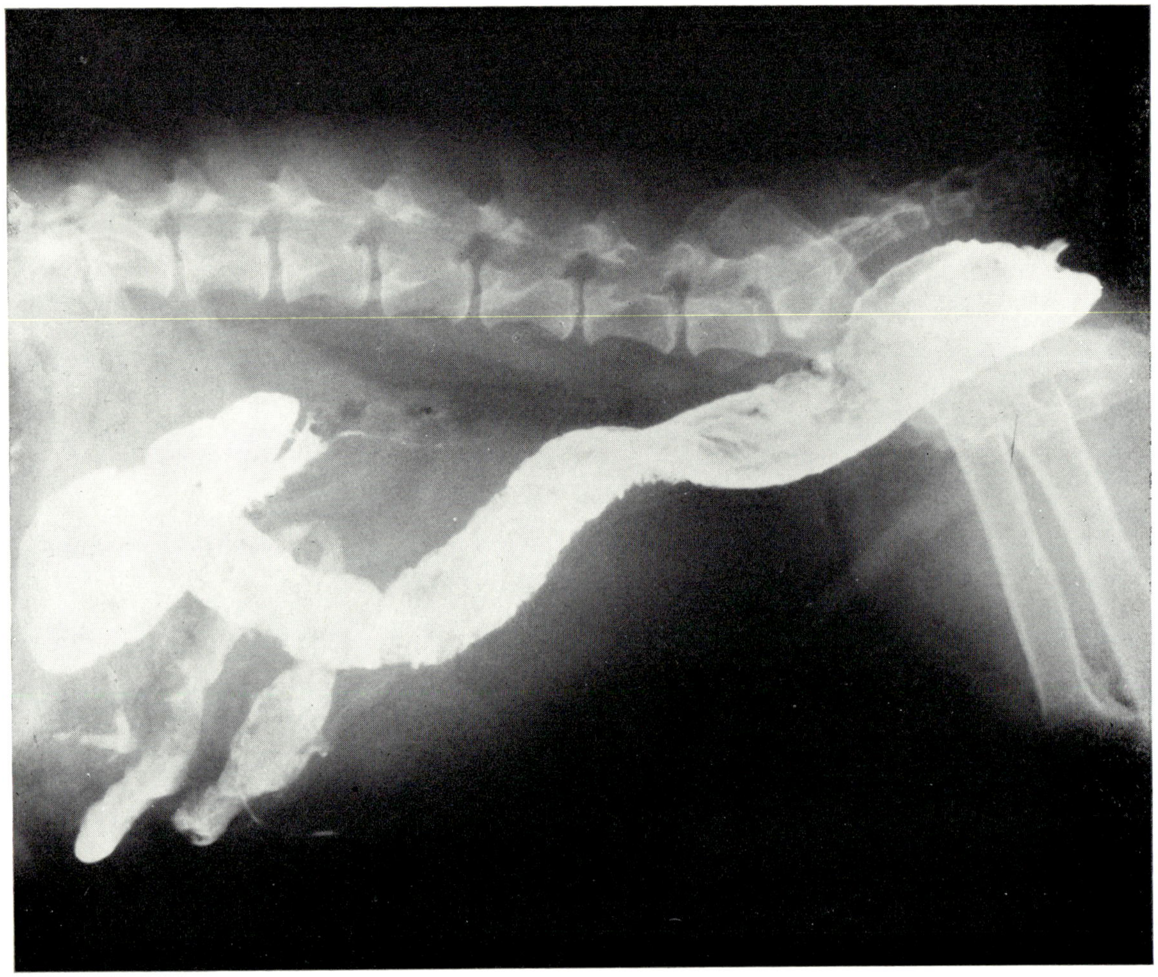

E

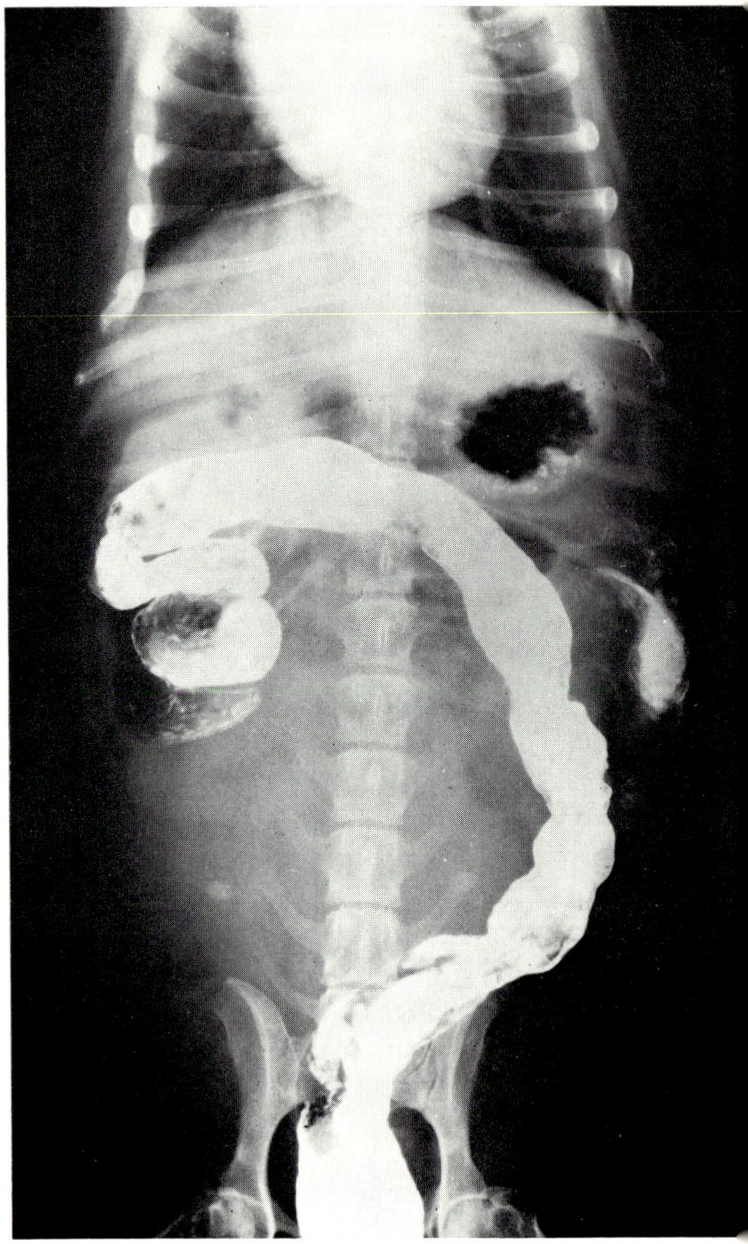

F

Case 26. **E** and **F,** After 24 hours, only a small amount of the barium remains in the small bowel. Most of it is close to or adheres to the foreign body. The bulk of the barium is in the large bowel. The urinary bladder is markedly distended.

Diagnosis: Sub-ileus due to a foreign body with sharp edges.

Case 27

Cocker spaniel, female, 7 years old. After 3 days of listlessness and anorexia, this dog began vomiting. After a day of intense vomiting, it was brought to the clinic. On examination it was found to be dehydrated and in poor general condition. Its abdomen was painful on palpation. Radiographs of the abdomen revealed several distended, gas-filled bowel loops, but no foreign body was apparent. Four hours after a barium swallow was given the radiographic examination was repeated. This time the diagnosis of obstructive ileus due to a peach seed could be made. The dog was operated on. Recovery was rapid and uneventful.

Differential Diagnosis: The diagnosis of ileus was made on the basis of the first radiographs. However, since no foreign body could be observed, a barium swallow was given. The radiographs made subsequently confirmed the diagnosis of ileus. Because of its irregular shape and hollow center the foreign object was identified as a peach seed. Such seeds are relatively common foreign bodies in dogs. Swallowed hazelnuts are also common causes of ileus in dogs. They are of low radiopacity, have a somewhat granular appearing nucleus, and often gas is seen between the nucleus and the shell.

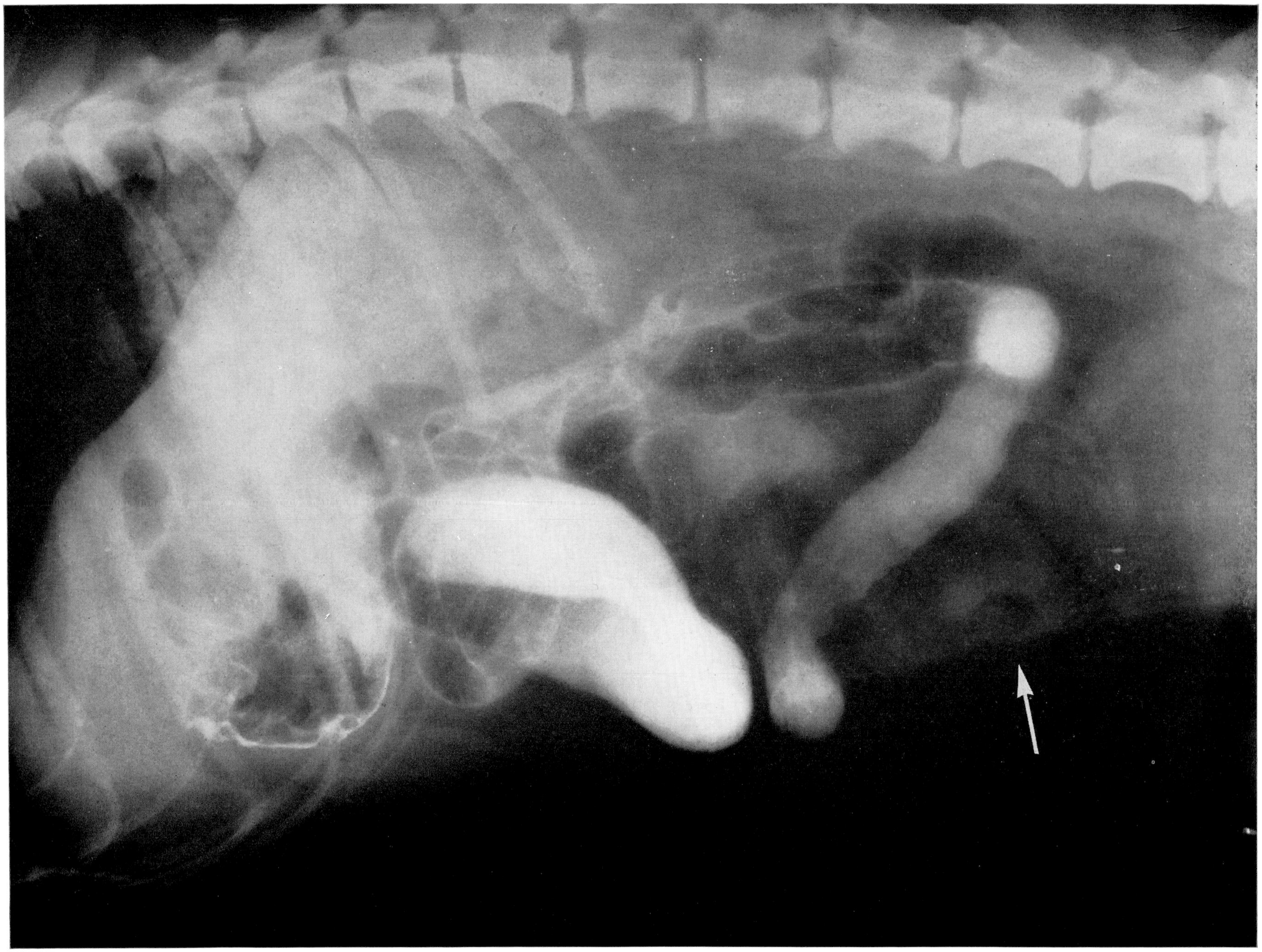

Case 27. **A,** Lateral radiograph made 4 hours after oral administration of meglumine diatrizoate. A considerable amount of the contrast medium is still in the stomach. The pyloric antrum is slightly distended and filled with gas. One slightly distended bowel loop is filled partly with gas and partly with contrast medium. Another bowel loop is more distended and packed with meglumine diatrizoate. Ventrally in the abdomen just cranial to the urinary bladder, there is a foreign body with a core of low density (arrow). This has the typical radiographic appearance of a peach seed.

Case 27. **B,** In this ventrodorsal radiograph the gas-filled pyloric antrum, the distended bowel loops filled with gas or contrast medium, and the foreign body (arrow) are even better demonstrated than in the lateral radiograph. It is noteworthy that the duodenum is of normal width and that the foreign body is lodged in a bowel loop which contains only very little contrast medium.

Diagnosis: Ileus caused by an obstructing foreign body. The ileus is of the "high" type, the foreign body being lodged in the cranial part of the jejunum. The foreign body is a peach seed.

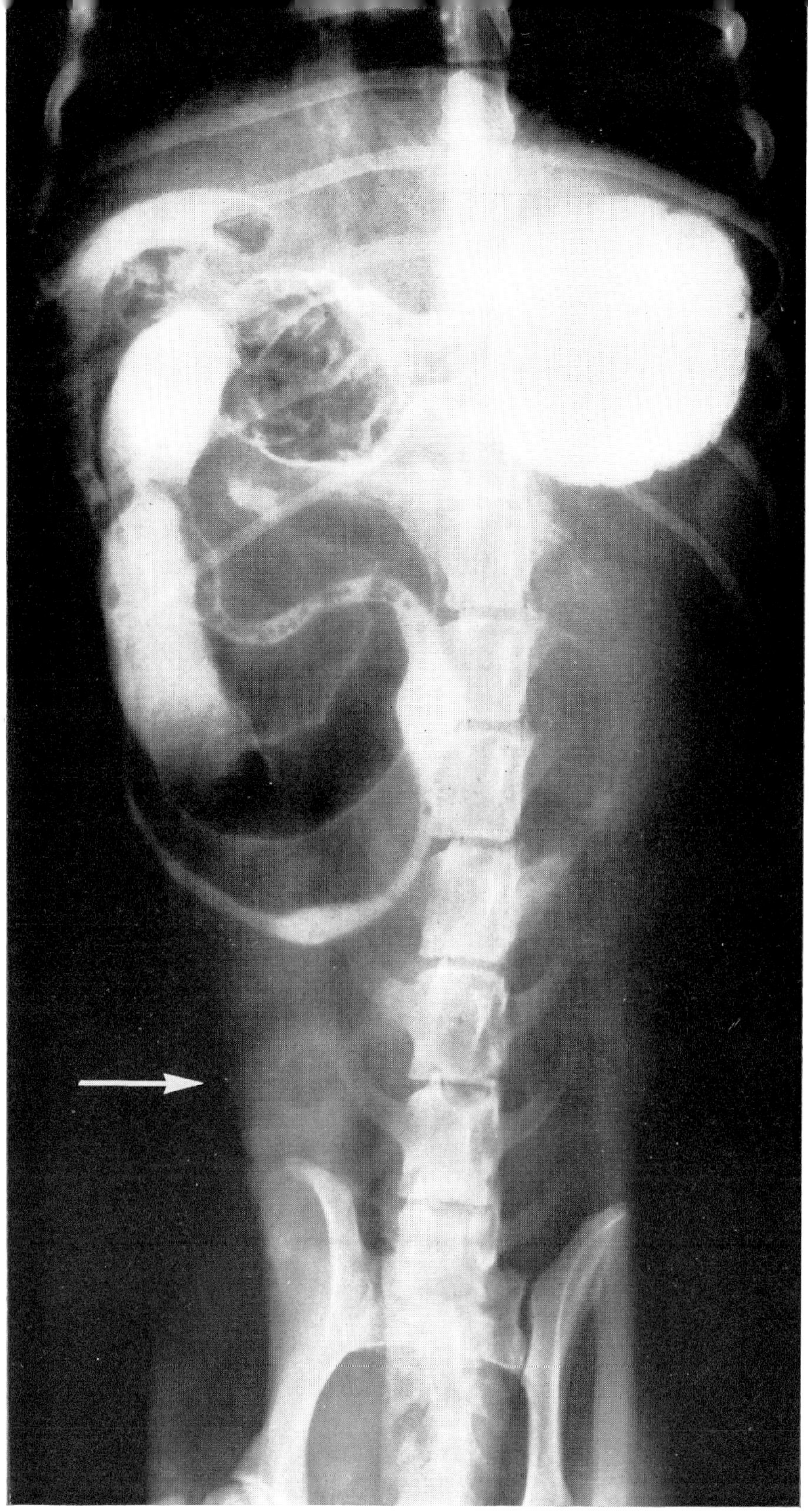

Case 28

Poodle, male, 9 years old. This dog had vomited repeatedly for about 24 hours when it was brought to the clinic. On admission it was listless and evidenced considerable pain when its abdomen was palpated. The most obvious signs of pain were obtained when pressure was exerted on a mass located cranially in the abdomen. Radiographs revealed a lump of ingesta in the mid abdomen. Cranial to this lump there was a distended and gas-filled bowel loop. The dog was given transfusions. The radiographic examination was repeated the following day. At this time, more distended and gas-filled bowel loops were noted. The impaction of ingesta could still be seen.

Radiographs made 4 hours after the administration of meglumine diatrizoate revealed that most of the medium was still in the stomach. Several loops of the small bowel were filled with the contrast medium. Close to the impaction, however, only a minimal amount of the contrast medium was present in gas-filled and distended loops.

At operation an impaction was found in the ileum and cecum. The impaction in the ileum was caused by a stenosis of the first part of the colon. The stenotic segment was resected. Biopsy revealed that the stenosis was due to to a granuloma. The dog made a rapid recovery.

Differential Diagnosis: Impaction of ingesta in the small bowel occurs occasionally after large bone meals. In these instances the impaction consists of very radiopaque material. This was not the case in this dog. The cause of impaction and obstruction could not be demonstrated radiographically. The overwhelming majority of cases of obstructive ileus in dogs are caused by foreign bodies. Intussusceptions, neoplasms, and granulomas are other possibilities which should be kept in mind.

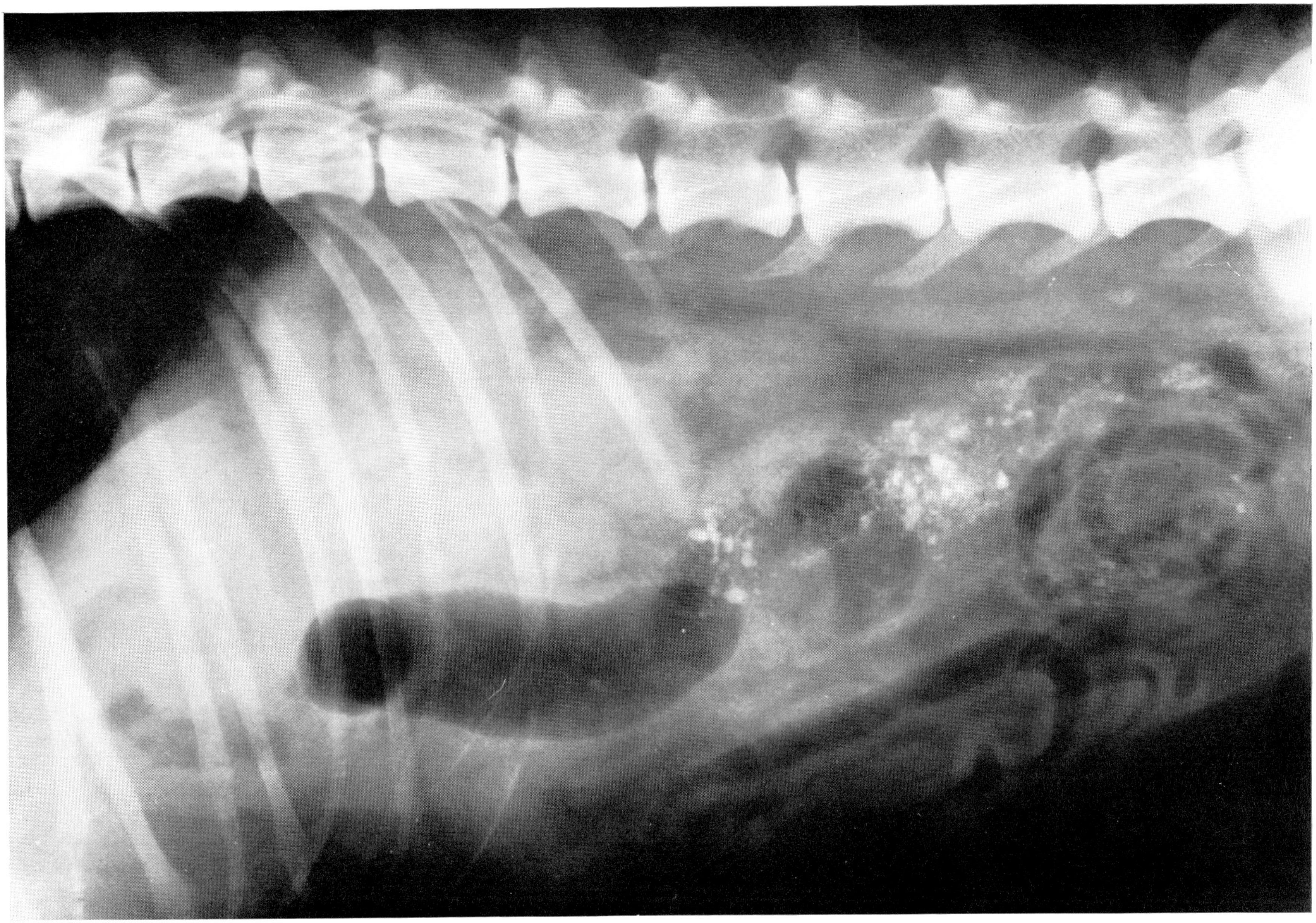

Case 28. **A,** Lateral radiograph made on admission. In the mid abdomen there is an impaction of ingesta. Cranial to the impaction a distended and gas-filled bowel loop is noted. (It was seen on the ventrodorsal radiograph that this bowel loop was not a part of the large bowel.)

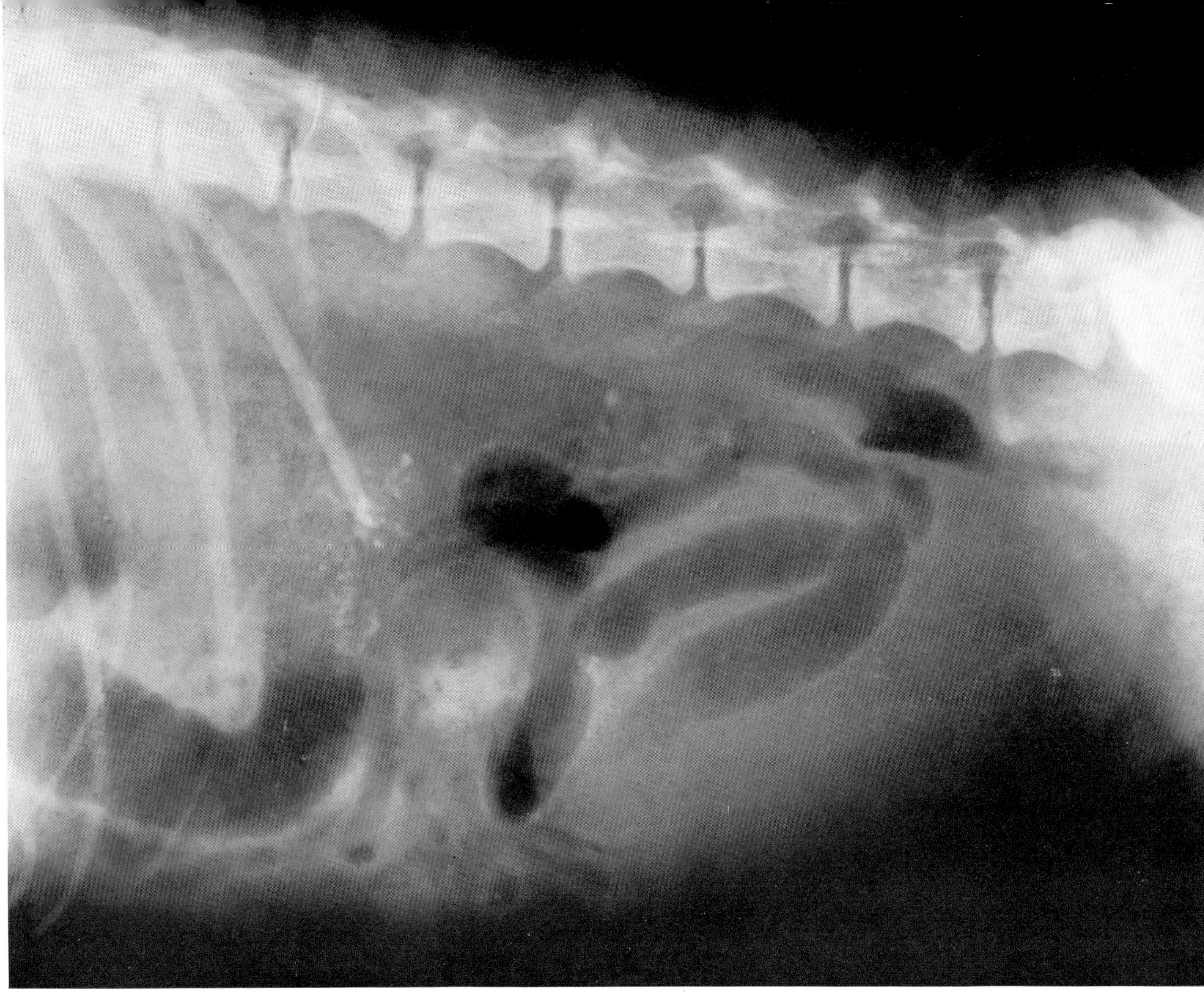

Case 28. **B,** Lateral radiograph made one day after admission. There is still impaction of ingesta in the mid abdomen. The bowel loop cranial to this impaction is more distended than on the previous radiograph. There are now other bowel loops which are distended and gas-filled. The urinary bladder is large.

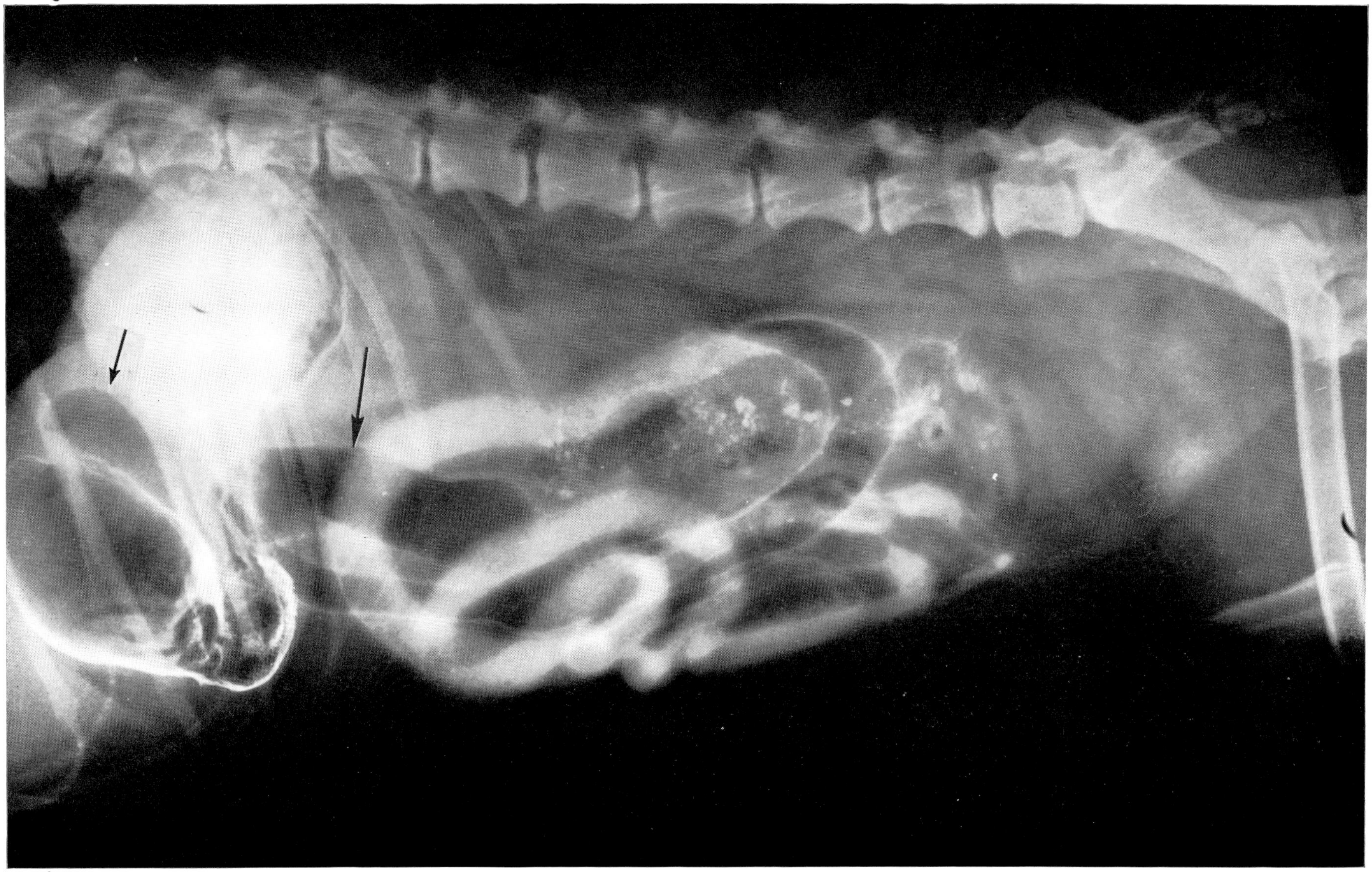

Case 28. **C,** Radiograph made 4 hours after oral administration of meglumine diatrizoate. A great portion of the meglumine diatrizoate is still in the stomach. The pyloric antrum and the duodenum (small arrow) are gas-filled and distended. Most of the jejunum is filled by meglumine diatrizoate, but closer to the impaction the bowel contains less contrast medium and becomes more distended (large arrow).

Diagnosis: Obstructive lesion (granuloma) in the ascending colon causing impaction of ingesta in the ileum and clinical and radiographic signs of ileus.

Case 29

Dachshund, female, 10 years old. About 24 hours prior to admission to the clinic the dog began to vomit. On examination it was found to be in poor general condition. It was dehydrated and two painful masses could be palpated in the mid abdomen. On radiographic examination these masses appeared to be impactions of dense ingesta. With all probability they were the remains of a heavy bone meal. One of the masses, which consisted of the largest pieces of bone, was apparently lodged in the small bowel. Because of the dog's severe dehydration, electrolyte and fluid therapy was instituted. Following the oral administration of a large amount of paraffin oil the dog's condition improved considerably and its bowel movements were normal. Radiographic examination revealed that the bony masses had passed out to the large bowel and some of them had been defecated. The dog left the clinic fully recovered.

Differential Diagnosis: Small bowel "constipation" (impaction of ingesta) should be recognized as a separate entity. It should not be confused with "regular" large-bowel obstipation. In the present case it was obvious from the location of the mass containing the largest chunks of bone that the impaction was not in the large bowel. In cases of impaction, an underlying cause should always be suspected (see Cases 28, 34, 35, and 36). In the present case it was obvious that the heavy bone meal was enough to explain why the impaction had occurred.

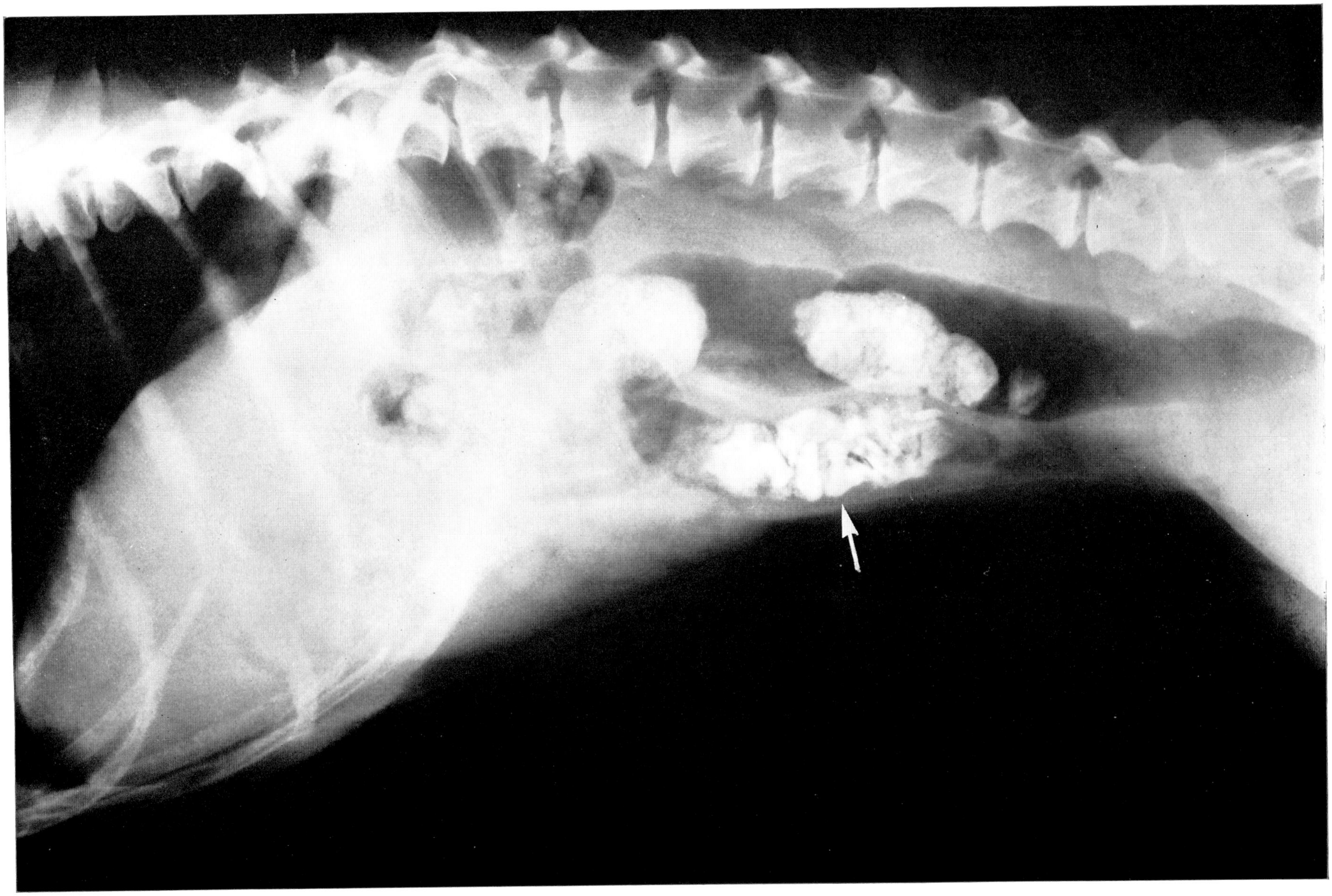

Case 29. **A,** Lateral radiograph demonstrating several dense masses and gas in the bowel. Most of the gas and all lumps of ingesta except one are lodged in the large bowel. The mass containing the largest chunks of bone (arrow) seems to be lodged in the ileum. There is little sign of ileus in spite of the impaction of ingesta.

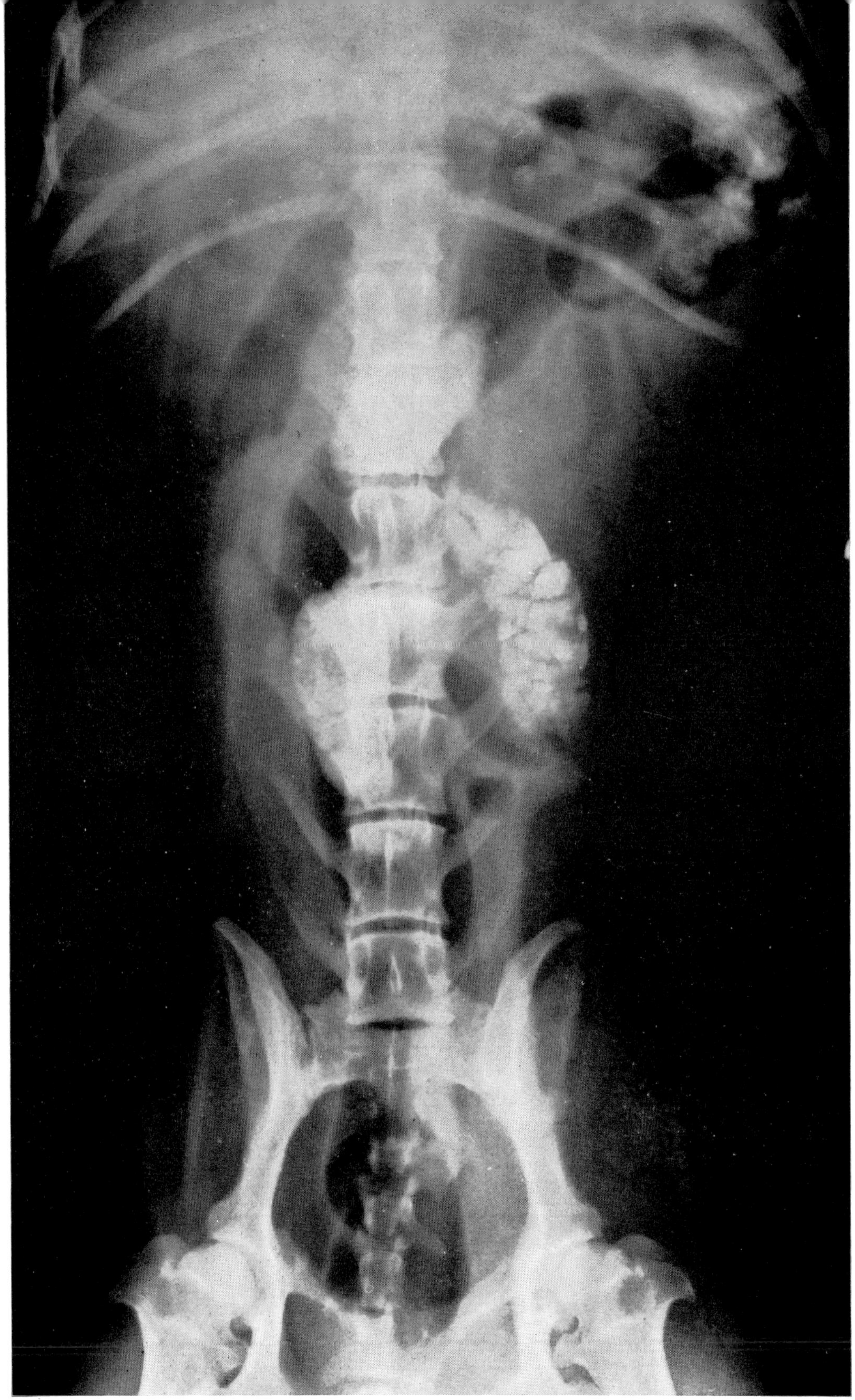

Case 29. **B,** In this ventrodorsal radiograph it is as obvious as in the lateral radiograph that "the lump of bony chunks" is lodged in the small bowel. The descending colon (which holds two lumps of ingesta) and the rectum are gas-filled and easily distinguished from the small bowel.

Diagnosis: Impaction of ingesta in the ileum.

Case 30

Irish setter, male 10 years old. This dog developed anorexia and vomited repeatedly. Its condition deteriorated rapidly. After several days of illness it was brought to the clinic in a miserable condition. The animal was dehydrated. Palpation of the abdomen revealed marked rigidity of the abdominal muscles and produced extreme pain.

Radiographs revealed a severe ileus with many bowel loops "pulled together" in the mid abdomen. A string or a stocking was suspected as the cause of the ileus.

At laparotomy a nylon stocking was found to have perforated the small bowel in several places, at the insertion of the mesentery. The bowel was threaded onto the stocking. The heel of the stocking completely obstructed a loop of the cranial portion of the jejunum. Because prognosis was considered poor the dog was put to sleep. Necropsy was not performed.

Differential Diagnosis: On this radiograph the typical appearance of the bowel threaded onto a string or stocking is demonstrated. This radiographic appearance is pathognomonic for this type of foreign object.

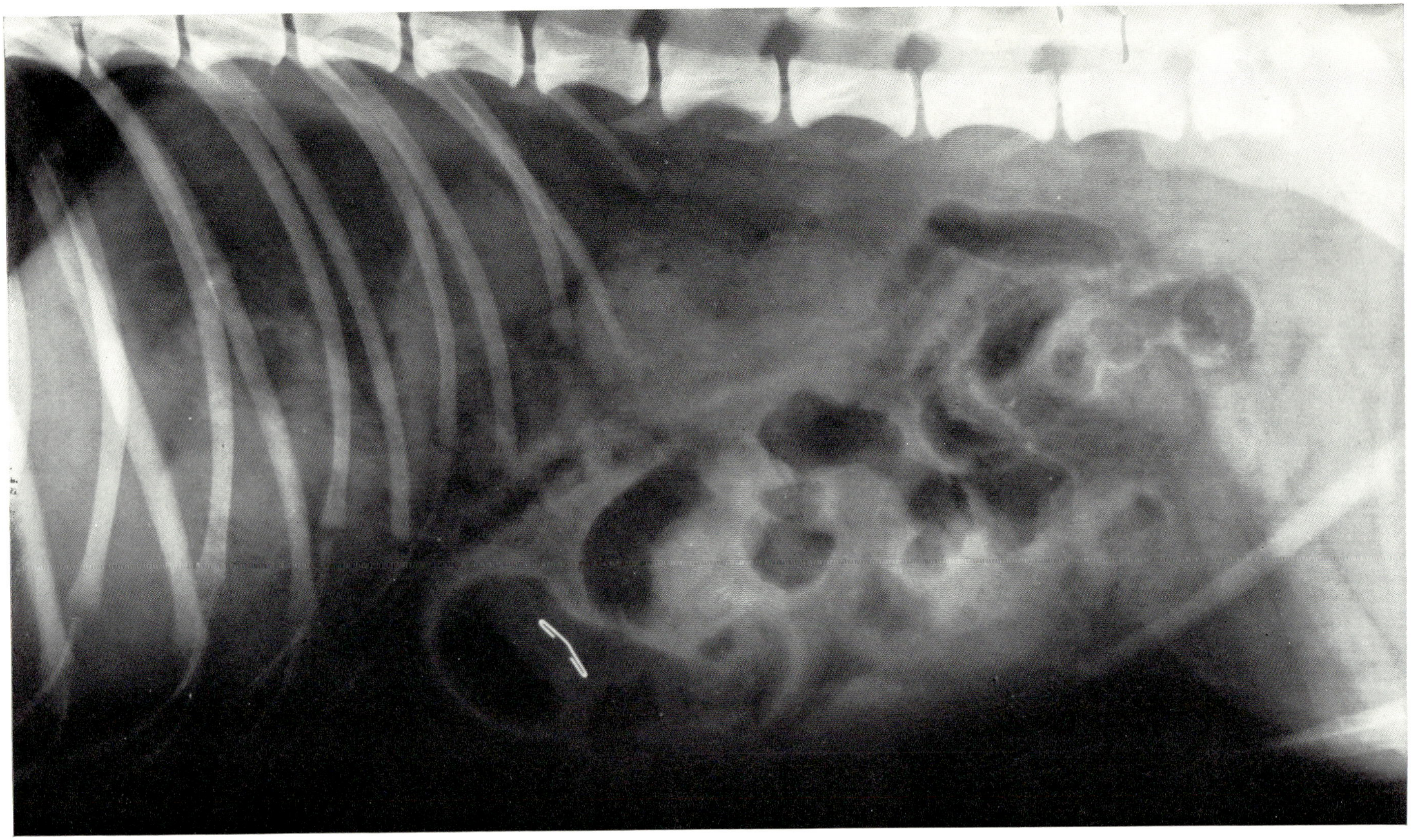

Case 30. Many gas-filled and distended bowel loops are pulled together in the mid abdomen. This gives rise to a wrinkled pattern or a "gathered flounce." There is a staple in one of the gas-filled bowel loops.

Diagnosis: Obstructive ileus. Nylon stocking onto which the bowel is threaded.

Case 31

Cat, male, 10 weeks old. This cat had played with a piece of string. The string could then not be retrieved. One day later the cat became ill and vomited several times.

On admission to the clinic the cat was listless but showed no other physical signs of illness. A few gas-filled and somewhat distended bowel loops could be seen on radiographs. Barium was administered orally and additional radiographs were made 2 hours later. At this time the diagnosis was evident. The small bowel had the typical "gathered-flounce" pattern, indicating that the foreign body was a piece of string or a similar object.

The cat made a rapid recovery following surgical treatment.

Differential Diagnosis: The "gathered-flounce" pattern is pathognomonic for an ileus caused by a piece of string or an object of similar shape. The bowel becomes threaded onto the foreign body and frequently a perforation occurs at the insertion of the mesentery. The present case presented no problem in differential diagnosis.

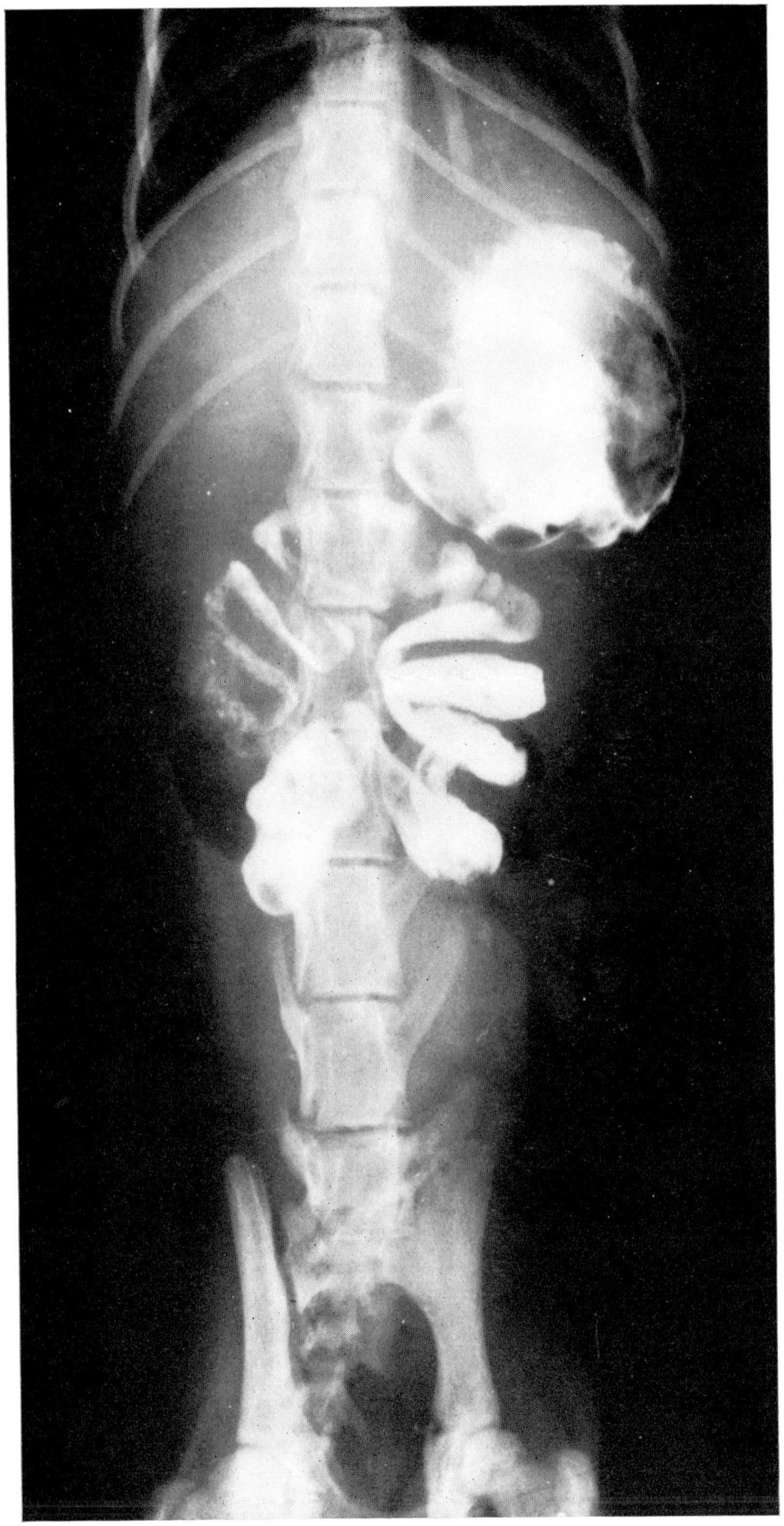

Case 31. Ventrodorsal radiograph made 2 hours after the oral administration of barium. The contrast medium is in the stomach and in several loops of the small bowel. These bowel loops are arranged like a "gathered flounce," which indicates that the bowel is threaded onto a piece of string, stocking, or similar foreign object.

Diagnosis: Ileus caused by a string.

Case 32

Lakeland terrier, female, 1 year old. When this dog was 10 months old it developed anorexia, vomited, and became very listless and somewhat dehydrated. A local veterinarian radiographed the dog. Nothing definite was found. Laparotomy was performed but no abnormality was detected.

The animal's condition improved somewhat after the operation, but a week later intensive vomiting and diarrhea occurred. The vomiting of fecal matter ensued and the diarrhea became increasingly more hemorrhagic. Hemoglobin and hematocrit values decreased. Probably the dog survived only because of intensive transfusions with blood and electrolyte solutions. It was also given various antibiotics. After more than a month of this treatment, the animal was lethargic and also suffered several episodes of rectal prolapse. It was brought to the clinic in this miserable condition. There was a palpable, elongated mass in the abdomen. It was clearly demonstrated on radiographs. The clinical history together with the findings indicated the presence of an intussusception. A barium enema given under fluoroscopic observation permitted visualization of a large intussusception. At operation it was found that the ileum was intussuscepted into the colon. Severe necrotic changes had taken place in the intussuscepted ileum. About 10 cm of ileum had to be resected. The dog made a complete recovery.

Differential Diagnosis: The radiographic appearance of an elongated mass in the abdomen combined with the clinical signs, such as vomiting and diarrhea, made the diagnosis of intussusception a likely one. The positive fluoroscopic findings confirmed the diagnosis.

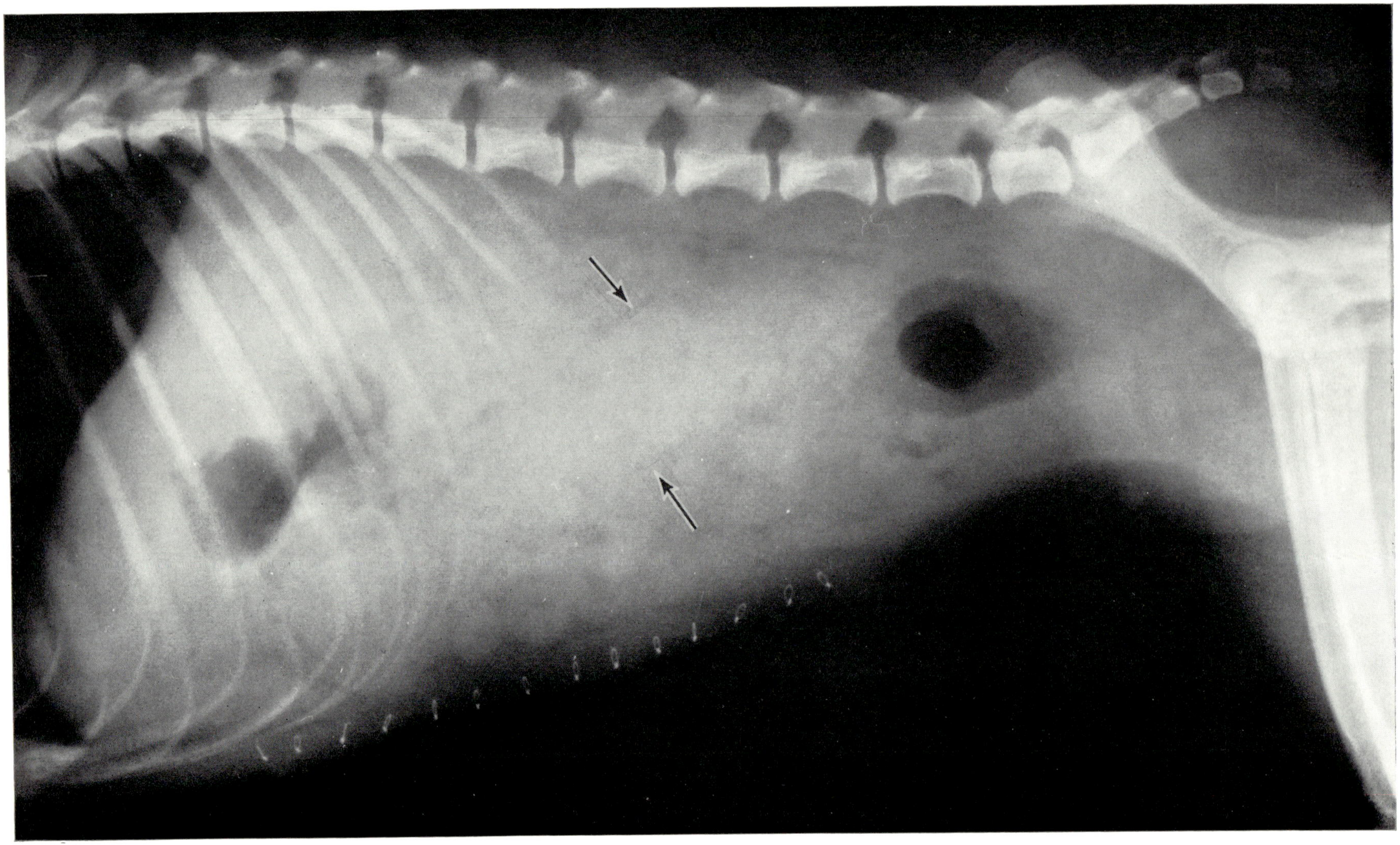

Case 32. **A,** Lateral radiograph made on admission. There is gas in the stomach and rectum and the most caudal portion of the descending colon. An ill-defined elongated mass (arrows) can be seen in the mid abdomen extending from the liver to the gas-filled part of the colon. There are metal sutures in the abdominal wall.

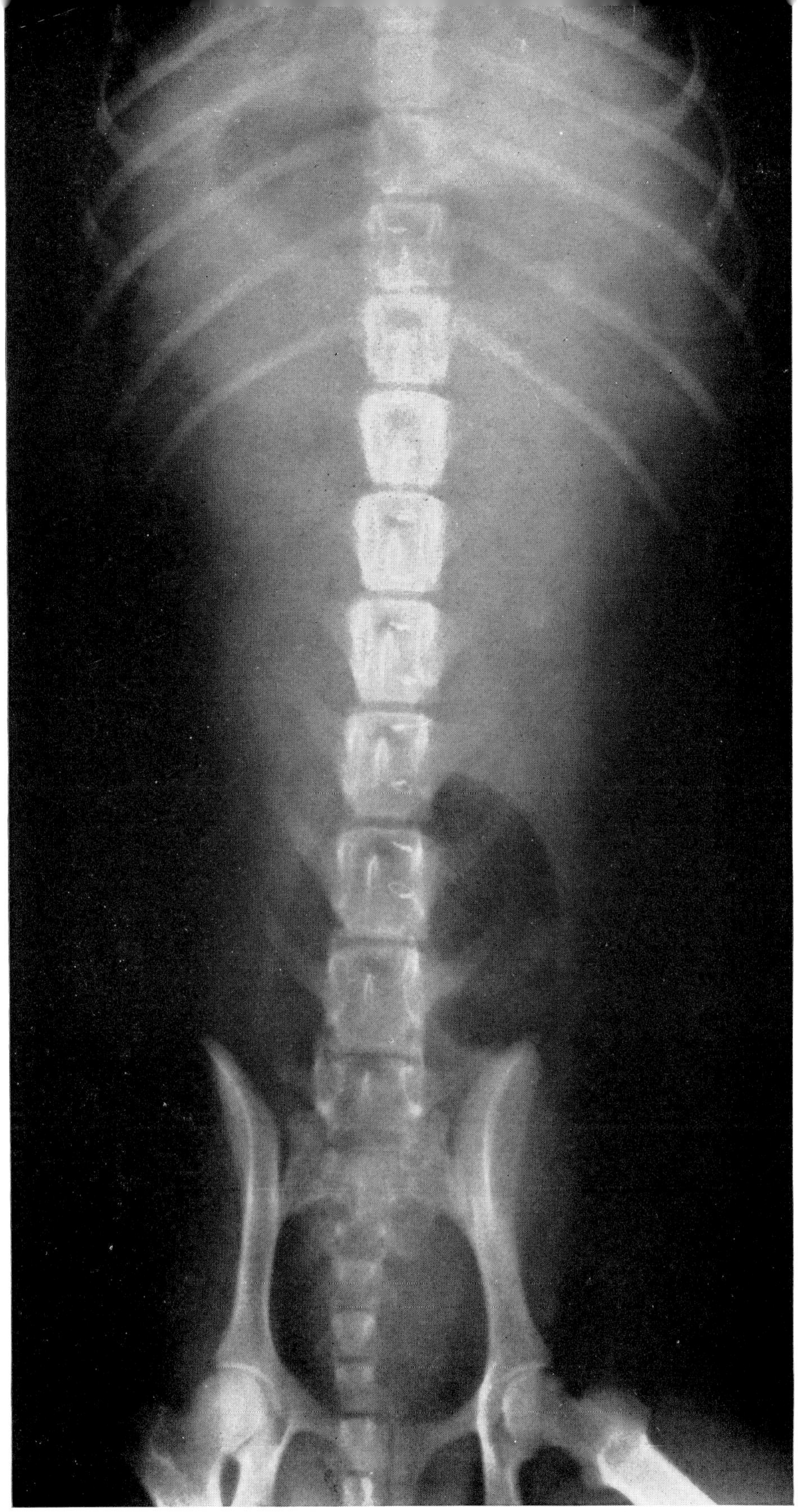

Case 32. **B,** In this ventrodorsal radiograph it is seen that the bowel loop containing gas has a sigmoid shape. The mass that is obvious on the lateral radiograph cannot be seen clearly in ventrodorsal projection.

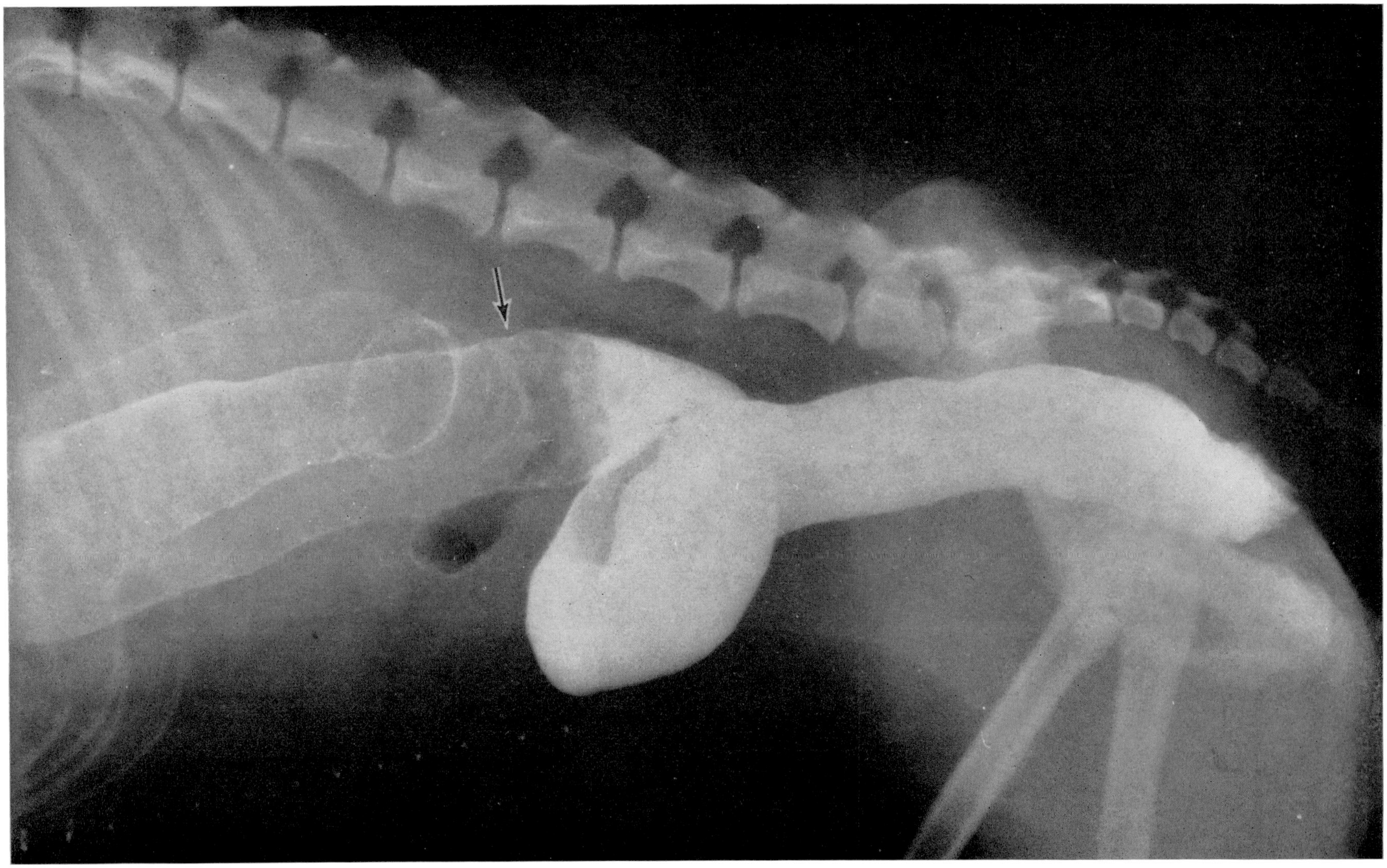

Case 32. **C,** As shown in this lateral radiograph, barium given as an enema reaches the intussuscepted part of the bowel lying cranial to the sigmoid loop of the colon. Only a minimal amount of contrast medium passes by the intussusception. This contrast medium appears as a line between the mucosa of the intussuscepting bowel loop and the intussuscepted part (arrow). The ascending, transverse, and descending portions of the colon are involved in the intussusception.

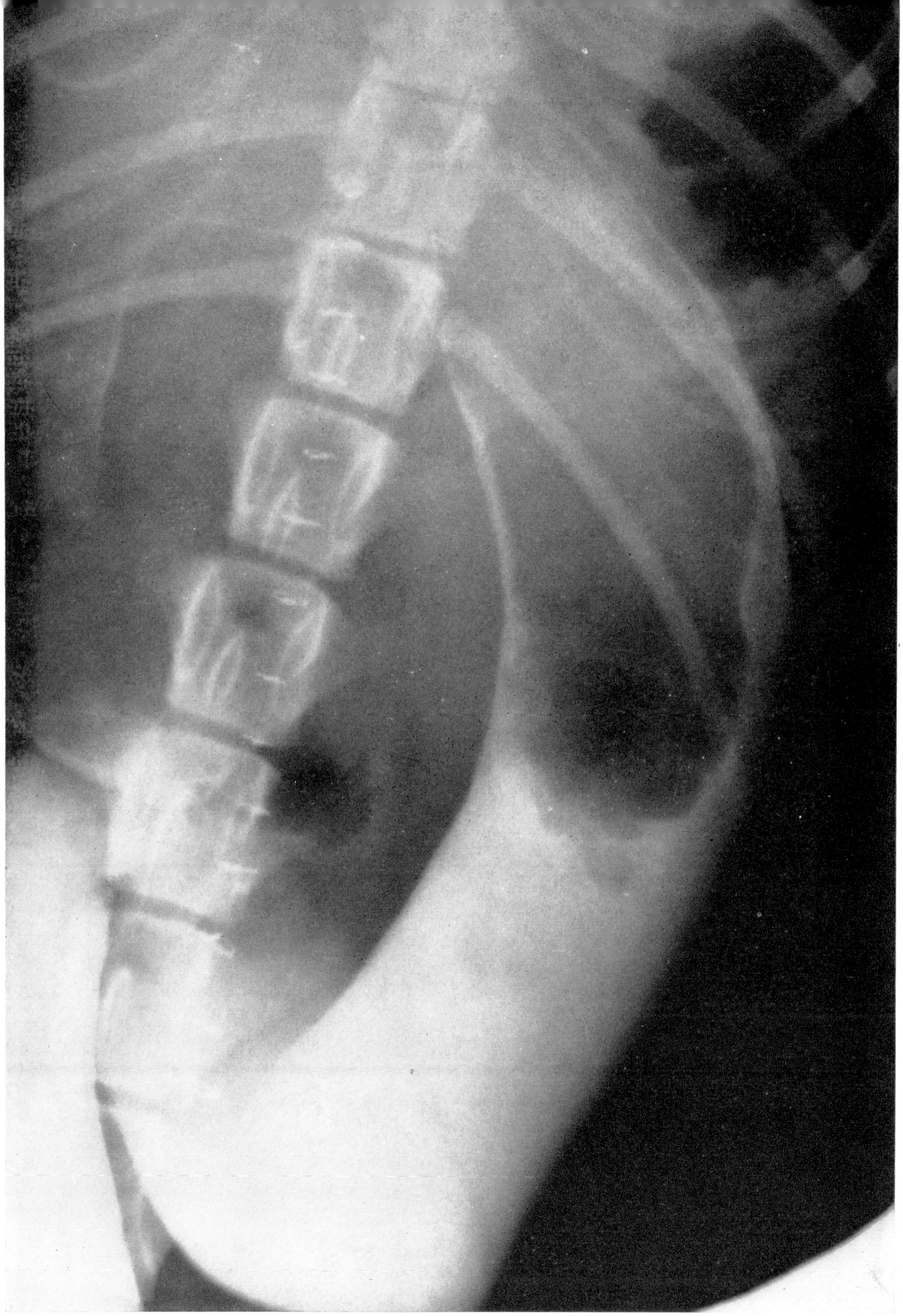

Case 32. **D,** Spot film made during fluoroscopy and administration of a barium enema. The caudal end of the intussuscepted bowel loop is clearly seen as a dark "bud" surrounded by contrast medium. The sigmoid colon is in the lower left corner.

Diagnosis: Intussusception of the ileum into the colon.

Case 33

Cat, male, 2 years old. For several days this cat had been listless. It had vomited and had also had bouts of diarrhea. At examination it was found to be slightly dehydrated and a small sausage-like mass could be palpated in the mid abdomen. Radiographs revealed a gas-filled bowel loop, to the right in the mid abdomen, containing something that appeared to be an intussuscepted loop of bowel.

Radiographs made 6 hours after the administration of meglumine diatrizoate showed the contrast medium in the cecum and rectum but only traces of the material in the colon. The colon was winding and it was difficult to determine which was the ascending and which was the upper part of the descending colon. The descending colon seemed to harbor a loop of intussuscepted bowel.

There was contrast medium in the urinary bladder, indicating a pathologic resorption of meglumine diatrizoate from the gut. At operation the radiologic diagnosis was confirmed and the intussuscepted ileum was reduced. The animal made a rapid and complete recovery.

Differential Diagnosis: In this case the possibility of the presence of a foreign body could not be excluded. What was probably the ascending colon contained something that looked very much like an intussuscepted bowel loop. After oral administration of meglumine diatrizoate it seemed even more probable that an intussusception was the cause of the cat's problem. The radiographic findings in combination with the palpatory findings were considered to give enough evidence for the presence of an intussusception and hence for surgical intervention.

The fact that the contrast medium had leaked out through or been resorbed by the bowel wall was not in itself pathognomonic. Apparently any kind of damage to the intestinal mucosa seems to enhance resorption of the medium. Unfortunately such resorption can also take place through a seemingly normal mucosa.

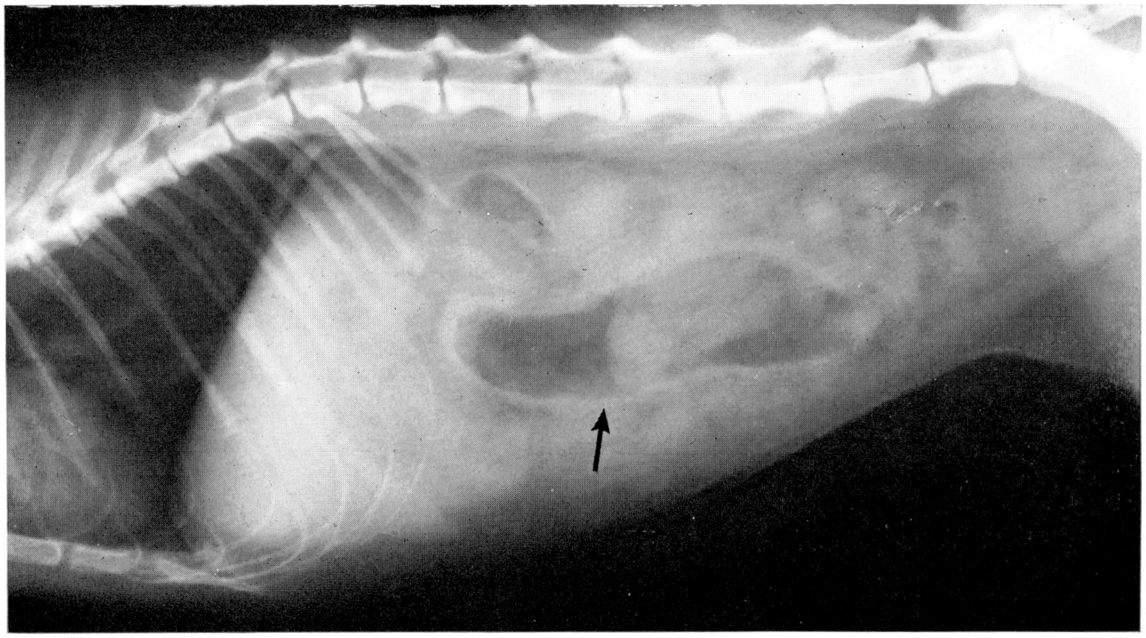

A

Case 33. **A,** Lateral radiograph. In mid abdomen is a bowel loop, distended by gas. Within or superimposed on this bowel loop is a mass which apparently is the one that can be palpated. Its cranial end is rounded (arrow).

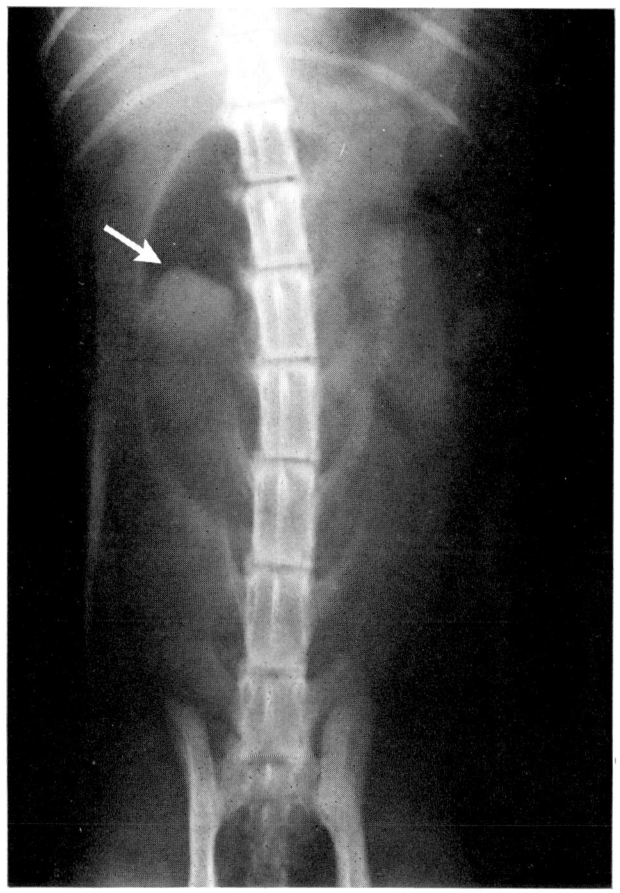

B

Case 33. **B,** The ventrodorsal radiograph indicates that the mass is actually lodged within the gas-filled bowel loop. The rounded cranial end is clearly seen (arrow).

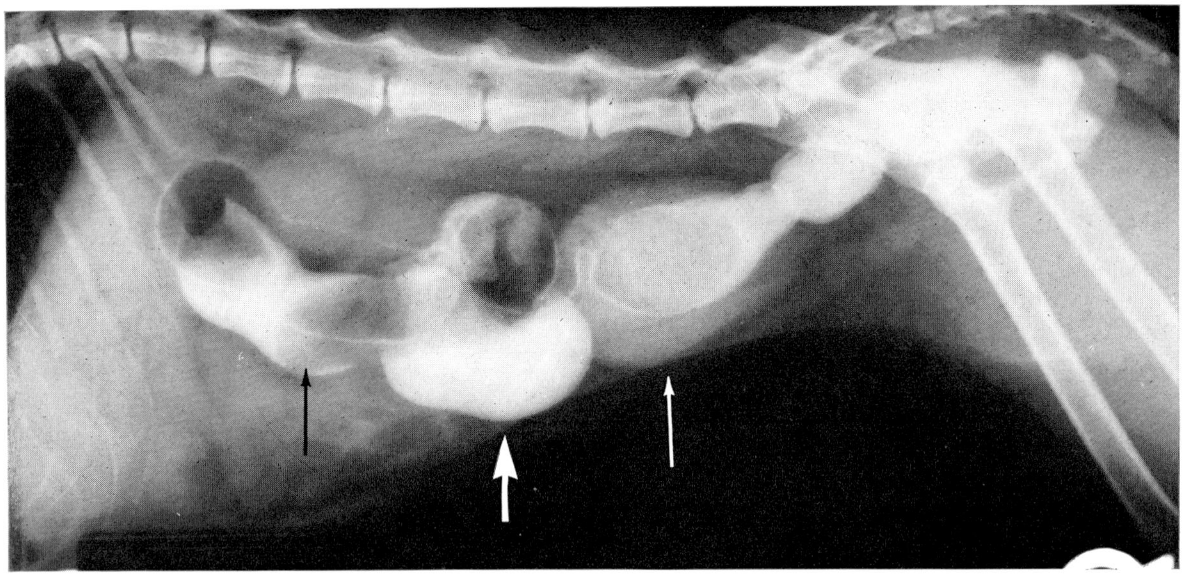

C

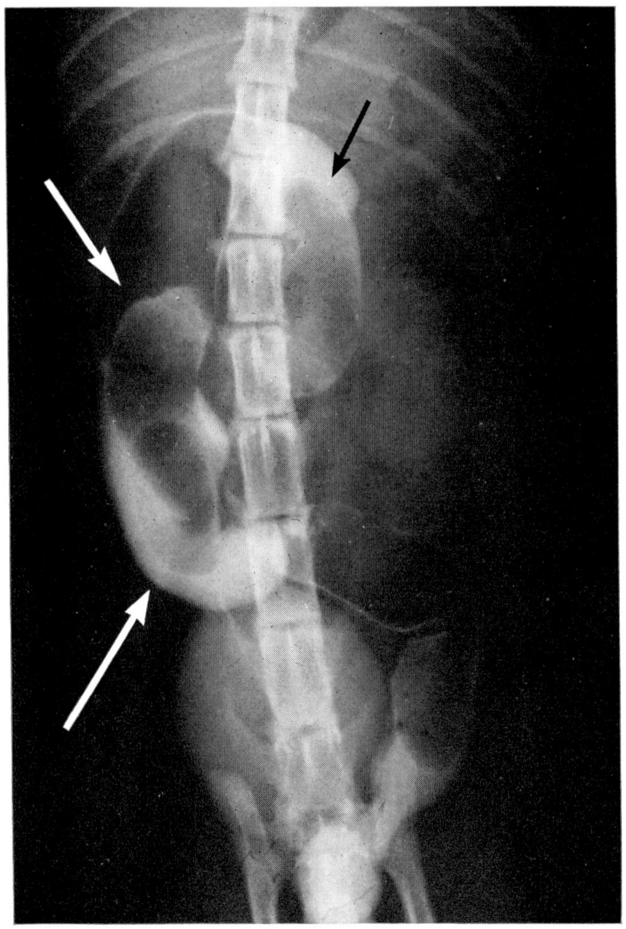

D

Case 33. **C,** Lateral radiograph made 6 hours after oral administration of meglumine diatrizoate. The cecum is filled with contrast medium (large white arrow). There are only traces of the medium in the colon while the rectum is filled with it. The urinary bladder contains contrast medium (thin white arrow). The intussuscepted bowel can be seen as a defect in the contrast medium in the ascending colon (black arrow).

Case 33. **D,** Ventrodorsal radiograph. The meglumine diatrizoate-filled cecum (long white arrow) is seen. The budlike, cranially protruding bowel loop (short white arrow) is probably the intussuscepted ileum. There is gas (black arrow) in the descending colon.

Diagnosis: Intussusception of ileum into the colon.

Case 34

Welsh corgi, male, 6 years old. This dog had become restless after a bone meal. The following day it showed difficulties in defecating and was unable to defecate during the following 2 days in spite of severe straining. The animal was admitted to the clinic when anorexia and vomiting complicated the picture. On examination, a long, hard mass could be palpated in the abdomen. Cranial to the pubic bones there was another mass which was round, hard, and painful.

Radiographs revealed impaction of bony fecal masses in the descending colon to a point where a large round mass, apparently the prostate gland, obstructed the passage to the pelvic inlet. Cranial to the impaction, there were masses of less radiopaque ingesta. A few loops of small bowel were gas-filled, but not distended to any degree.

The fecal impaction was dissolved by laxatives and enemas. The dog regained the ability to have normal bowel movements. Prostatitis was diagnosed as the probable cause of prostatic enlargement.

Differential Diagnosis: There was little question about the diagnosis. The possibility of impaction of bony material in the small bowel should, however, always be considered (see Case 29). In the present case it was obvious that the descending colon was involved. It is important always to ask why obstipation has occurred. In the present case the combination of a large bone meal and an enlarged prostate was the apparent cause of fecal impaction.

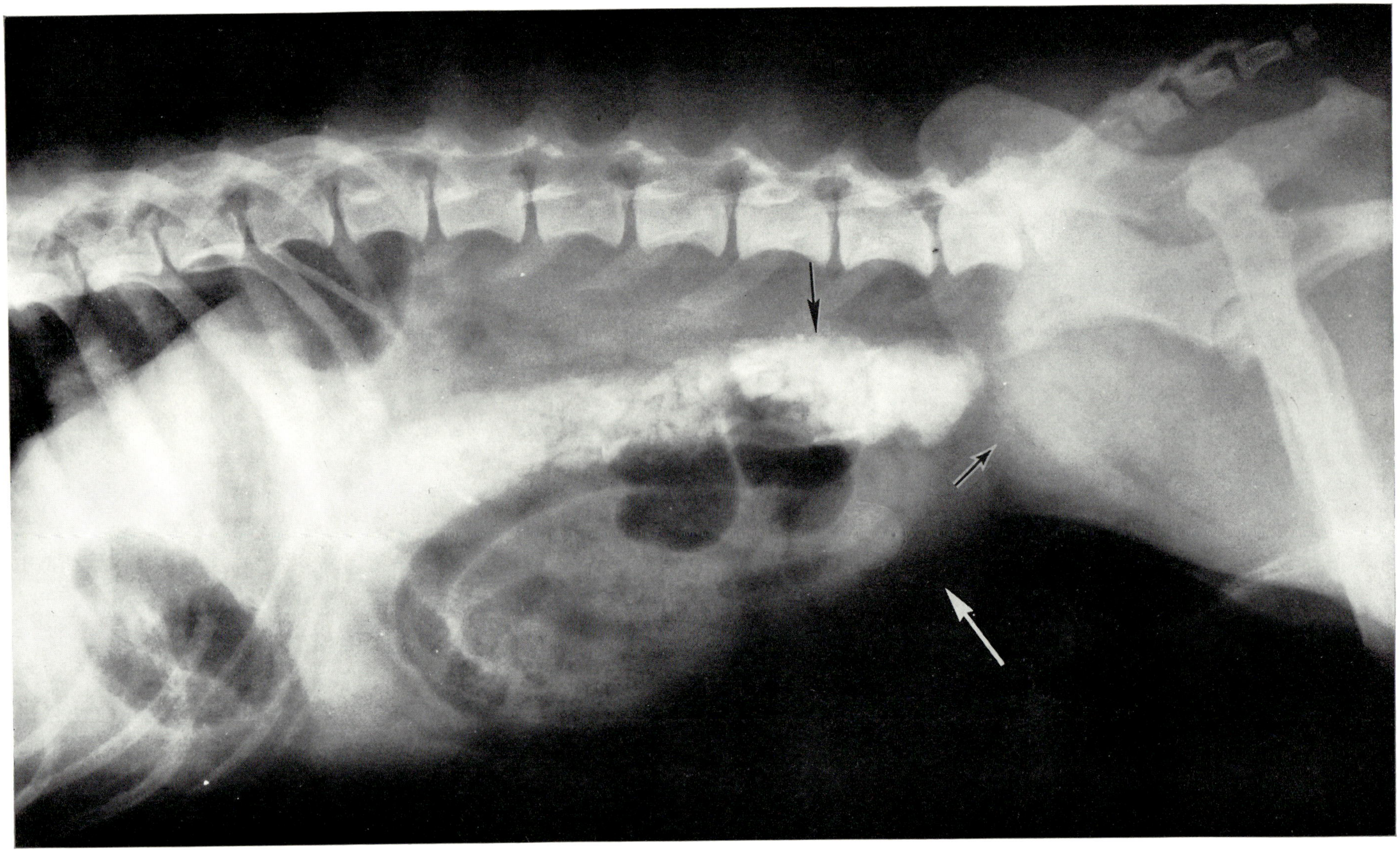

Case 34. **A,** The most obvious change in this lateral radiograph is the large amount of radiopaque material in a bowel loop (large black arrow). In all probability this bowel loop is the descending colon. Caudal to the impaction is a large, round, soft-tissue mass close to the pelvic inlet (small black arrow). This formation is most probably an enlarged prostate gland, since the urinary bladder can be seen cranial to it (white arrow). There is gas in the stomach as well as in some loops of the small bowel and in the cecum.

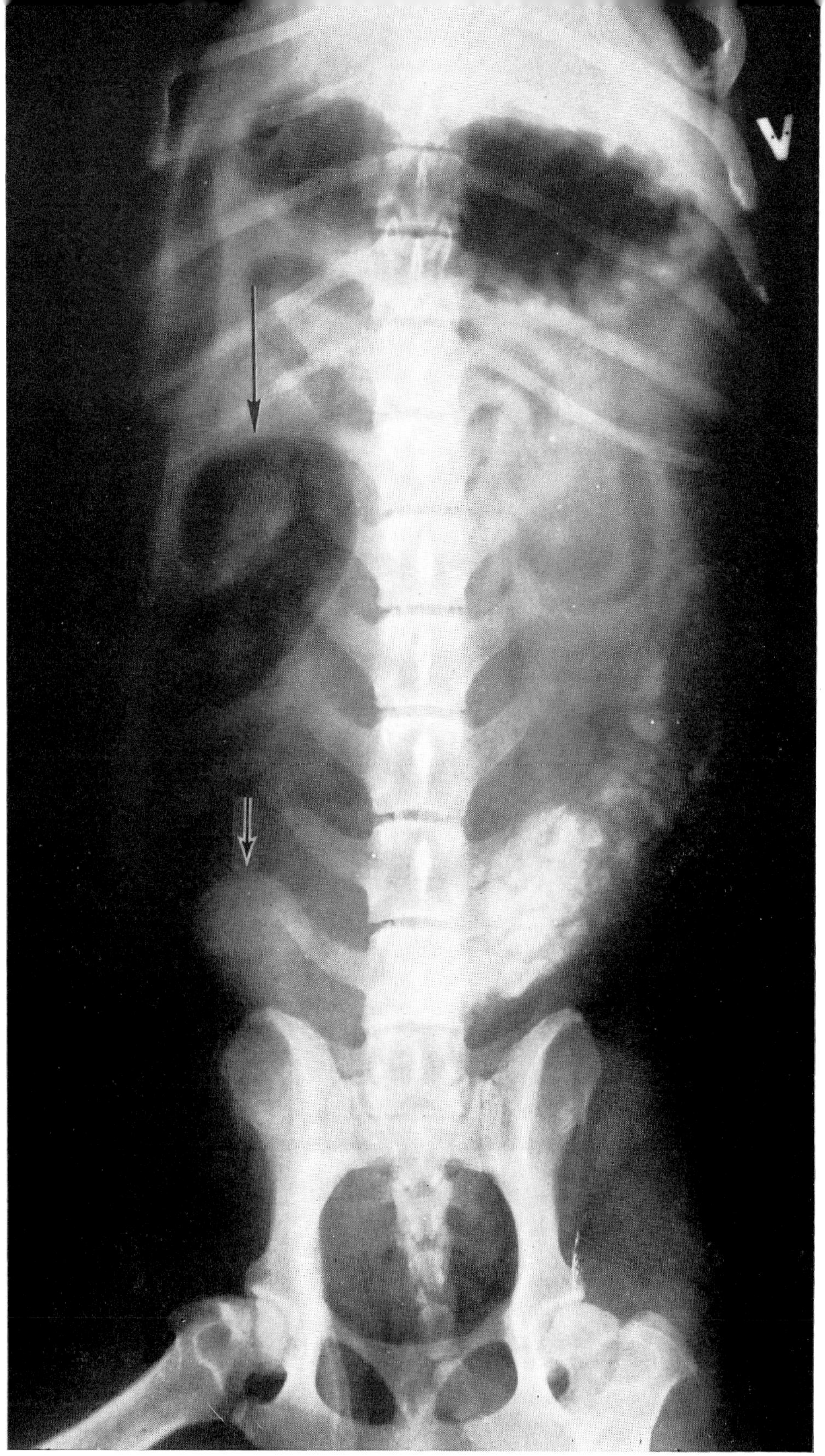

Case 34. **B,** On this ventrodorsal radiograph it is possible to demonstrate most of the changes seen on the lateral radiograph. The enlarged prostate gland, however, is obscured by the pelvis and the sacrum. It is noteworthy that the prepuce (short arrow) presents itself as a rounded shadow to the right just cranial to the right iliac crest. It is important not to mistake this shadow for something lying within the abdomen. The penile bone is seen projected on the right iliac bone, the obturator foramen, and the ischiatic bone. There is gas in the cecum (long arrow).

Diagnosis: Fecal impaction due to a large bone meal and enlarged prostate gland.

Case 35

Cat, female, 15 years old. For a week this cat had not defecated or urinated. At the time of admission to the clinic it was anorectic and vomited occasionally. At examination it was plainly evident that its abdomen was enlarged. A large urinary bladder and an ill-defined mass could be palpated in the lower abdomen.

Radiographs revealed a mass cranial to the pelvic inlet, fecal material in the descending colon, and a distended urinary bladder. The stomach and the small bowel were empty.

The mass which apparently obstructed both fecal and urinary passages did not have any distinct borders. It was interpreted as a malignant tumor, most probably originating from the uterus.

Laparotomy was performed. An inoperable tumor was found surrounding the neck of the enlarged uterus. The cat was put to sleep.

Necropsy: The tumor was found to be an infiltrating adenocarcinoma of the cervix of the uterus.

Differential Diagnosis: A mass at the location as in this case in a female animal could be a large tumor in the cranial portion of the vagina. Such a tumor, however, is usually well defined. A malignant tumor at this site (with diffuse borders radiographically) most probably originates from the cervix of the uterus.

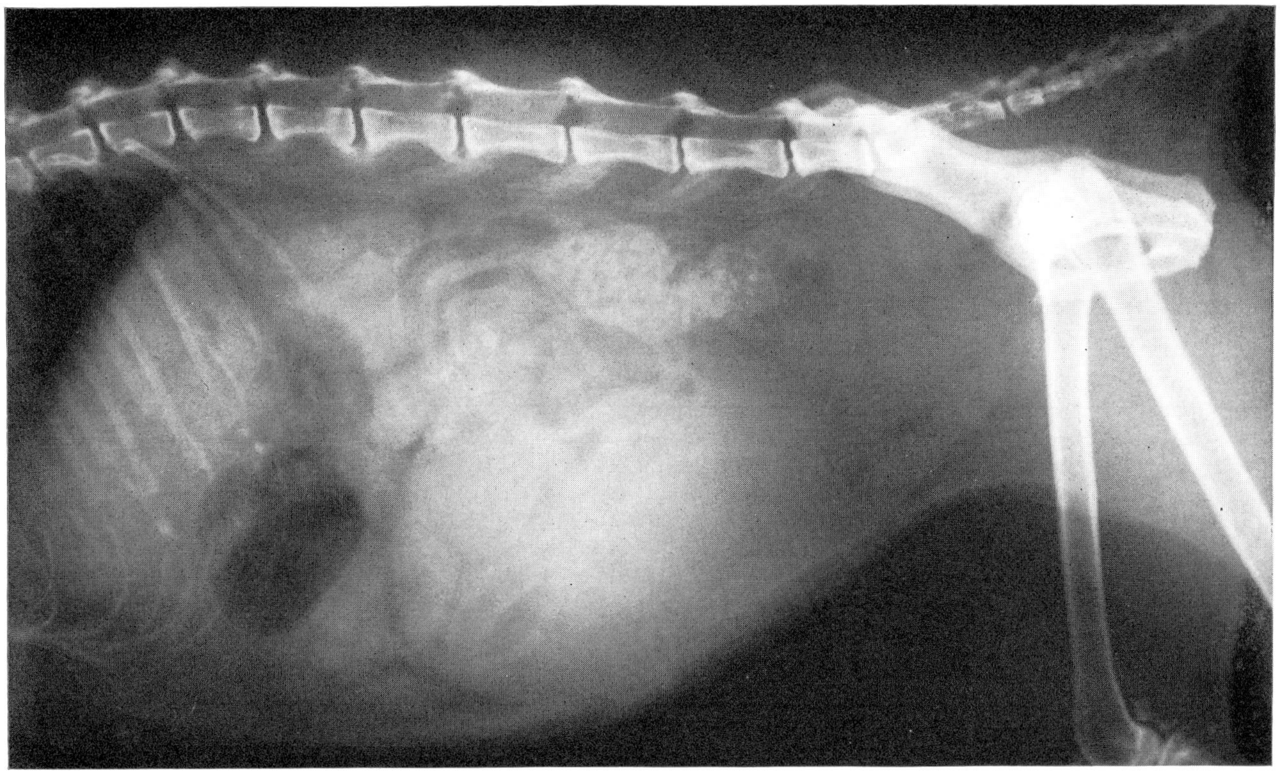

Case 35. The most obvious pathologic feature on this lateral radiograph is an irregular mass with ill-defined borders. It is localized to the pelvic inlet and apparently obstructs both fecal and urinary passages. There is some fecal material in the descending colon and the urinary bladder is distended. Within or superimposed on the bladder can be seen an increased density somewhat difficult to delineate. There is reason to believe that this could be an enlarged uterus. The stomach is gas-filled, but contains no fluid. There is spondylosis at L2-L3 and L3-L4.

Diagnosis: Adenocarcinoma of the cervix of the uterus blocking the passage of feces, urine, and discharge from the uterus.

Case 36

Cat, spayed female, 3 years old. This animal was brought to the clinic by its owner who had noticed that it unsuccessfully had strained for defecation for several days. At examination a long, hard mass could be palpated in the abdomen. Radiographs revealed fecal impaction in the descending colon and in the cranial part of the rectum extending to the pelvic inlet, which was narrower than normal.

The cat recovered after treatment with laxatives and enemas.

Differential Diagnosis: As is often the case, the diagnosis of fecal impaction in this animal was easily made.

The cause of impaction should always be looked for. An animal may have been given too much bone to eat and this alone or in combination with some hindrance to normal passage may produce impaction. In the male animal an enlarged prostate is often the cause (see Case 34). An example of an obstruction in a female animal is presented in Case 35. Other causes may be tumors in the rectum and perineal hernia with a diverticulum of the rectum.

In the present case the cause of obstruction apparently is a deformation of the pelvis. The dorsally convex pelvis in combination with a healed fracture of one femur suggests that this animal has suffered from nutritional calcium deficiency during adolescence, giving rise to secondary hyperparathyroidism with a softening of the skeleton.

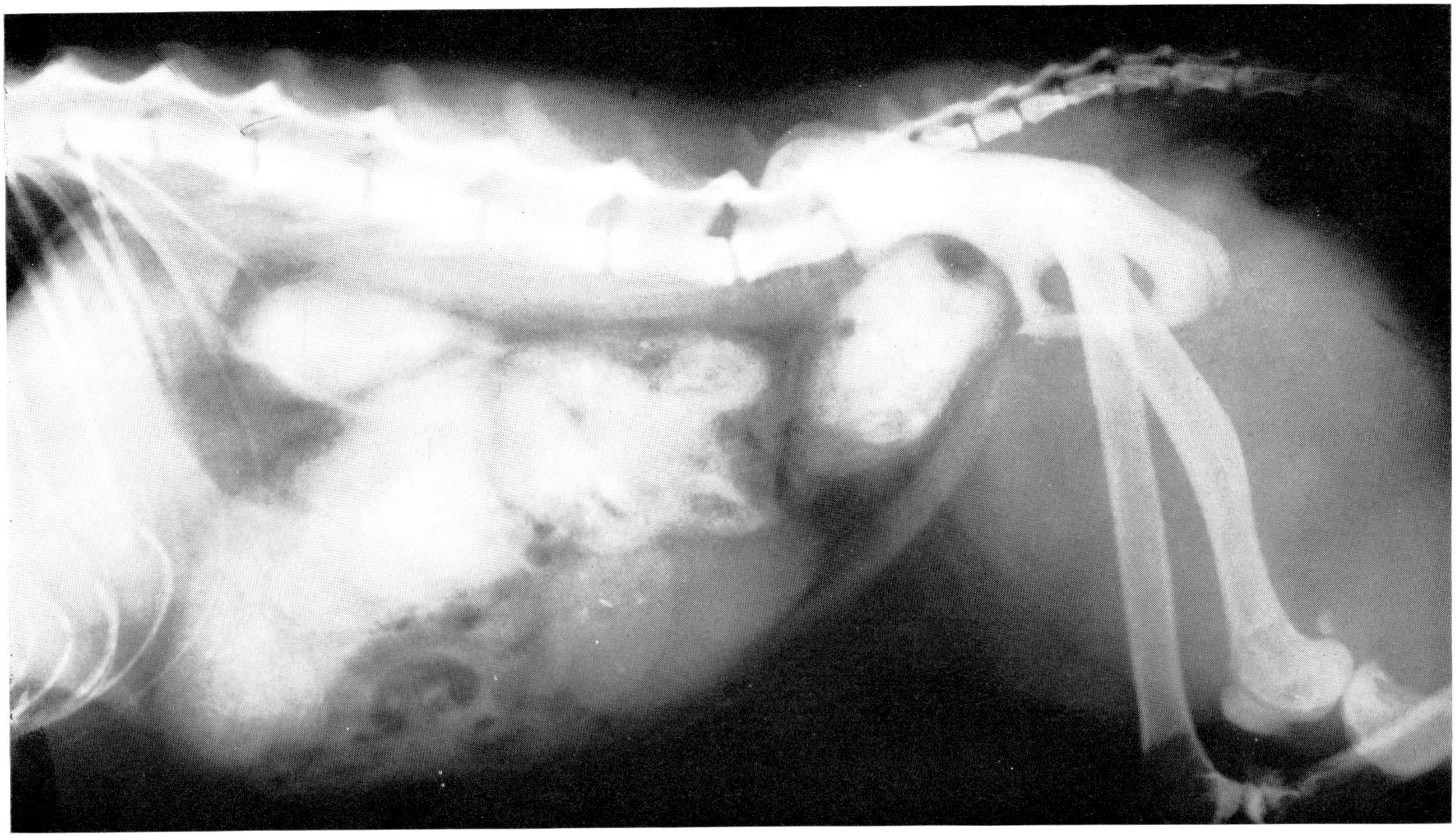

Case 36. This lateral radiograph demonstrates the massive impaction of fecal material in the colon and the cranial portion of the rectum. The neck of the urinary bladder is elongated and the bladder itself is positioned almost in the mid abdomen. The pelvis has an abnormal shape, making a dorsal curve, thus narrowing the pelvic inlet. There is an angulation of one of the femurs as a result of a fracture which is now completely healed.

Diagnosis: Fecal impaction in colon and rectum. Contributing cause: pelvic deformation probably due to nutritional secondary hyperparathyroidism in adolescence.

Case 37

Dachshund, female, 7 years old. This dog did not defecate for 3 days after a heavy bone meal. It was brought to the clinic and the diagnosis of bony impaction in the descending colon and the rectum was made. Several enemas were given and a large amount of feces was removed. The following day the dog was listless and was standing with an arched back, apparently because of pain in the abdomen. Palpation of the abdomen produced pain. Radiographs revealed diffused contours of the abdominal organs, and free gas in the abdominal cavity. The diagnosis of bowel perforation and peritonitis was made. At laparotomy a rupture of the rectum was found. The rupture had apparently been caused by the efforts to remove fecal material that obstructed the rectum. The rupture was sutured and the dog made an uneventful recovery.

Differential Diagnosis: A diffuse outline of the abdominal organs, caused by a slightly increased density, and a mottled appearance are characteristic of peritonitis. These signs and free gas in the abdominal cavity are pathognomonic for intestinal rupture or perforation, or a wound in the abdominal wall.

Free gas in the abdominal cavity is best demonstrated by using a horizontal beam with the animal in the erect position, standing on its hind legs. The free gas will collect under the diaphragm and is easily demonstrable. In the present case it was not considered necessary to make such a radiograph. There was enough gas between the diaphragm and the liver with the dog in the ventrodorsal recumbent position to make the diagnosis.

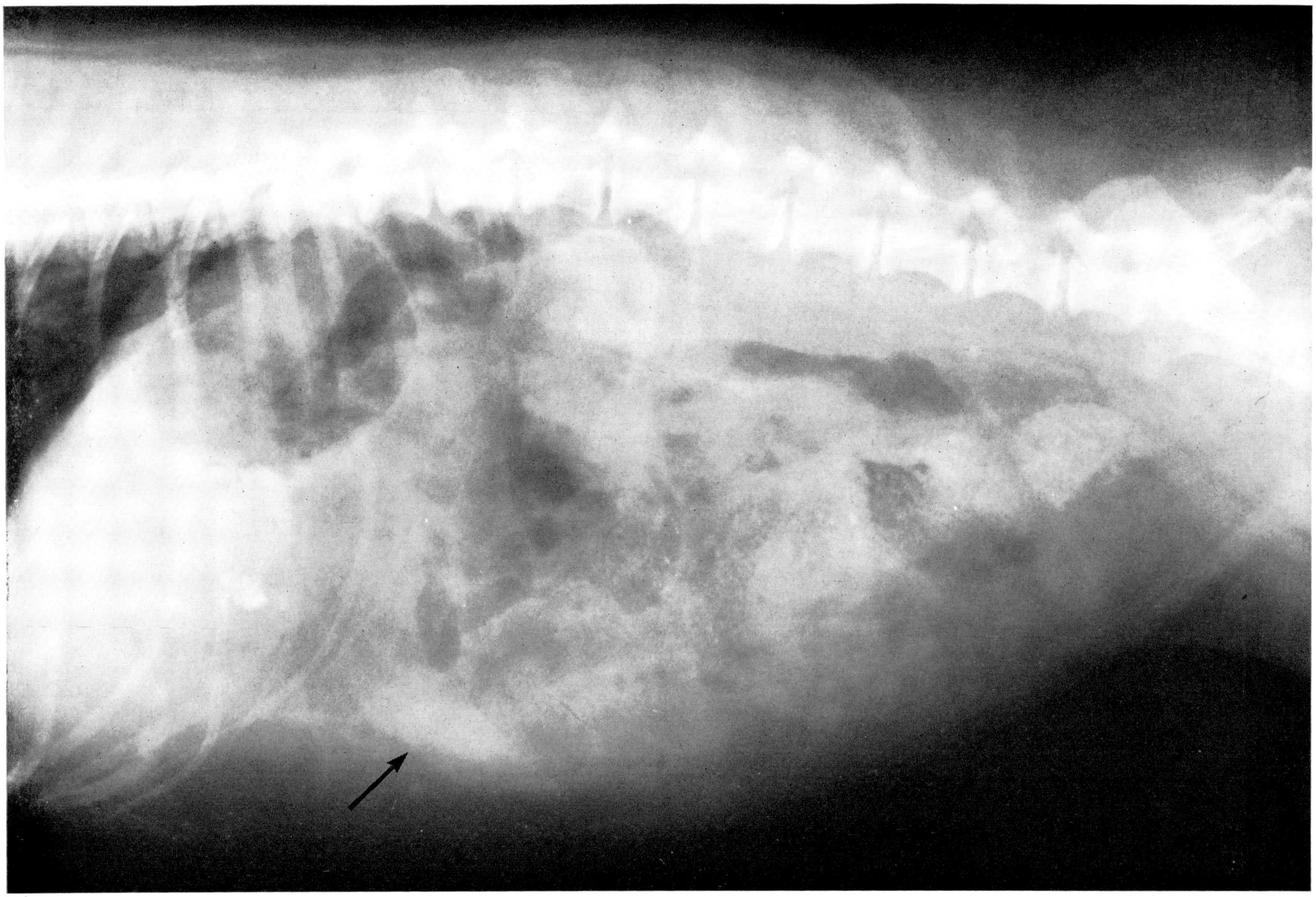

Case 37. **A,** There is a diffuse, slightly mottled density and diffuse contours of thc abdominal organs on this lateral radiograph. Also gas pockets which are apparently not within bowel loops are present. Ingesta having diffuse borders are seen in the descending colon. The contours of the bowel are most diffuse in the ventral part of the abdomen. The lower end of the spleen can be seen (arrow), but its borders are diffuse.

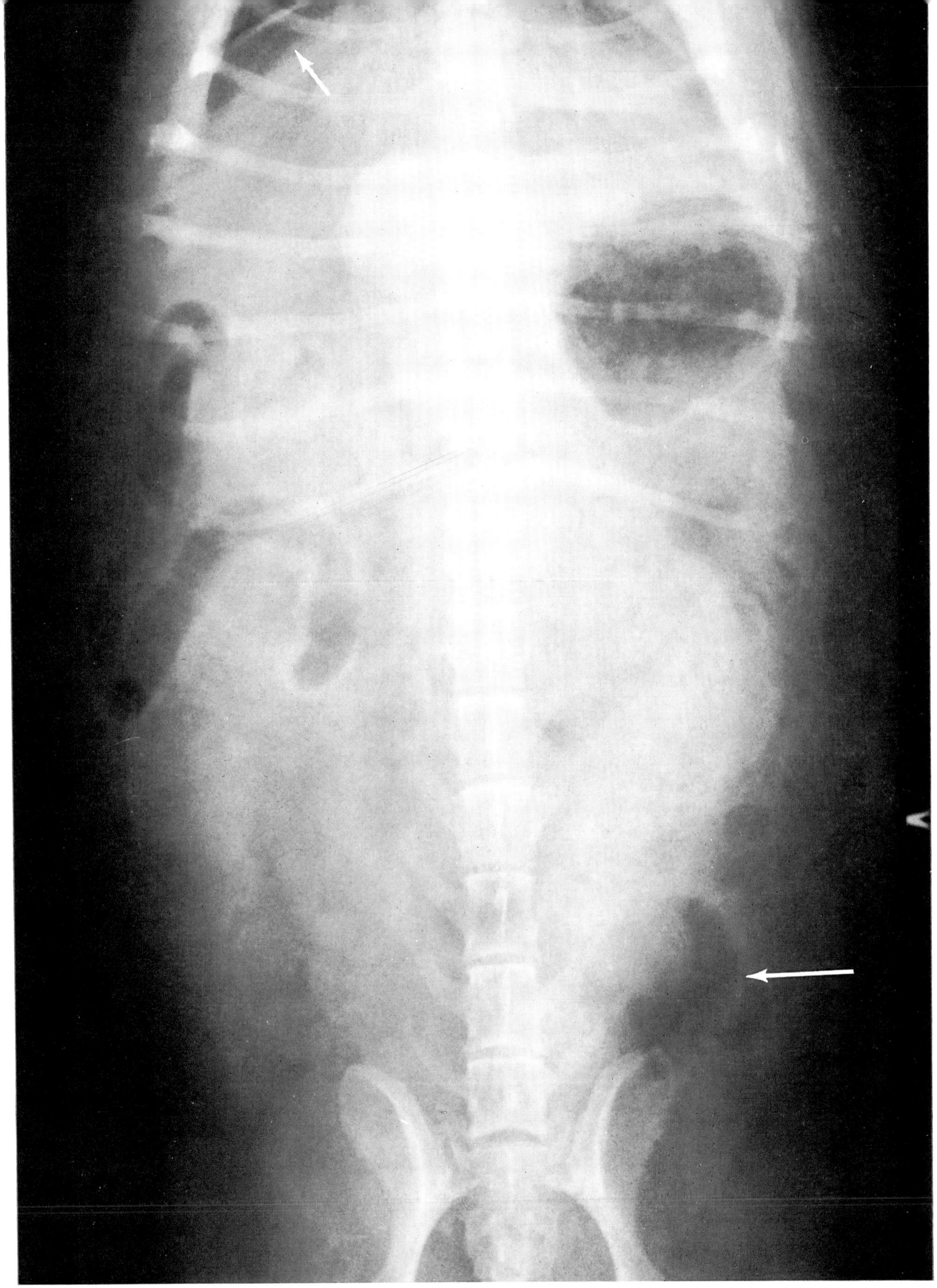

Case 37. **B,** On this ventrodorsal radiograph the increased density in the mid abdomen is evident. No distinct borders between the abdominal organs can be seen. There is a gas pocket cranial to the left iliac crest (long arrow). The most obvious sign of free gas in the abdominal cavity is that of a gas pocket between the liver and the diaphragm (short arrow).

Diagnosis: Perforation of the rectum giving rise to peritonitis with free gas in the abdomen.

Case 38

Beagle, male, 10 months old. This dog was hit by a car. It was able to run from the site of the accident, but became listless and anorectic after a while. A veterinarian who was consulted noticed that the dog's abdomen and pelvis were painful on palpation. Radiographs were made but they gave no clue to the diagnosis. The dog's condition slowly deteriorated, vomiting occurred, and abdominal tenseness increased.

On admission to the clinic a week after the accident the dog was very weak and dehydrated. A painful, rather soft mass could be palpated in the abdomen. The dog's condition improved following treatment with tetracycline, cortisone, electrolytes, and fluid. Radiographs at this time revealed diffuse density in the abdomen, with several fluid-filled bowel loops containing gas bubbles. These bowel loops were found close to a diffuse density in the mid abdomen. No obvious sign of free gas in the abdomen was noted. The sacrum was fractured.

Additional radiographs were made 8 hours following the administration of a barium swallow. The passage of barium was found to be delayed. The wall of some bowel loops was corrugated. Radiographs made with a horizontal beam, with the dog in erect position, standing on its hind legs, showed gas trapped between the stomach and the liver. This was interpreted as an indication of the presence of free gas within the omental bursa.

On the basis of these findings a diagnosis of intestinal rupture was made. Laparotomy confirmed this diagnosis.

There was a longitudinal rupture of the jejunum opposite to the insertion of the mesentery. The omentum had formed a pocket around the ruptured bowel. This pocket contained ingesta and some gas. There was only a minimal reaction in the peritoneum outside this pocket.

About 15 cm of the bowel were resected. The dog made a complete recovery.

Differential Diagnosis: Severe damage to the abdominal cavity was obvious clinically a few day after the accident and was evident radiographically at the time of admission. The diffuse density in mid abdomen with blurring of the borders of the abdominal organs was an indication of inflammatory reaction. Because considerable time had elapsed since the accident it was not conceivable that this density could be explained as the result of an uncomplicated hemorrhage. Such a hemorrhage would have been resorbed within a week following the accident. The possibility of a rupture of the urinary bladder was kept in mind, but the dog had urinated several times since the accident and a bladder rupture of long-standing would have produced more fluid than was present in the abdominal cavity. The slow passage of contrast medium and the corrugated wall of the small bowel were indications of peritonitis and ileus. The final proof of rupture of the bowel was obtained by radiographic examination with the dog in the erect position. Gas pockets outside the digestive tract could be demonstrated between the stomach and the liver. This showed that gas was trapped within the omental bursa since gas outside this bursa would have been trapped directly beneath the diaphragm.

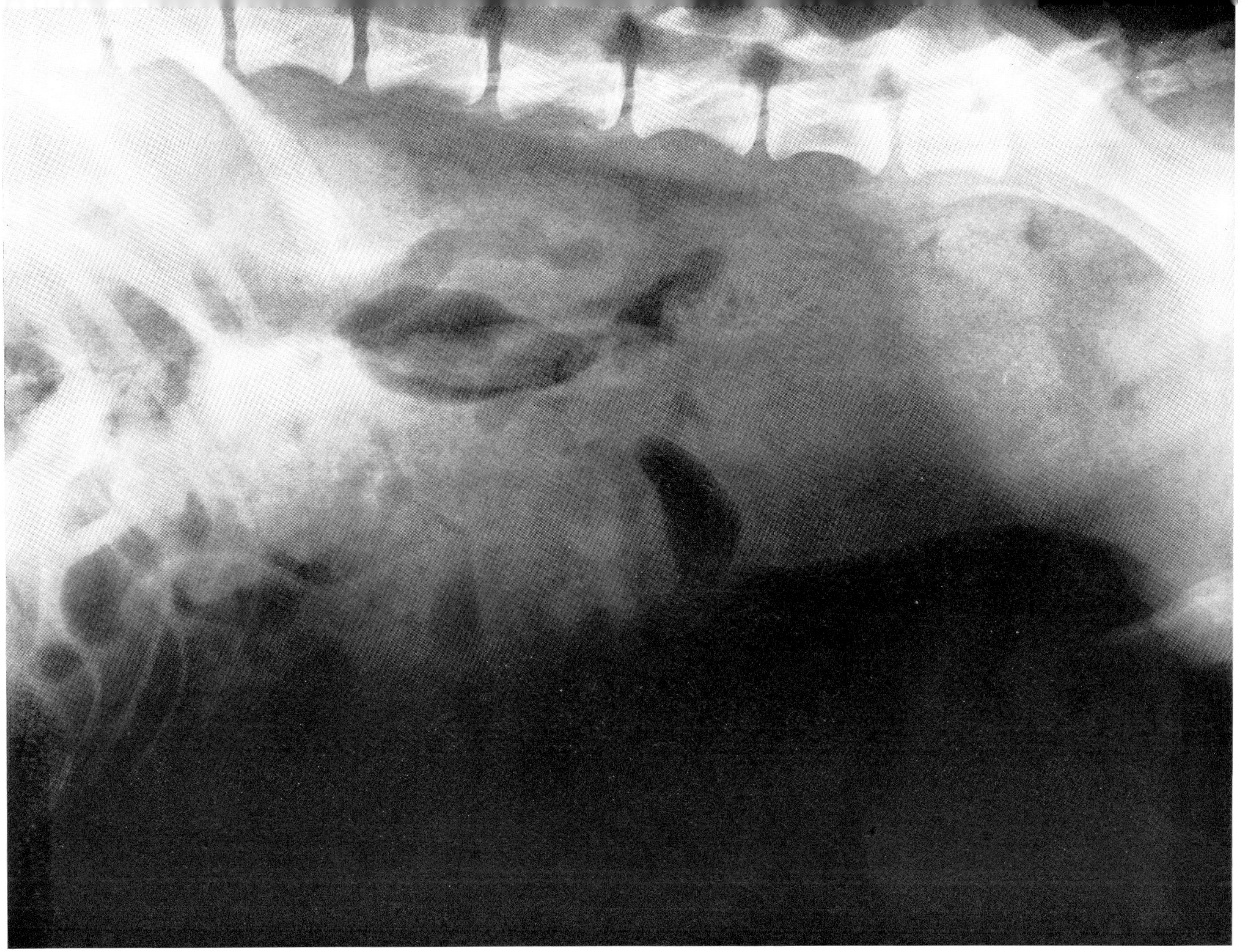

Case 38. **A,** Increased density with diffuse outline of the abdominal organs and a number of gas-filled small bowel loops are characteristics of this lateral radiograph. It is not possible to determine whether or not gas is present outside the bowel. The urinary bladder appears to be filled, but no distinct outline of the bladder can be seen. Rupture of an abdominal organ, hemorrhage, or peritonitis should be suspected on the basis of this radiograph.

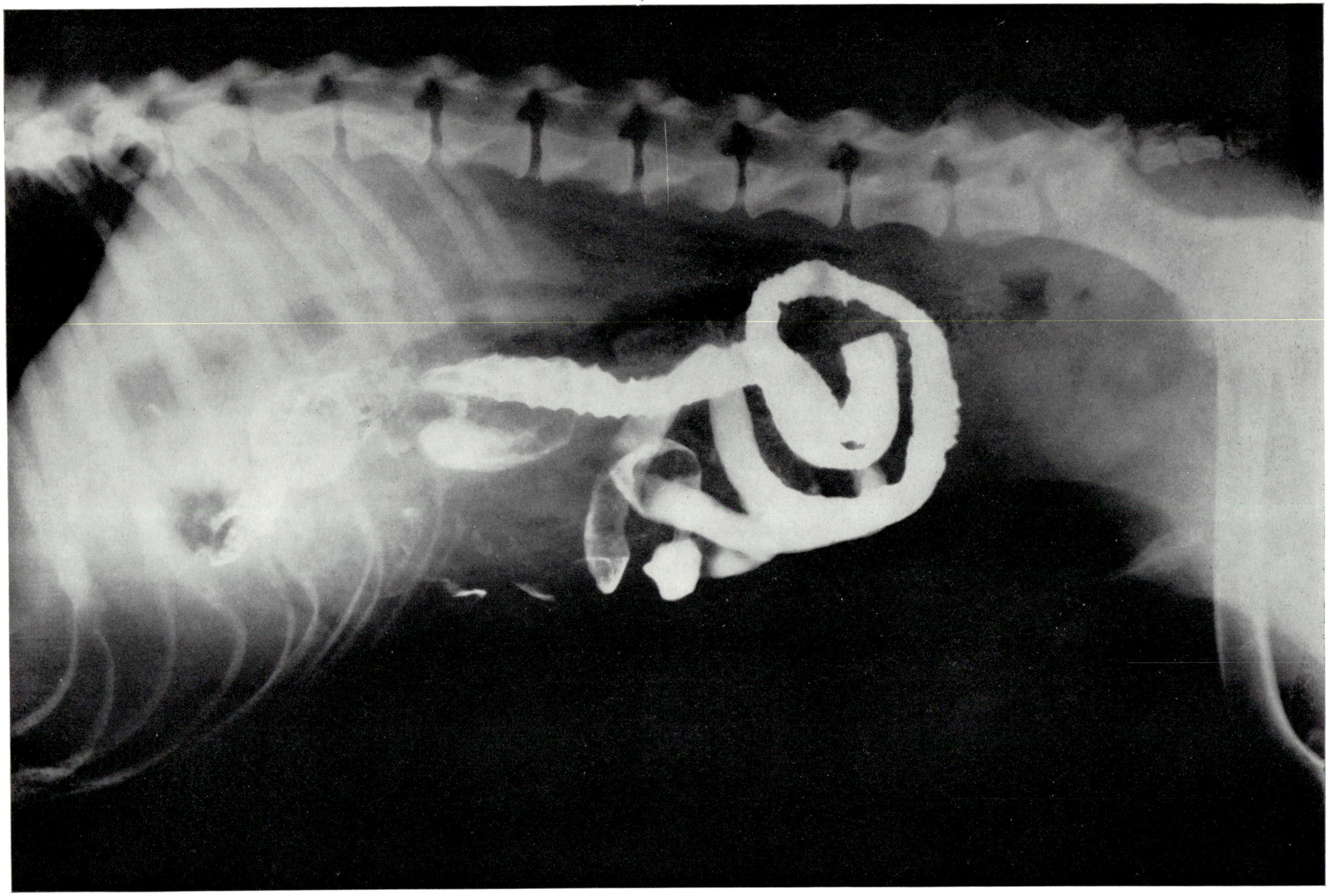

Case 38. **B,** Lateral radiograph made 8 hours after a barium swallow. Barium has not reached the large bowel. Instead, it is lodged in the jejunum, some loops of which have a corrugated wall.

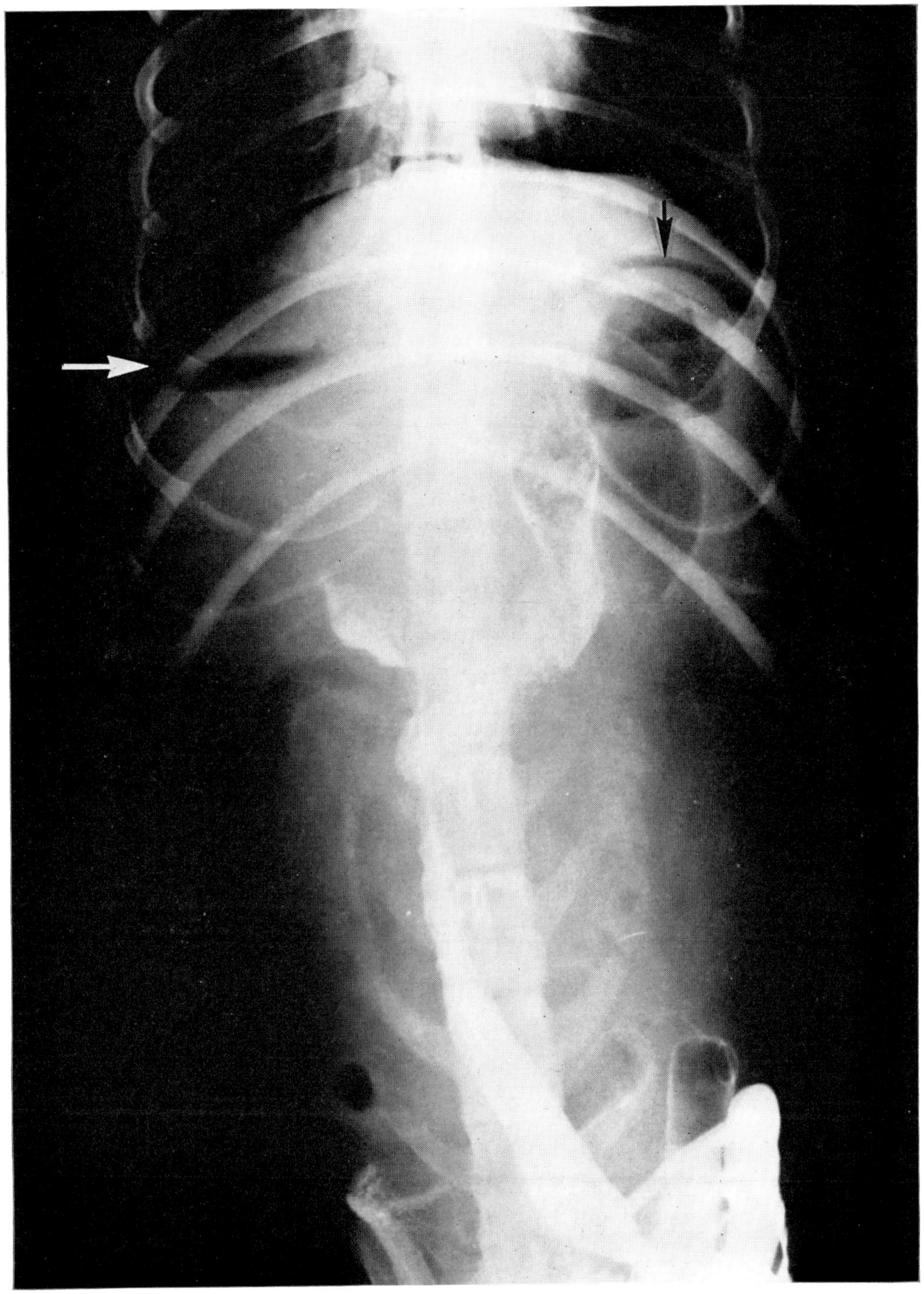

Case 38. **C,** Ventrodorsal radiograph made with the dog in the erect position. The beam is horizontal. Gas is trapped under the liver. On the left side the gas (black arrow) outlines the cranial contour of the stomach, and on the right side it is lodged between the liver and the pylorus (white arrow). The location of the gas pockets indicates that the gas is in the omental bursa.

Diagnosis: Rupture of the small intestine with a localized peritonitis and gas trapped in the omental bursa.

Case 39

Mongrel dog, male, 8 months old. This dog was brought to the clinic after being hit by a car. On admission, it was in a state of light shock. The mucous membranes were pale. The animal refused to walk or to put weight on its hind legs. It had, however, normal pain sensation and was able to move its hind limbs. The pelvic region was asymmetric. Respiration was strained. Radiographs revealed increased density in the abdomen and some gas-filled bowel loops. The left hip joint was luxated. The contours of the urinary bladder were not seen. For this reason, a retrograde urocystogram was made. The bladder was found to be intact.

The dog's condition improved slightly. Radiographs were made 20 to 24 hours following administration of a barium swallow. Some barium was found to be still lodged in the stomach, but most of it had reached the large bowel. The descending colon had a corrugated wall indicating irritation of the peritoneum. The borders between the abdominal organs were rather diffuse. Blood or fluid was not obtained by paracentesis.

Because of the persisting signs of peritonitis, laparotomy was performed. A rupture of the mesentery was found. This rupture had occurred along and close to the bowel, leaving about 40 cm of the gut without sufficient blood supply. Hemorrhagic infarction of the intestinal wall had followed. This dark-red portion of the jejunum was resected. The dog made a complete recovery.

Differential Diagnosis: Acute hemorrhage and peritonitis, developing during the first 24 hours after the accident, pointed to bowel damage. One of the most difficult diagnoses to make is infarction of the bowel. Hemorrhage can be minimal, peritonitis develops rather slowly, the bowel wall looks normal, and for some days a rather normal contrast passage can be maintained. Clinically, the initial abdominal signs are not alarming. Early resection of the affected part of the intestine is essential for recovery. In the present case, the differential diagnosis lay between uncomplicated intraabdominal hemorrhage and a tear in the mesentery. It is noteworthy that barium passed through the severely damaged small bowel loop. The slowly developing radiographic sign of peritonitis was in this case a warning signal indicating that laparotomy was necessary. The dog also developed impaction of ingesta in a segment of the small bowel.

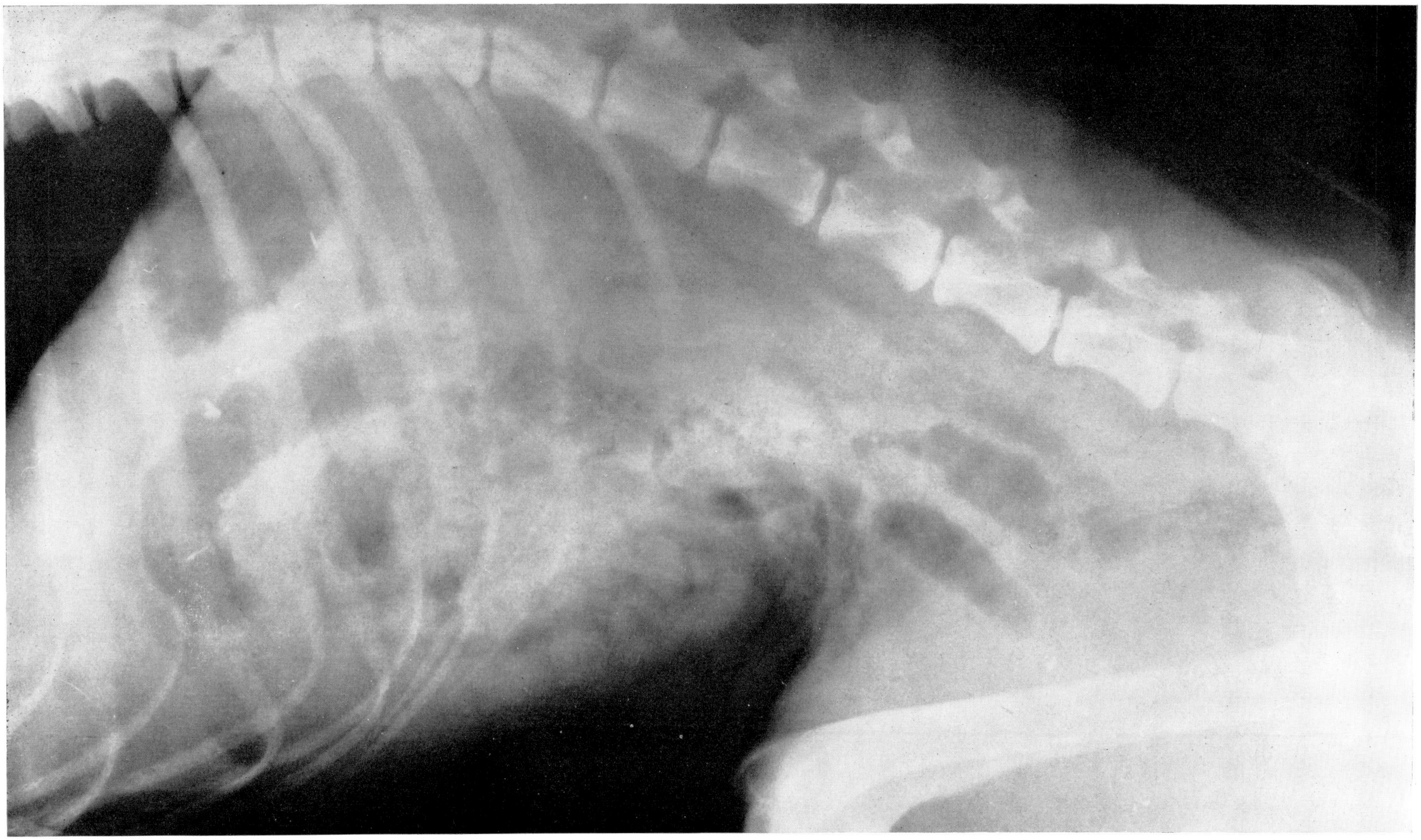

Case 39. **A,** Lateral radiographs made 2 hours after the accident. Because of pain from the luxated hip, the hind legs could not be properly extended during exposure. There is a slight increase in density and blurring of the contours in the abdomen. Some of the bowel loops are gas-filled.

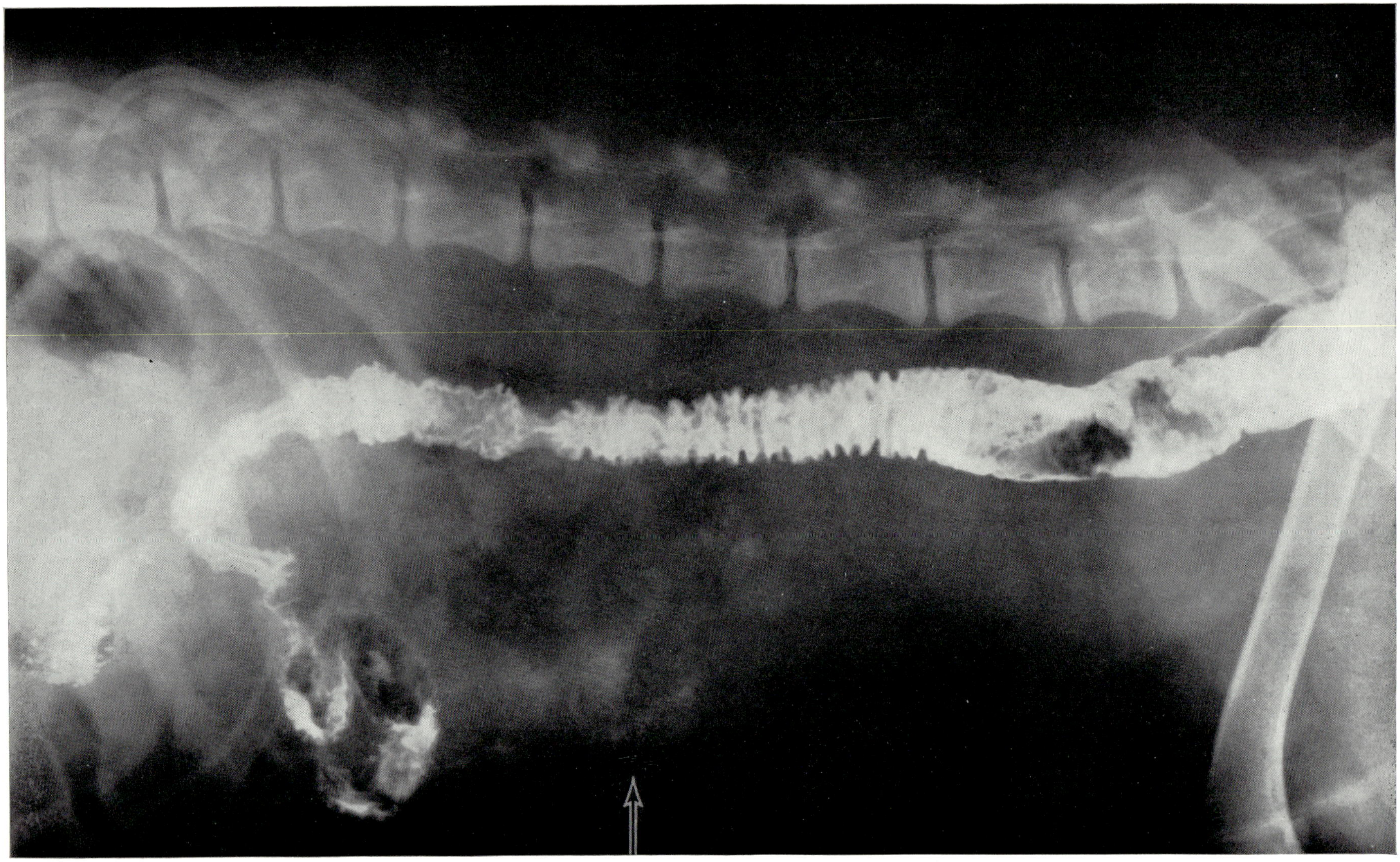

Case 39. **B,** Lateral radiographs made 25 hours after a barium swallow. There is some contrast medium left in the stomach. Ingesta apparently mixed with traces of contrast medium are present in a loop of the small bowel (arrow). This is a definite pathologic finding. The descending colon and the rectum contain most of the contrast medium. The descending colon has a very corrugated wall indicating irritation, probably due to peritonitis. The contours of the bowel are blurred in the mid abdomen.

Diagnosis: Rupture of the mesentery causing hemorrhagic infarction of a loop of the jejunum. Peritonitis.

Case 40

Cat, female, 11 months old. This cat fell a distance of four stories. On admission to the clinic it was conscious, but paralyzed in its hind quarters. The spinal reflexes were intact. There was a bloody discharge from the nostrils. Radiographs revealed intrapulmonary hemorrhage and pneumothorax. The twelfth thoracic vertebra was the site of a compression fracture. A diffuse patchy density in the mid abdomen blurring the contours of the bowel was interpreted as due to hemorrhage. The animal's condition improved slowly. Ten days after the accident it was returned to its owner who was instructed to empty the animal's bladder by external pressure. Two months later it was again brought to the clinic. This time it could walk, but with a very wobbly gait and it had urinary incontinence. The animal was euthanatized at the owner's request. Necropsy was not performed.

Differential Diagnosis: The changes in the thoracic cavity and in the spine were indisputable. The changes in the abdomen presented the only differential diagnostic problem. The diffuse patchy density blurring the abdominal organs could be due to an uncomplicated hemorrhage. Rupture of the urinary bladder or gallbladder and bile duct also had to be considered.

The urinary bladder was seen on the radiograph. It could easily be emptied by external pressure. Since there was no blood in the urine, bladder rupture was considered an unlikely possibility. The cat was carefully watched for several days, and because its condition improved and the radiographic appearance of the abdomen gradually returned to normal, the diagnosis of uncomplicated hemorrhage was confirmed.

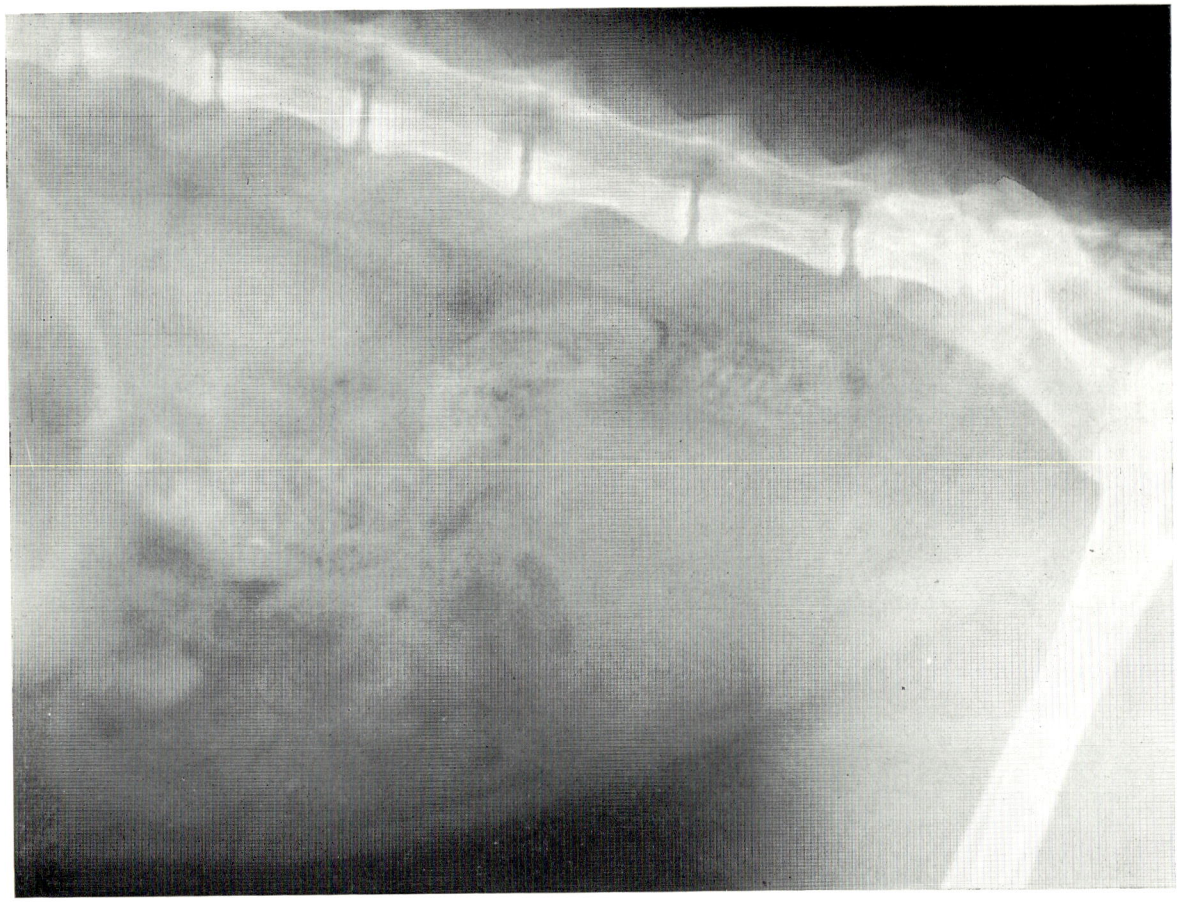

Case 40. Lateral radiograph of mid and caudal part of the abdomen made a few hours after the accident. The kidneys, the urinary bladder, and the descending colon, which is filled with fecal material, are seen. In the lower mid abdomen there is a blurring of the contours of the bowel caused by a patchy irregular density.

Diagnosis: Uncomplicated intraabdominal hemorrhage.

Case 41

Dachshund, male, 9 years old. This previously healthy dog was kicked by its owner. It soon became listless and was brought to a veterinarian who made the diagnosis of intraabdominal hemorrhage, due most likely to rupture of a pathologic spleen. The dog was referred to the clinic for surgical treatment.

On admission to the clinic the dog was in a state of shock. It had very pale mucous membranes. A painful mass could be palpated in the mid abdomen. The abdominal wall was rigid. Paracentesis of the abdomen yielded no abnormal material. Radiographs revealed a round mass in the mid abdomen apparently adhering to the spleen. The bowel contours were blurred, apparently by fluid causing a diffuse, slightly flaky density. Since the radiographic examination confirmed the clinical diagnosis of ruptured tumor of the spleen, blood transfusion was started and laparotomy performed.

There was a large amount of blood in the abdomen. A splenic tumor the size of a tennis ball had ruptured. Splenectomy was performed. Recovery was rapid and uneventful.

Differential Diagnosis: The diagnosis of intraabdominal hemorrhage was easily made on the basis of the history of acute trauma. In the absence of such information a tumor with metastases to the peritoneum (peritoneal carcinomatosis) would have to be considered. Hemorrhage, peritonitis, and carcinomatosis are very similar in radiographic appearance. However, the latter usually has a somewhat more nodular appearance. In the present case the location of the tumor indicated that its origin was in the spleen. The possibility of a malignant tumor of the omentum could not be completely excluded. It is noteworthy that paracentesis of the abdomen yielded no abnormal material. This negative finding is not uncommon in association with intraabdominal hemorrhages.

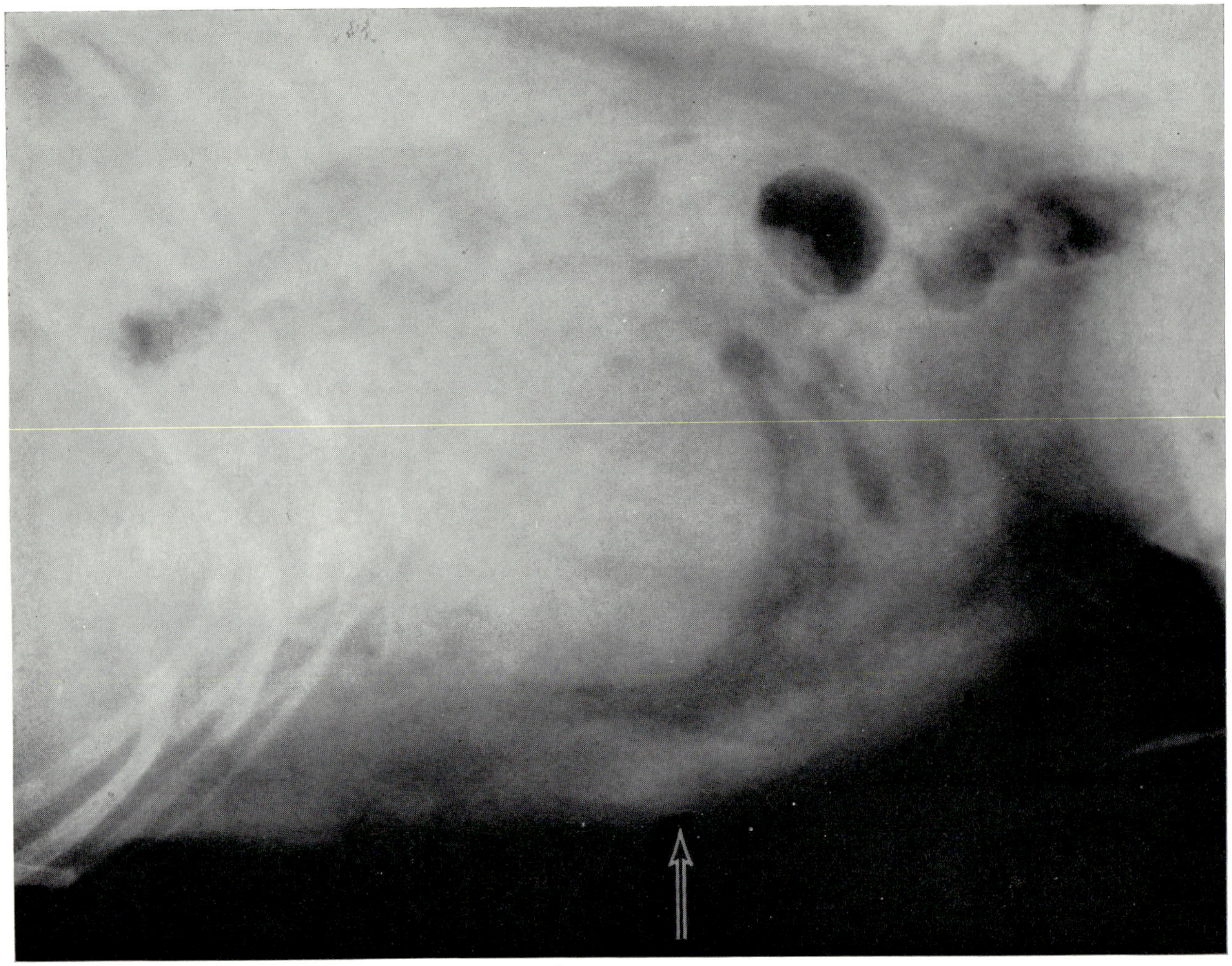

Case 41. There is increased density in the entire abdomen. Just caudal to the costal arch is a round, partly ill-defined mass the size of a tennis ball. The ventral end of the spleen (arrow) is seen lying on the ventral abdominal wall just below the mass. There are some gas-filled bowel loops. There is diffuse density blurring the outline of the tumor of the spleen and of the bowel. The cranial part of the urinary bladder can be seen to the right of the picture.

Diagnosis: Splenic tumor, ruptured by trauma to the abdomen. Intraabdominal hemorrhage.

Case 42

Doberman, female, 9 years old. Previously this dog had always been healthy. One morning it refused to leave its bed, and when forced it moved slowly with a dragging, wobbly gait. It had been out for a walk the night before and had appeared to be completely normal at that time.

The dog was brought to the clinic. At examination it was found to have very pale mucous membranes, rigid abdominal muscles, and apparent pain on palpation of its abdomen. There was a clear, slightly yellowish discharge from the vulva. Radiographic examination revealed increased density in the abdominal cavity. The contours of the organs were blurred. The descending colon was close to the ventral abdominal wall and the retroperitoneal space seemed to be widened.

Radiographs were made 30 and 90 minutes after a mixture of meglumine diatrizoate and barium had been given orally. The meglumine diatrizoate passed rather quickly to the large bowel, but barium was slow in leaving the stomach. Radiographs made 17 hours following the administration of the contrast media showed that barium still remained in the stomach and the small bowel.

The dog's condition improved somewhat and it accepted some food. Blood tests showed no abnormality. After 3 days the dog again turned pale and became almost lethargic. Radiographs at this time revealed a large area of diffuse density appearing cranial to the urinary bladder. No contrast media remained in the digestive tract. The area of slight diffuse density in the ventral part of the abdomen that was seen on all the previous radiographs had become more marked.

The increased density was interpreted as indicative of a continuous oozing of blood into the abdominal cavity. Against advice, the owner of the dog postponed surgical treatment, but on the fourth day gave his consent to laparotomy, which was immediately performed.

The abdomen was full of blood. Almost every abdominal organ was infiltrated by small tumors, many of them oozing blood. The diagnosis of hemangioendotheliomatosis was made. The dog was euthanatized.

Necropsy: The diagnosis of hemangioendotheliomatosis was confirmed.

Differential Diagnosis: The sudden onset of the clinical signs and the appearance of radiographic signs of hemorrhage and peritoneal irritation pointed towards rupture of an abdominal organ. There was, however, no history of trauma. For this reason, and because of lack of demonstrable enlargement of any of the abdominal organs the cause of the intraabdominal hemorrhage could not be determined.

Indication for laparotomy was evident. The operation was, however, postponed on the owner's request.

In retrospect it may be said that in cases like the present one in which no other sign of disease is present and in which there is no history of trauma, spontaneous ruptures of hemangioendotheliomas should be considered as a possible diagnosis.

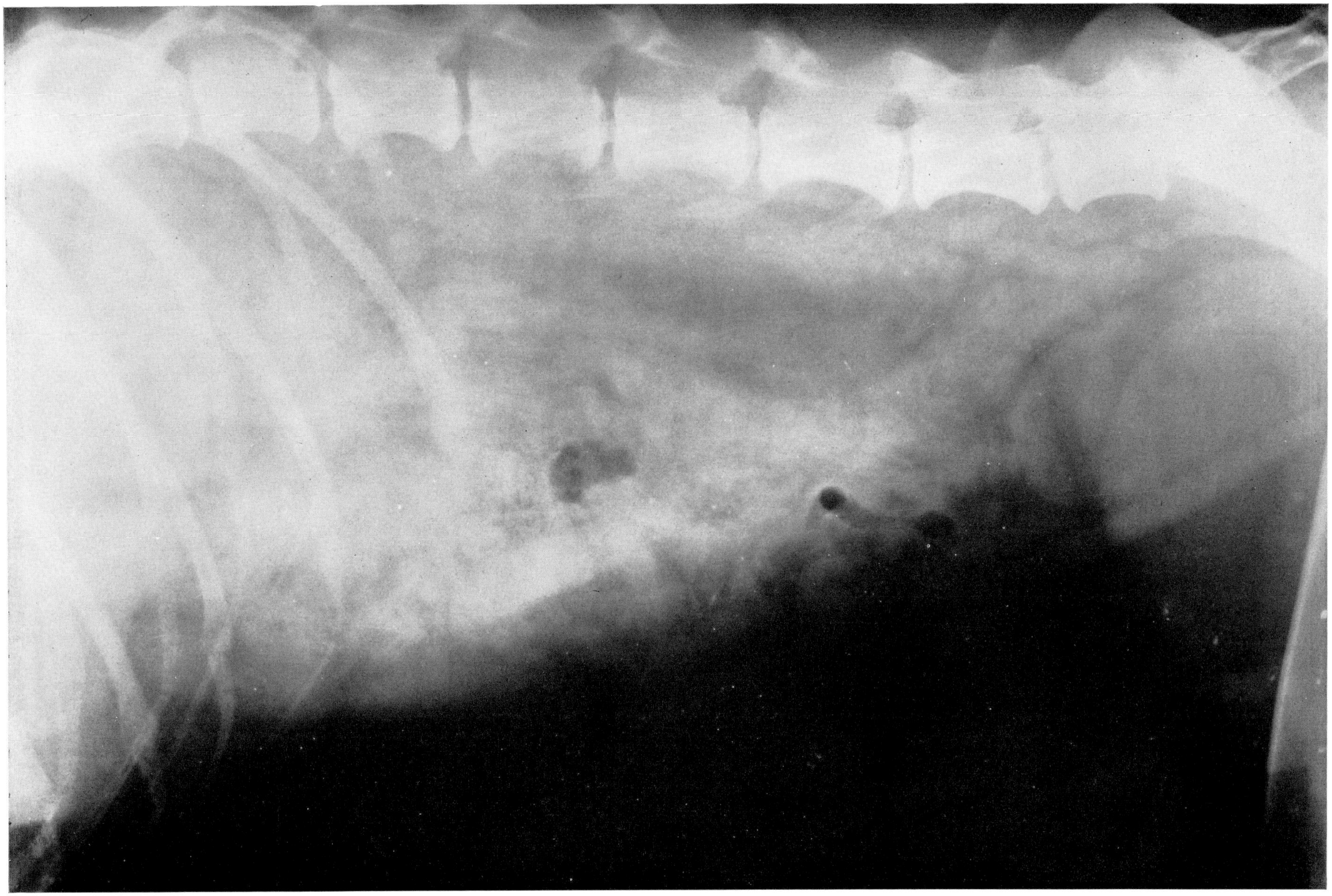

Case 42. **A,** Lateral radiograph made on the first day of illness. There is a slightly diffuse density in the ventral portion of the abdomen. The bowel loops are not well delineated. The descending colon and rectum are filled with a rather radiopaque ingesta. Cranial to the urinary bladder the colon seems to be pressed in a ventral direction.

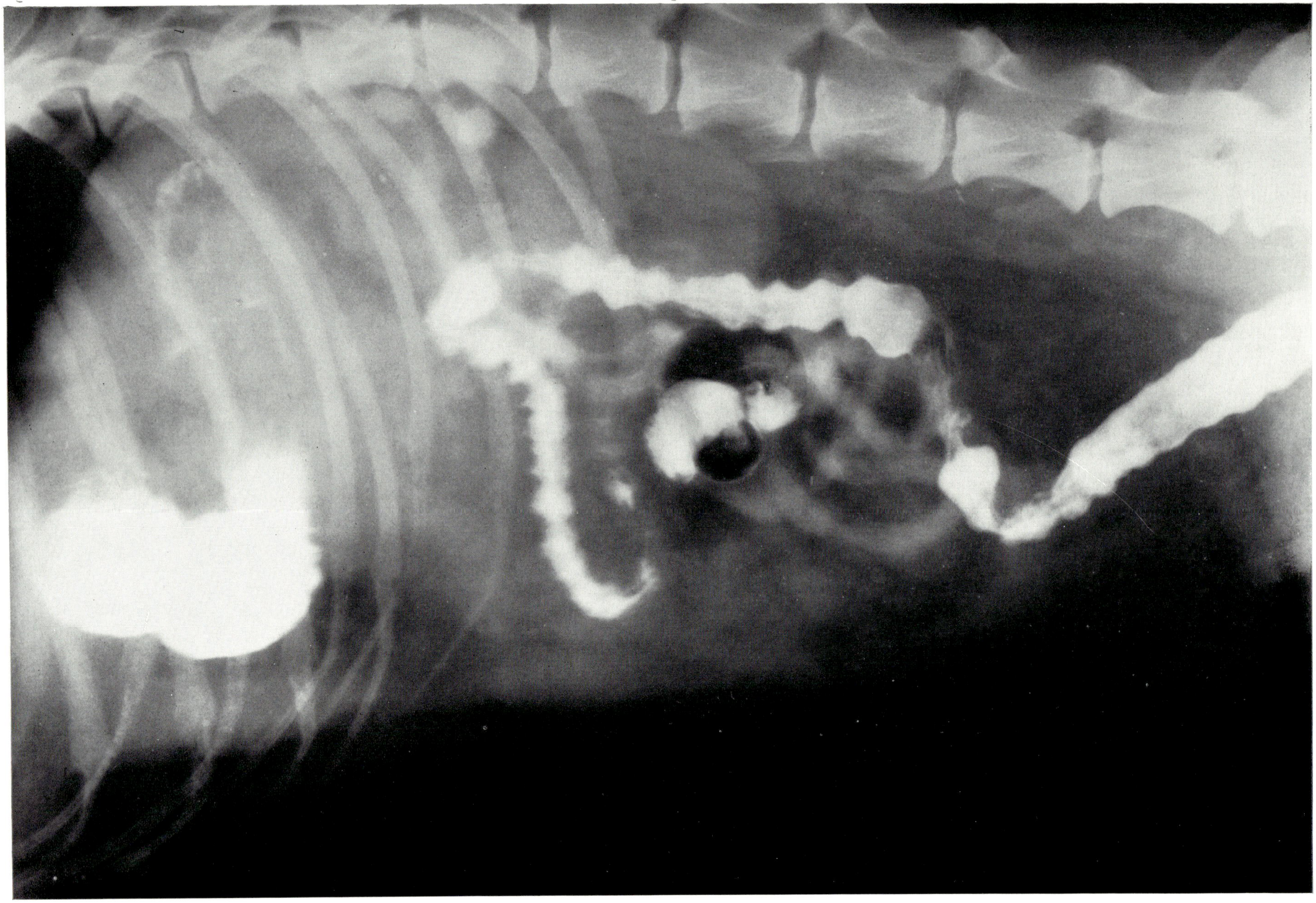

Case 42. **B,** Lateral radiograph made 90 minutes after oral administration of barium and meglumine diatrizoate. Barium remains in the stomach while meglumine diatrizoate has reached the rectum. There is some meglumine diatrizoate in the small bowel and some in the cecum and colon. The large bowel has a corrugated appearance, indicating a peritoneal irritation. The caudal part of the descending colon is deviating ventrally. There is a diffuse density over the whole abdomen most pronounced in its ventral part. The left kidney and the spleen can be seen, the latter especially is surrounded by an area of diffuse patchy density.

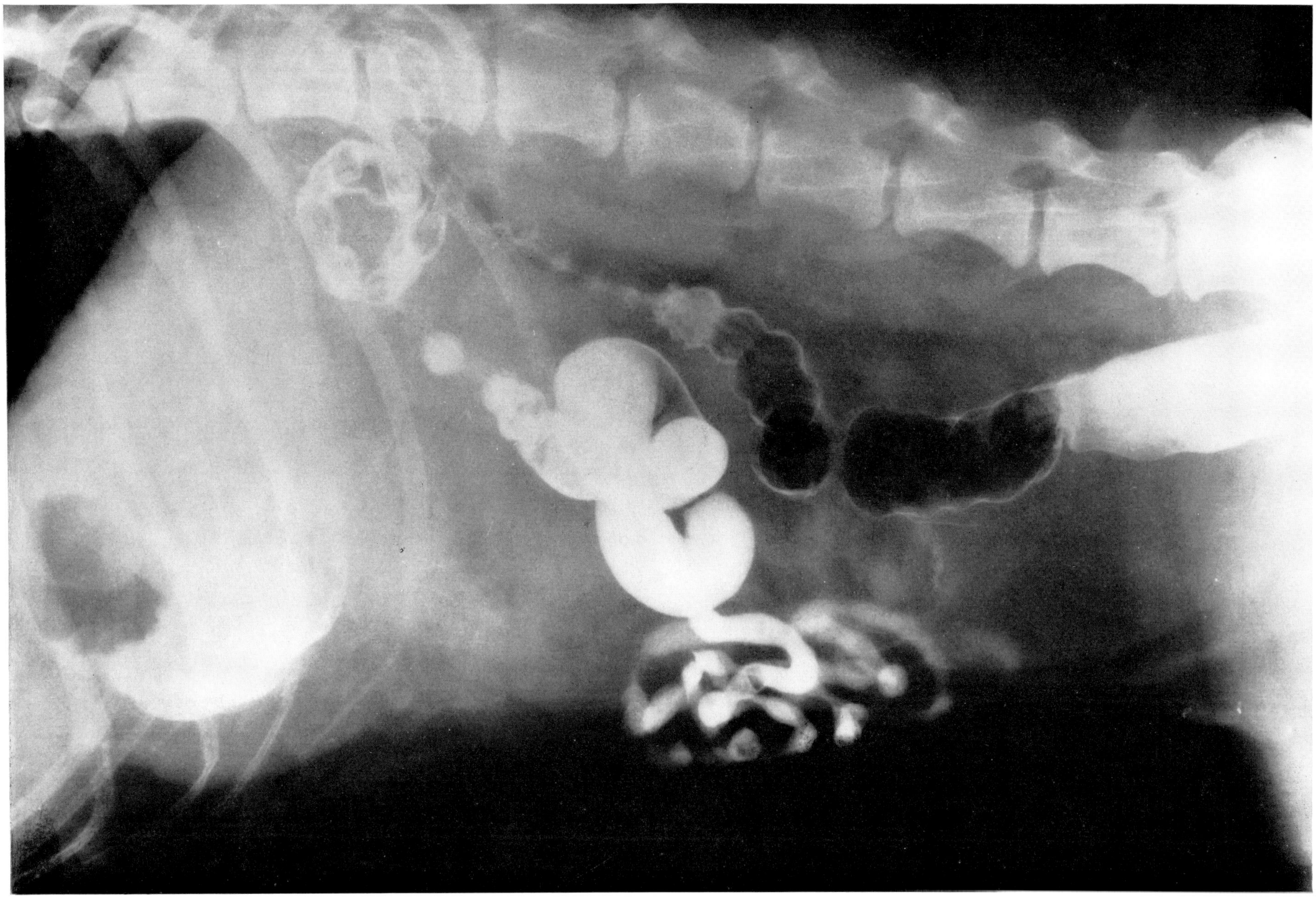

Case 42. **C,** Lateral radiograph made 17 hours after oral administration of meglumine diatrizoate and barium. Some barium is retained in the stomach. Most of it is in the small bowel and cecum. The colon shows segmental contractions and is almost void of contrast media, while the rectum is filled with the media. The descending colon and rectum are in a more normal position than on the previous two radiographs. The pyloric antrum is distended. This was noted also in the previous radiograph. There is still a diffuse patchy density in the entire abdomen.

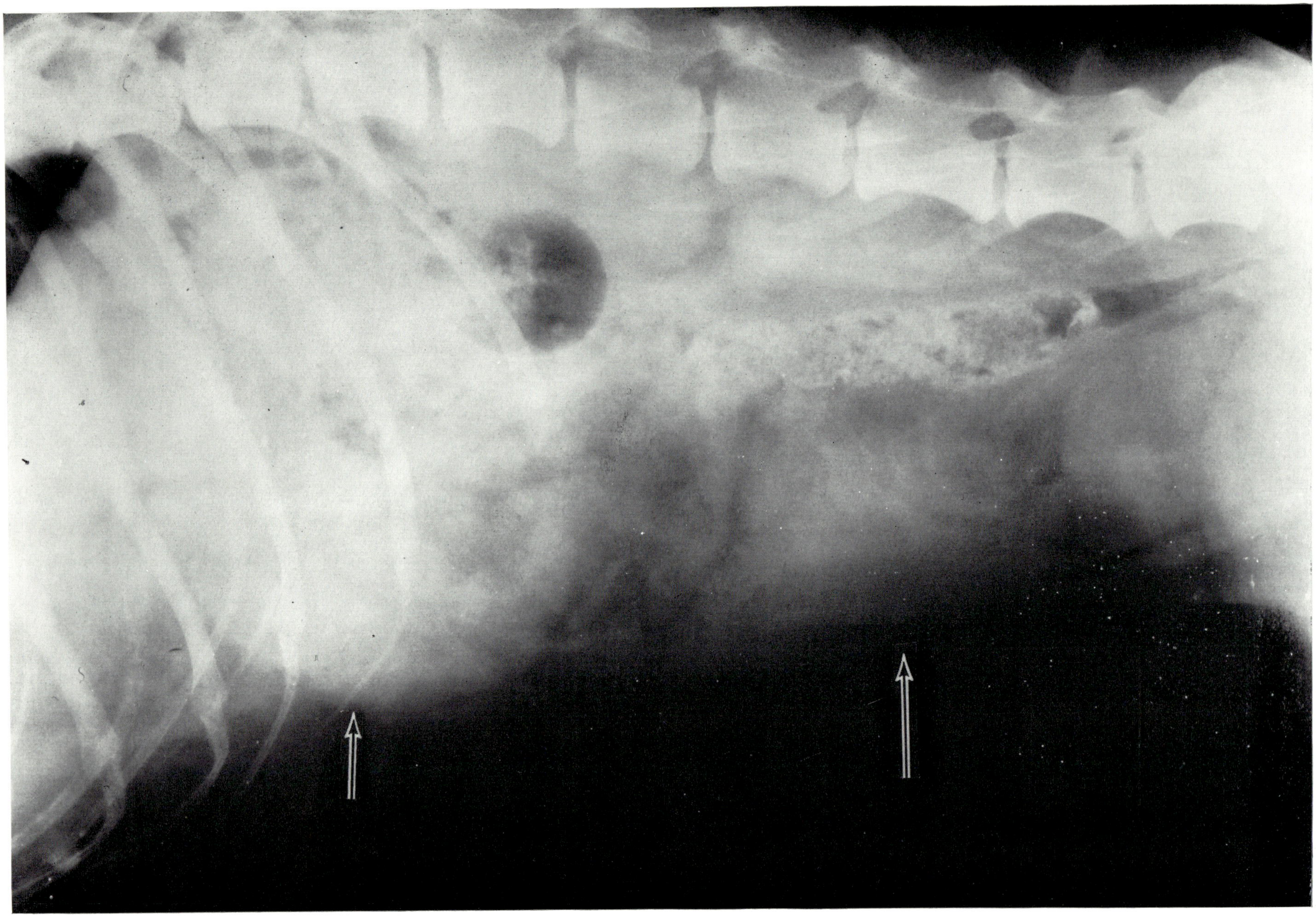

Case 42. **D,** Lateral radiograph made on the third day of illness. The contrast media have left the digestive tract. In addition to the rather homogenous density surrounding the spleen (small arrow) there is another area of density cranial to the bladder (large arrow). This density was interpreted as being due to a large clot of blood.

Diagnosis: Hemangioendotheliomatosis. Spontaneous ruptures of several tumors. Intraabdominal hemorrhage.

Case 43

Welsh corgi, male, 5 years old. This previously healthy dog suddenly began to vomit, became very listless, and refused to eat. A veterinarian was consulted. Radiographs were made, but no abnormality was demonstrated and no diagnosis was made. The dog was referred to the clinic after 3 days of illness. At examination it was noted to be extremely listless and slightly dehydrated. Its temperature was subnormal. Abdominal palpation produced pain. Radiographs revealed no definite abnormality, but there was a slight, diffuse density caudal to the stomach. The dog's condition deteriorated. It vomited violently after intake of water. Oral administration of barium initiated vomiting. Fluoroscopic examination revealed that not even a trace of barium left the stomach and entered the small bowel. On the fifth day of illness, radiographs were again made. The previously observed density was now more marked. On the basis of the radiographic findings, pancreatitis was suspected, but the clinician in charge insisted on an exploratory laparotomy.

At operation the pancreas was found to be the site of a severe inflammatory reaction with ecchymoses. There was also rather widespread peritonitis. Surprisingly the dog survived the operation. Its condition improved slowly. Eventually it recovered completely.

Differential Diagnosis: Acute pancreatitis is difficult to diagnose radiographically. In the initial phase there may not be any radiographic signs, and later only a diffuse density due to the reaction from the peritoneum will be found. Usually the peritonitis is localized to the anterior part of the abdomen. Violent vomiting after oral administration of contrast medium often occurs. In the present case the signs of peritonitis did not develop until after several days.

The combination of vomiting, no or very slow passage of contrast medium from the stomach to the duodenum, and a slight diffuse peritonitis in the cranial portion of the abdomen should always be regarded as possible signs of pancreatitis. In addition the duodenum may have an unusual location. It may even have a fixed position and an irritated corrugated wall.

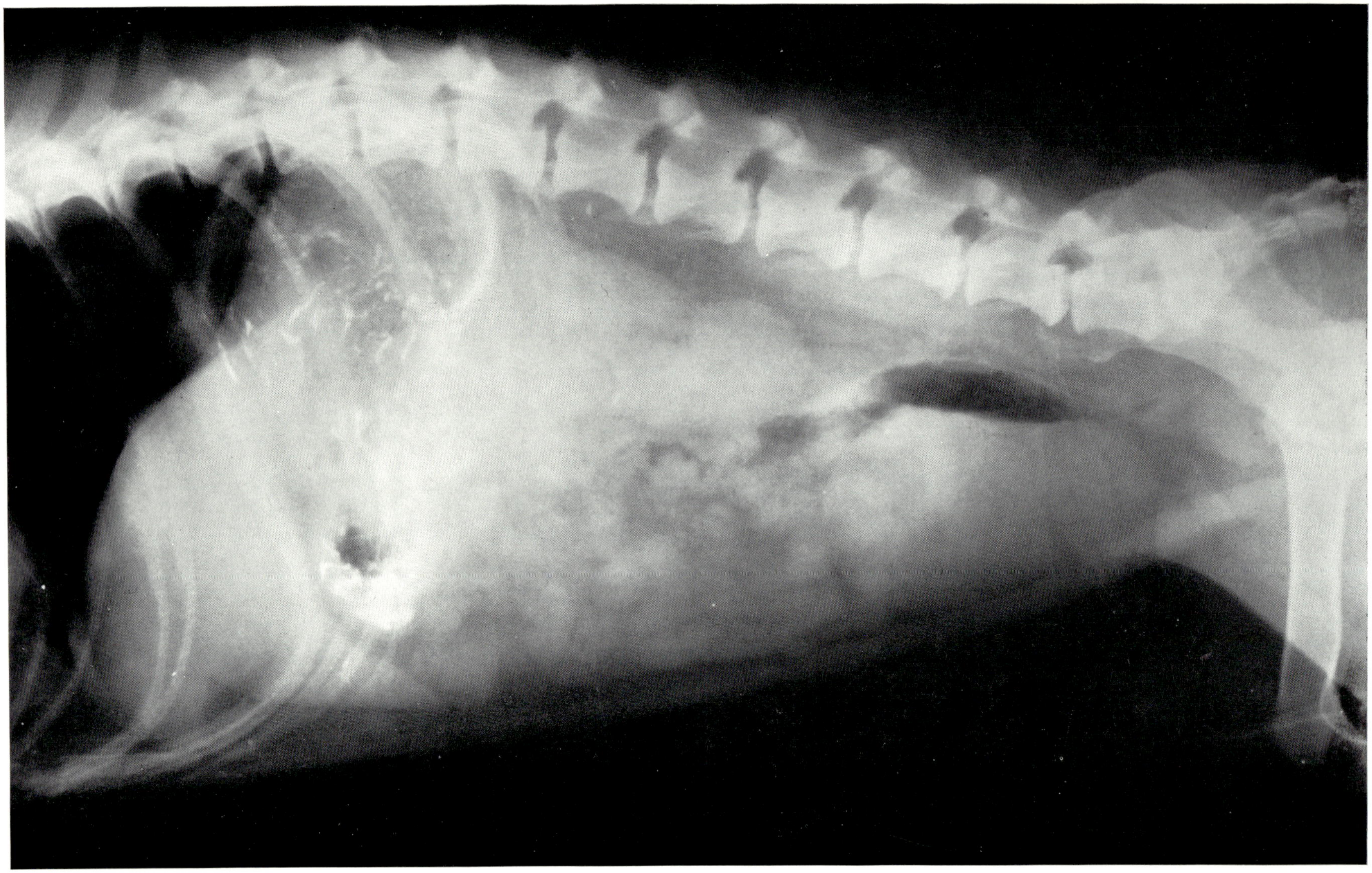

Case 43. Lateral radiograph made 1 hour after the oral administration of barium on the third day of illness. The dog has thrown up most of the contrast medium. The barium has not entered the bowel. The small bowel is empty, contains no gas or fluid, and its contours are somewhat obscured by areas of slight, diffuse density. This density is most obvious close to the stomach.

Diagnosis: Acute pancreatitis and peritonitis.

Case 44

Cat, female, 1½ years old. This animal was brought to the clinic immediately after having fallen a distance of eight stories. It was bleeding from the nostrils and its palate was split. Radiographs of the thorax and abdomen revealed pneumothorax and a slight blurring of the contours in the area caudal to the stomach. A retrograde urocystogram showed the bladder to be intact. The condition of the animal slowly deteriorated and on the third day it had fever and the abdomen was more tender and tense than before. Radiographs revealed a mottled, flaky density in the mid abdomen typical of hemorrhage or peritonitis. The diagnosis of traumatic peritonitis was made. The finding of a high serum lipase level supported this diagnosis. After another 3 days, radiographs indicated that the peritonitis had spread over the entire abdomen. Laparotomy was performed. Hemorrhagic pancreatitis and multiple areas of fat necrosis were seen. The cat was euthanatized.

Necropsy: The diagnosis of hemorrhagic pancreatitis was confirmed.

Differential Diagnosis: In this case, peritonitis (with or without necrosis of fat) and hemorrhage were the only two conditions for consideration in determination of the diagnosis since the bladder was intact and bile duct or gallbladder rupture could be ruled out for two reasons: no bile-tinged fluid could be obtained on paracentesis and the animal did not become icteric. Hemorrhage alone was not considered compatible with the slow development of the changes and anemia did not develop. The high serum lipase value in combination with the radiographic signs of peritonitis confirmed the diagnosis.

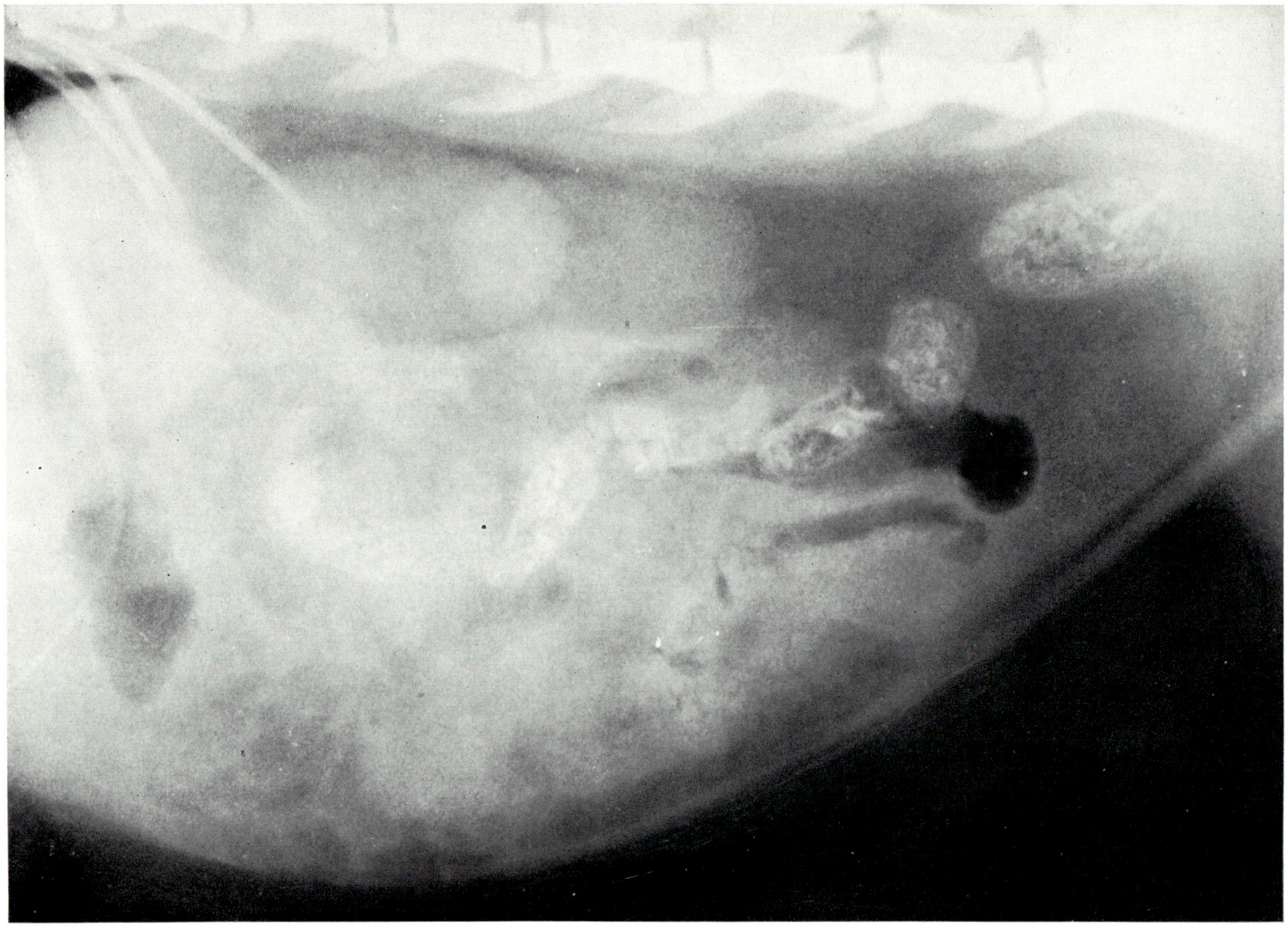

Case 44. Lateral radiograph made 6 days after the animal had fallen eight stories. There is a diffuse, mottled flaky density in the abdomen. The most caudal part is less involved than the remainder of the abdomen. The contours of the liver, stomach, spleen, and bowel are blurred.

Diagnosis: Traumatic, hemorrhagic pancreatitis with necrosis of fat. Peritonitis.

Case 45

Tibetan terrier, male, 5 months old. This dog had been vomiting occasionally for several days. It continued to have normal appetite and normal stools. On admission to the clinic it appeared alert. Although palpation of the abdomen revealed no abnormality it did produce evident pain. Radiographs revealed that a needle was lodged in the mid abdomen. There were no signs of peritonitis. The vomiting subsided. The dog was kept under observation to see if the needle would be eliminated normally. However, this did not happen; instead the signs of abdominal pain seemed to increase. The dog began to stand with an arched back. It was reexamined radiographically. This time there were signs that the needle had perforated the intestinal wall although it was still in the same location. Around the tip of the needle some slightly dense material had collected and the contours of the bowel were more diffuse than on the previous radiographs.

The dog was operated upon. The needle, which had penetrated the ileum, was removed. A slight peritonitis with some adhesions was present. The dog made an uneventful recovery.

Differential Diagnosis: The diagnosis of a radiopaque foreign body such as a needle is easily made. It is more difficult to determine whether or not an animal with such a foreign body should be operated upon immediately or if mere observation is required. Often a needle will pass through the entire bowel only to become stuck in the anal sphincter. From this position, however, it can be removed easily. In the present case, clinical signs as well as radiographic evidence of perforation made laparotomy necessary.

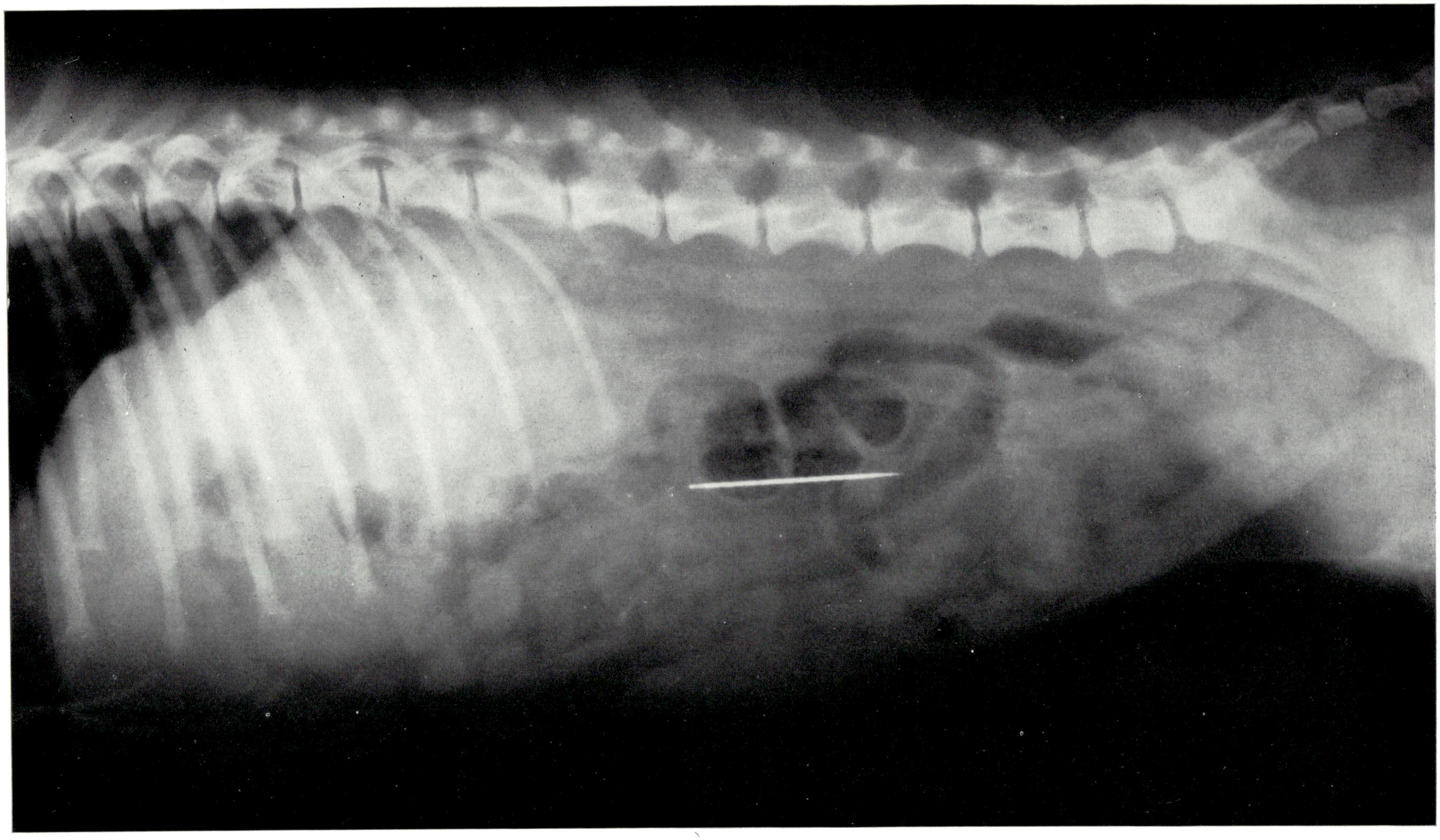

Case 45. **A,** Lateral radiograph made on day of admission. There is a needle in the mid abdomen. The stomach and the bowel are empty. This indicates that the animal has been either anorectic or has vomited. There is some gas in the stomach, in a loop of the small bowel, in the cecum, and in the descending colon.

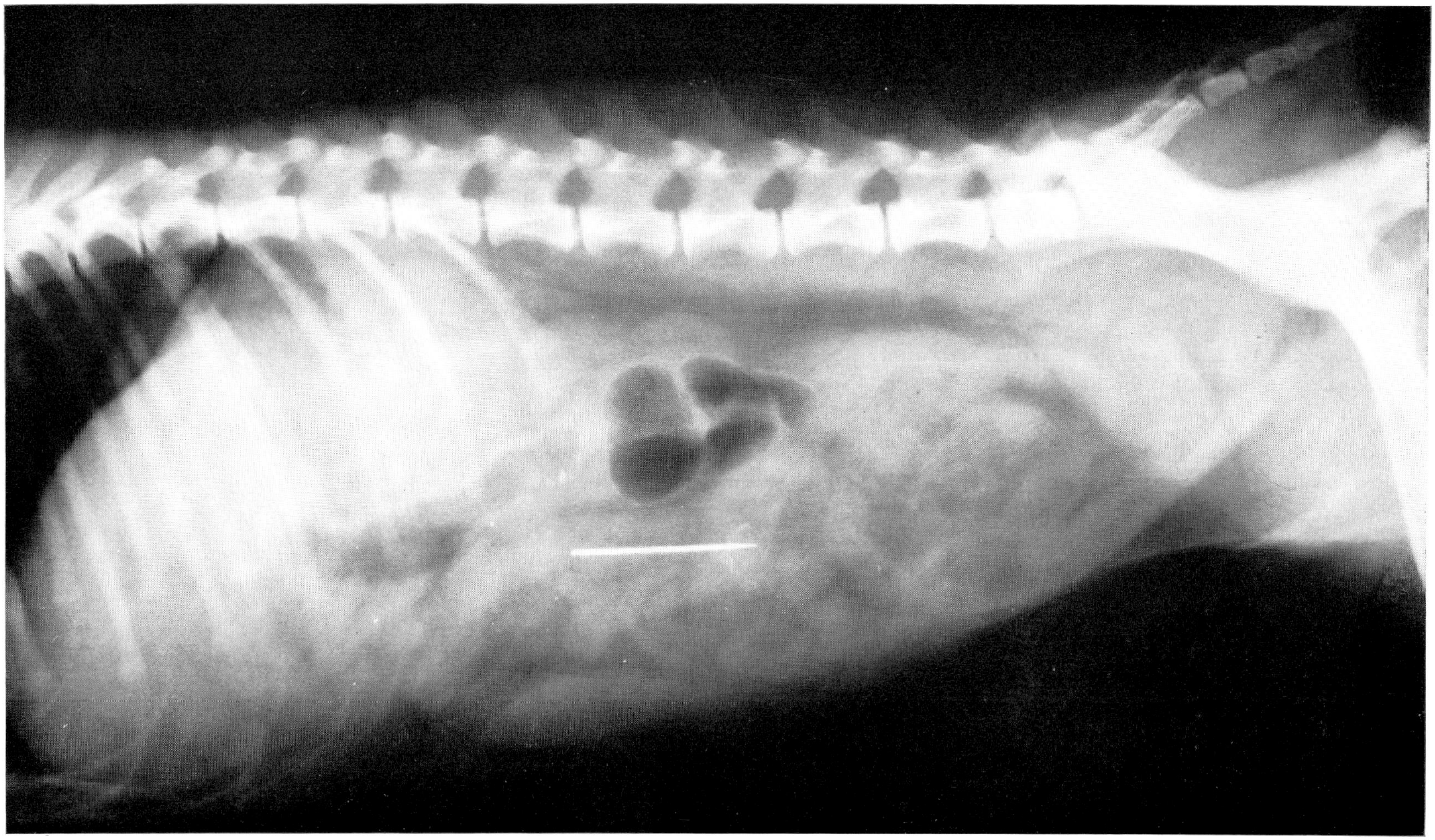

Case 45. **B,** Lateral radiograph made 3 days after that shown in **A.** The needle has not changed position to any great extent. A somewhat "cloudy" density has appeared around the tip of the needle and there is also a very slight, diffuse patchy density in the middle and caudal part of the abdomen. Because of this the contours of the bowel are less distinct than on the previous radiograph.

Diagnosis: Foreign body (needle) perforating the ileum and causing peritonitis.

Case 46

Collie, male, 9 years old. This dog had been out running for an hour. When it returned the owner noticed that it limped on its left hind leg. There was also a swelling the size of an orange to the left of the penis. On admission to the clinic these observations of the owner were confirmed. The swelling was painful and had apparently increased in size since the owner first noticed it. A traumatic hernia was suspected. Radiographs revealed that the swelling had a diffuse density indicating the presence of bowel loops. A puncture made through the wall of the swelling yielded some blood.

A barium swallow was given and the owner was asked to return the dog to the clinic the following day for another radiographic examination. At this examination, bowel loops containing contrast medium were found in the large soft-tissue mass, but there were no signs of incarceration such as distention of the bowel loops or impaction of contrast medium.

The acute inflammatory reaction was allowed to subside before the dog was operated upon. At operation performed about 10 days later, the bowel loops were reduced, the rupture in the abdominal wall was sutured, most of the hematoma was evacuated, and the surgical incision closed. At first, wound healing seemed normal, but after 5 days the swelling recurred. This time it was extremely painful and it also felt warm on palpation. The left testicle was swollen and warm. The dog was febrile. Radiographs revealed a large amount of subcutaneous gas but no bowel loops in the swollen area. Bacteriologic examination showed infection with Clostridium perfringens. Vigorous treatment with antibiotics was instituted, but the dog died 2 days later.

Necropsy: Death was found to be due to sepsis (Clostridium perfringens).

Differential Diagnosis: The diagnosis of hernia is usually based more upon clinical than radiologic findings. However, when it comes to deciding if there are bowel loops in the hernia, the radiographic examination is of great help. In the present case the definite diagnosis could not be made clinically, and only by means of the passage of contrast material could it be revealed that there were bowel loops in the hernia.

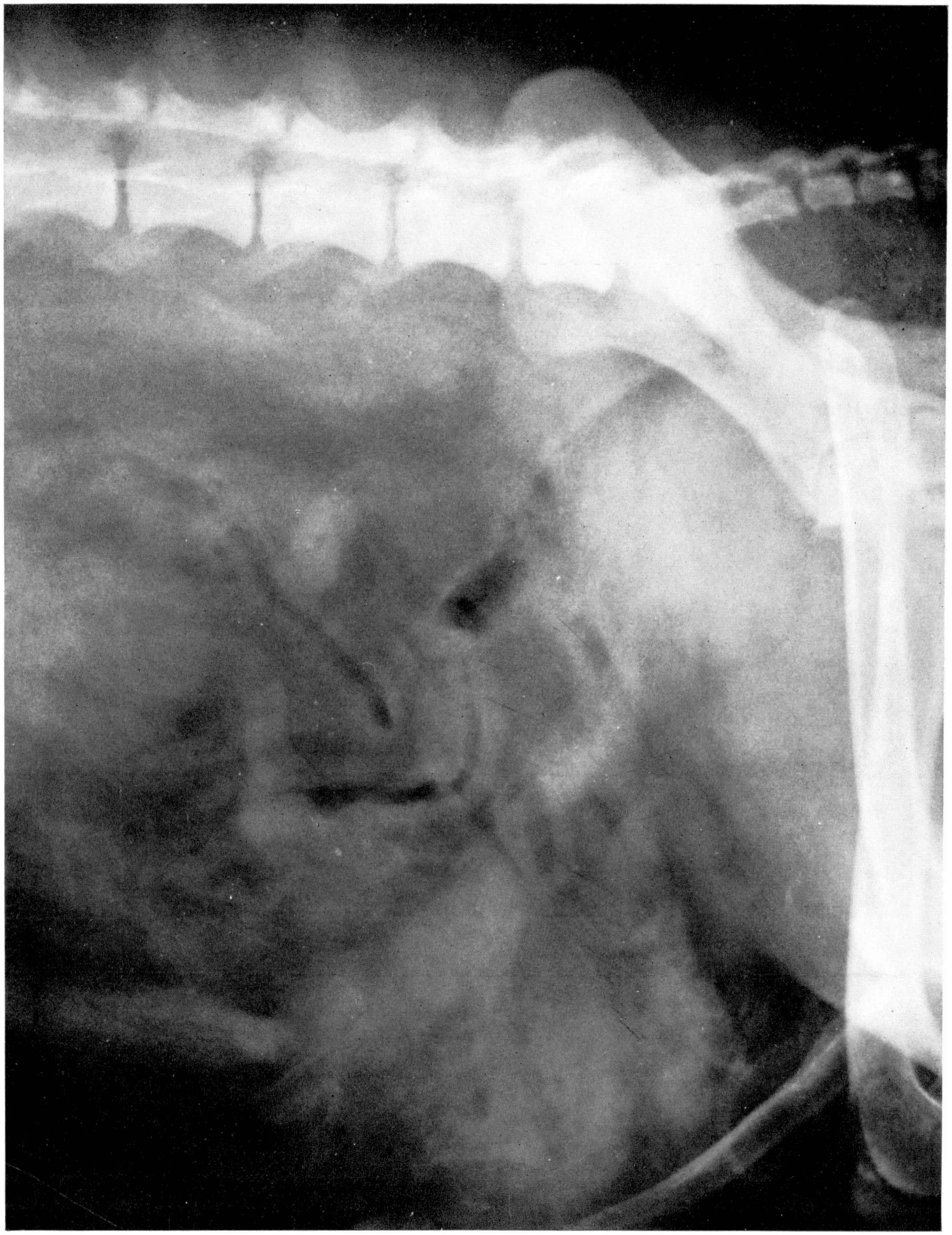

Case 46. **A,** Lateral radiograph of the caudal part of the abdomen. There is a diffuse soft-tissue mass between the abdominal wall and the penis. There are ill-defined soft-tissue structures in the mass. The contours are blurred because of a rather marked patchy density. There is a gas-filled bowel loop projected over the ventral abdominal wall.

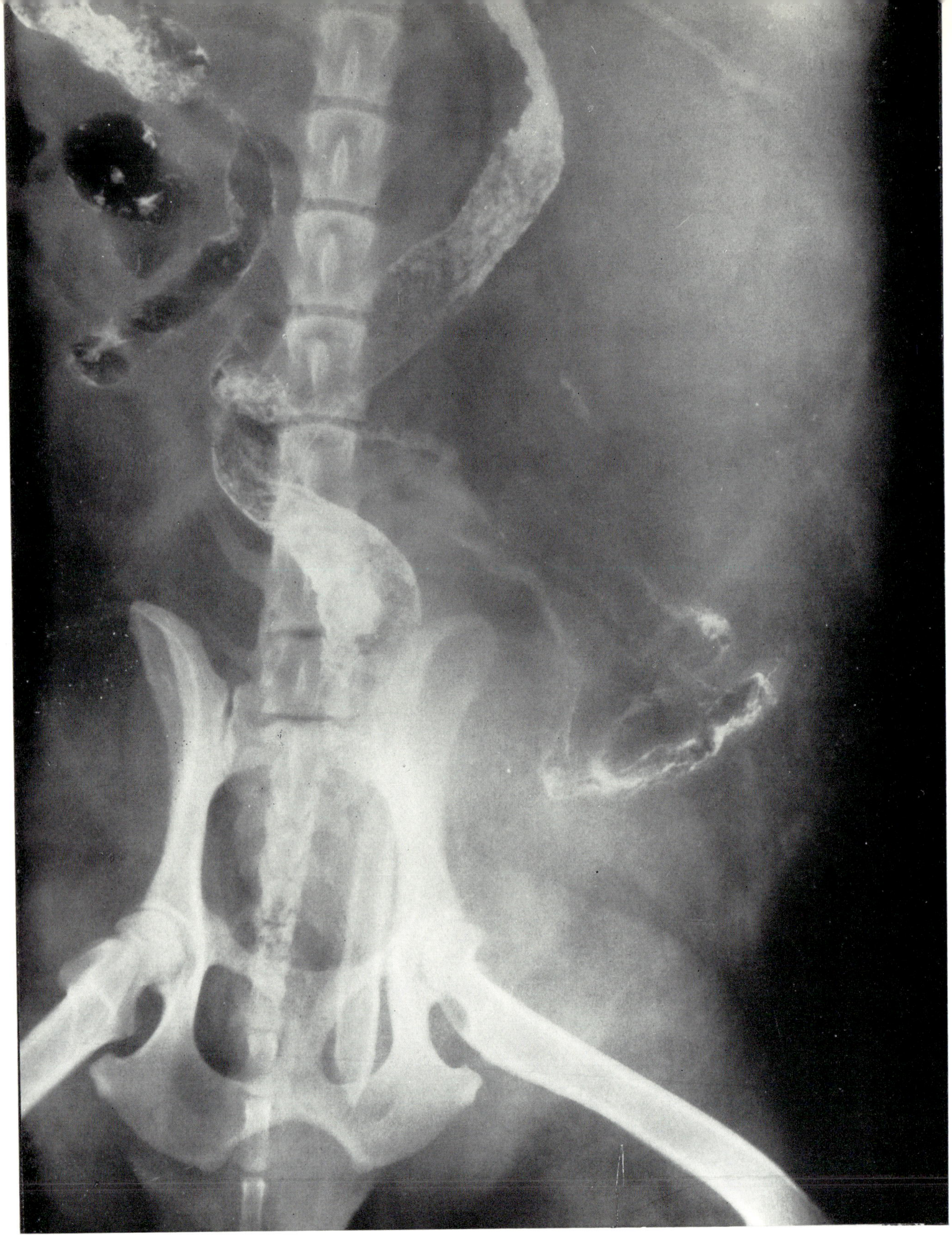

Case 46. **B,** Ventrodorsal radiograph made 14 hours after oral administration of barium. The contrast medium has reached the rectum, but traces of contrast medium in the small bowel show that bowel loops are lodged in the large soft-tissue swelling. This confirms the diagnosis of hernia. The mottled appearance of the diffuse density in the hernia is probably a sign of hemorrhage.

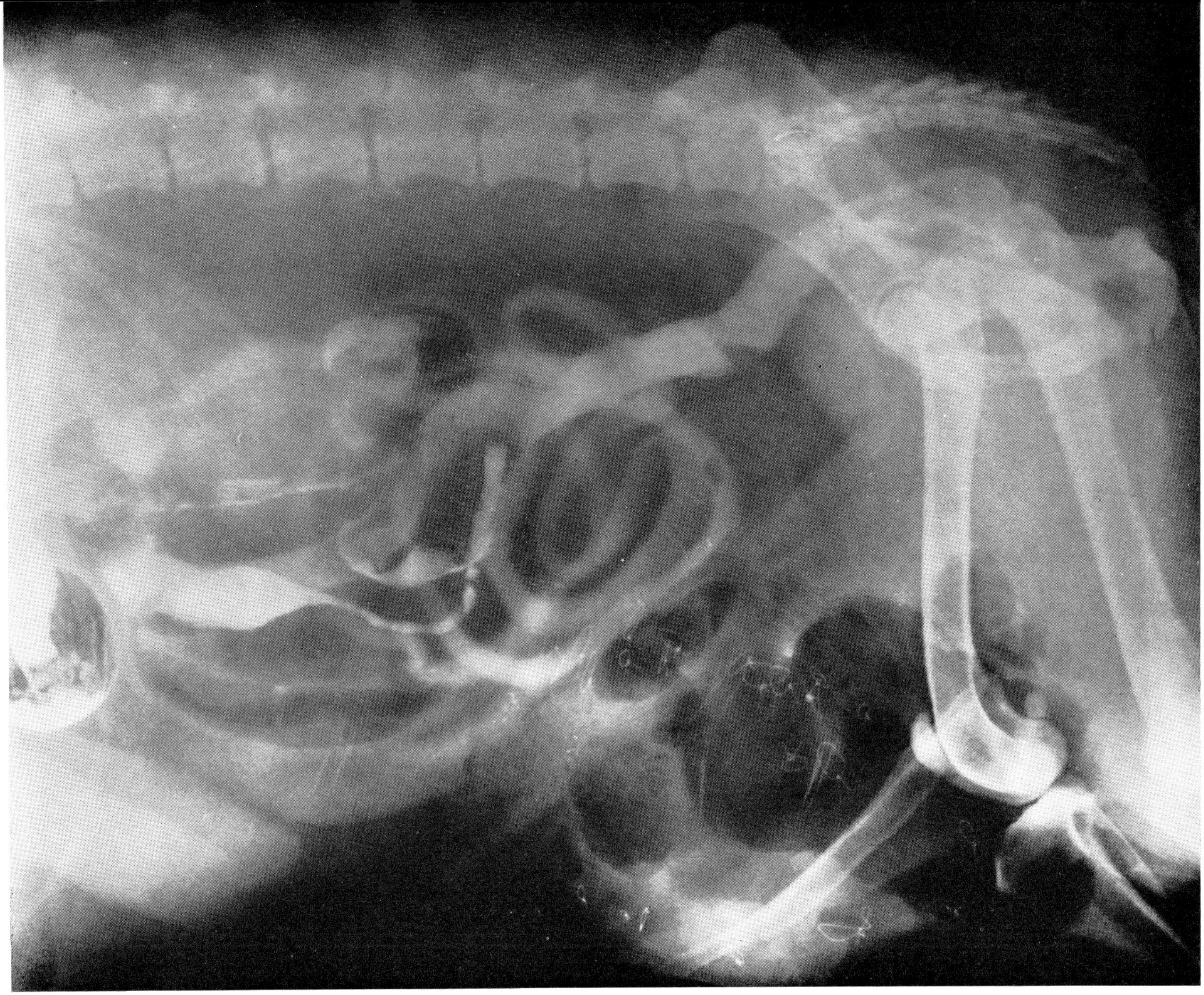

Case 46. **C,** Lateral radiograph made 5 days after the surgical repair of the hernia. Two hours prior to examination the dog had been given meglumine diatrizoate orally. There is a large amount of gas trapped in a swelling at the site of the previous hernia. There is evidently no recurrence of the hernia and bowel loops are not found in the swelling.

Diagnosis: Traumatic abdominal hernia with prolapse of the bowel. Surgical correction. Subsequent infection by Clostridium perfringens forming large gas pockets at the site of the previous hernia.

Case 47

Mongrel dog, female, 1 year old. This animal was hit by a car but apparently did not sustain any serious injury, judging from its behavior after the accident. After a day, however, it became listless and was brought to the clinic. Its general condition was fair, but it displayed some pain when its abdomen was palpated. Radiographs revealed fractures of the pubic and ischiatic bones and an increased intraabdominal density. Rupture of the urinary bladder was suspected. A retrograde urocystogram showed no abnormality and the bladder was intact. The owner was told to keep the dog under close observation and to return it to the clinic if there were any signs of continued illness.

The dog was not brought back to the clinic until 3 weeks later when it was in a miserable condition. It was unable to stand on its legs, it was very icteric, and its abdomen was enlarged. Radiographs revealed a large amount of fluid in the abdomen. At laparotomy, rupture of the gallbladder was found. The dog died before the operation was completed.

Necropsy: The diagnosis made at operation was confirmed.

Differential Diagnosis: Increased density in the abdomen after trauma is usually caused by hemorrhage or by leakage of urine or bile. In this patient, urine could be excluded as the cause. The bladder and urethra were intact and rupture of the ureters is extremely unusual. Blood from a ruptured organ or bile from a ruptured gallbladder or bile duct was therefore suspected as the cause of the diffuse density in this animal. Intravenous cholecystography may have been helpful in the differential diagnosis. A good outline of the gallbladder eliminates the suspicion of rupture of this organ. Failure to fill the gallbladder does not, however, confirm the diagnosis of rupture. If the dog had been kept in the clinic and carefully observed for a few days the fatal outcome should have been prevented. Bile accumulates fast in the abdomen when the gallbladder has ruptured. A few days following rupture of the gallbladder, a ground-glass appearance of the cranial part of the abdomen can be noted on radiographs and bile can be withdrawn from the peritoneal cavity.

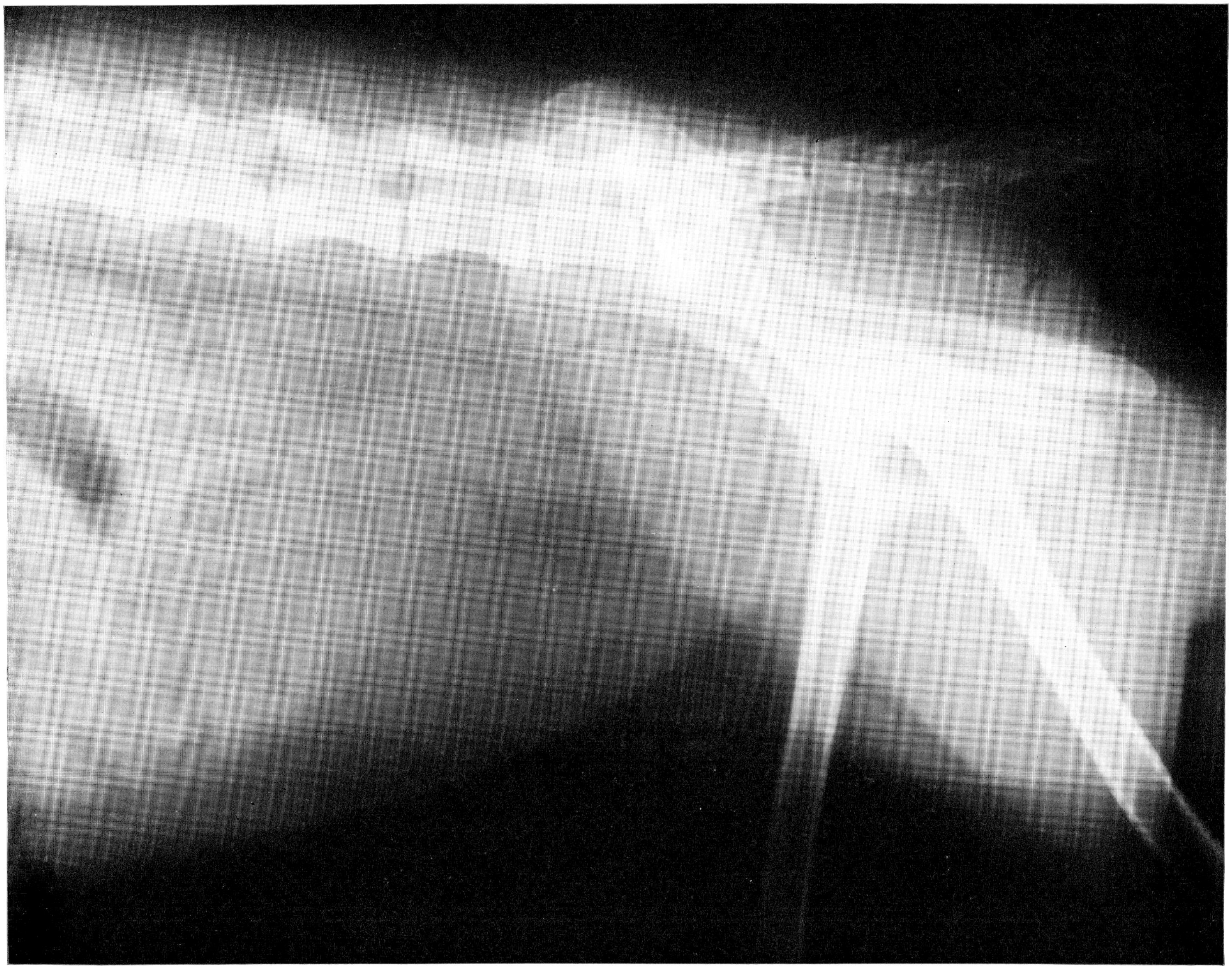

Case 47. **A,** Lateral radiograph of the caudal part of the abdomen including the pelvis. There is a diffuse density in the abdomen. The contour of the urinary bladder cannot be distinctly seen. (The pelvic fractures were demonstrable only on ventrodorsal radiographs.)

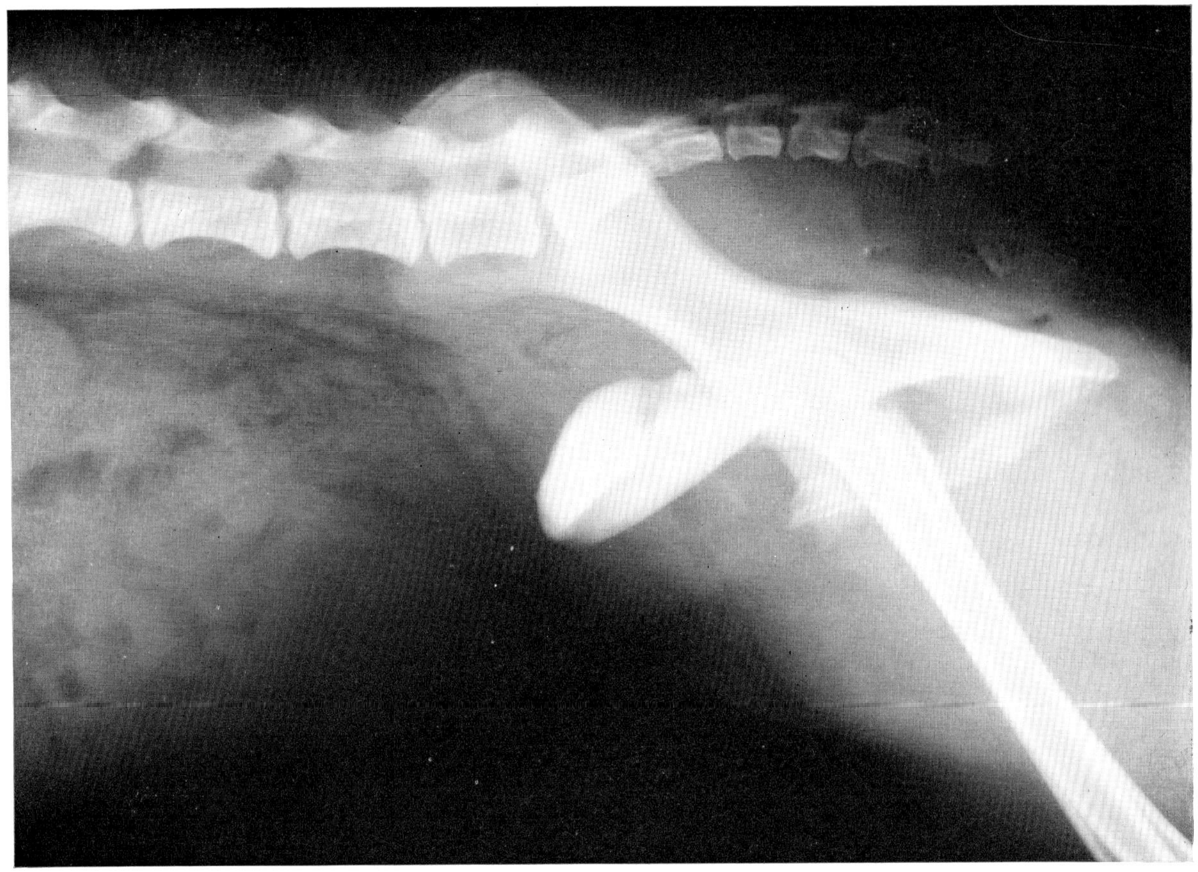

Case 47. **B,** Lateral retrograde urocystogram. There is no rupture of the urinary bladder.

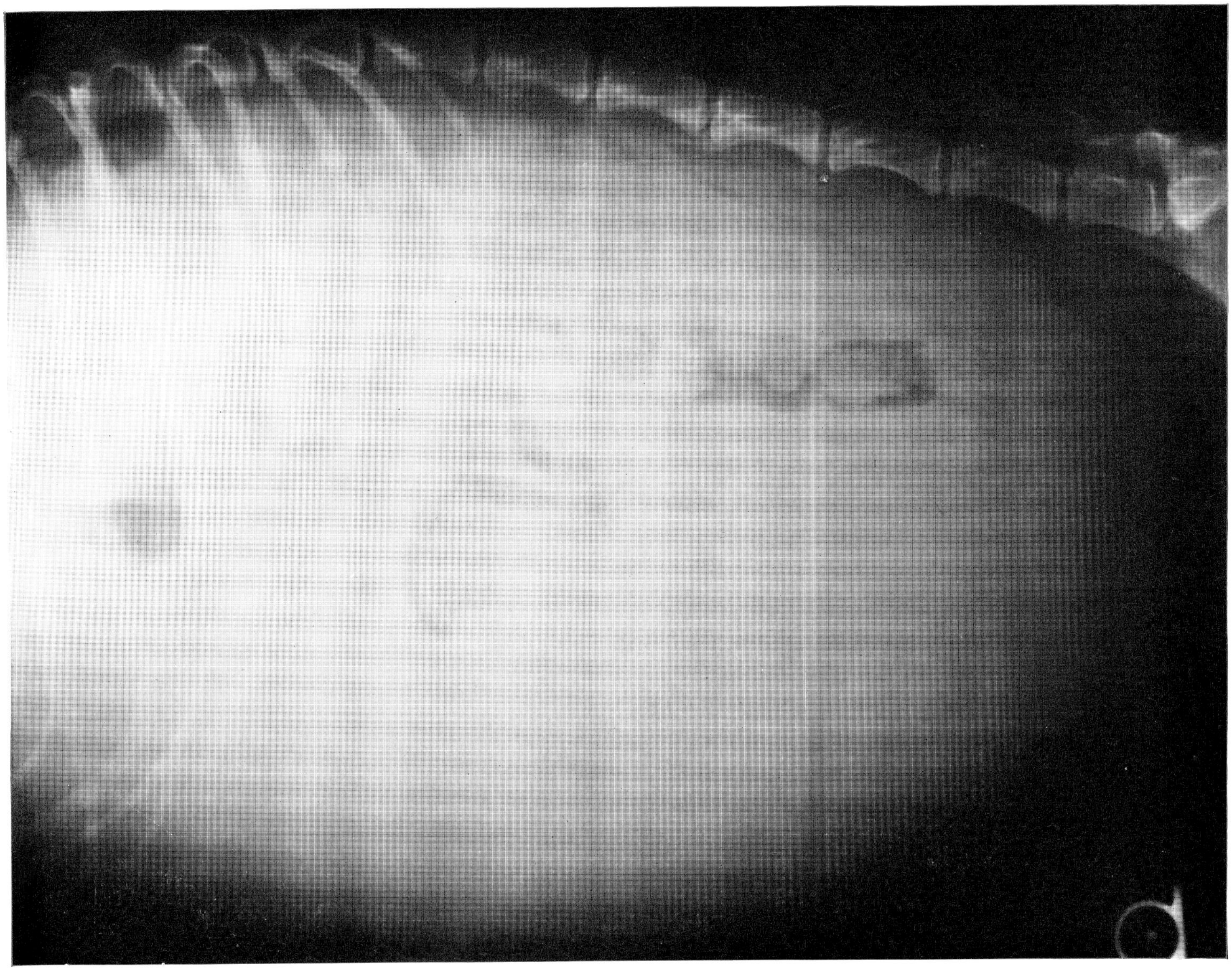

Case 47. **C,** Lateral radiograph made on second admission. The entire abdomen is very distended by fluid which completely obscures all details and gives most of the abdomen a ground-glass appearance.

Diagnosis: Traumatic rupture of the gallbladder.

Chapter 4

The Urogenital Tract

Illustrated in this chapter are the radiographic appearances of the following conditions: pyometra with and without complicating peritonitis, "false pyometra," prostatitis with and without peritonitis, torsion of a retained testicle, rupture of the urinary bladder and urethra, urolithiasis, retroflexion of the urinary bladder into a perineal hernia, dystocia, emphysematous endometritis and fetal death, physometra, postpartum endometritis, and peritonitis following hysterectomy.

It is desirable and sometimes necessary to empty the digestive tract by means of laxatives and enemas before making radiographic examination of the abdomen. If this is not done a urinary calculus may, for example, be obscured by ingesta. Under emergency conditions there is little time for such precautions and it should be kept in mind that errors on interpretation can be made under these circumstances.

A helpful technique for the demonstration of a slight enlargement of the uterus is that of applying compression on the caudal part of the abdomen. A large wooden spoon can be used for this purpose. By applying pressure over the caudal area of the abdomen with the spoon, the bowel loops and the urinary bladder will be pushed aside facilitating demonstration of the uterus.

The choice of contrast medium for retrograde urocystography should be based upon the aim of the examination. For demonstration of a rupture of the urinary bladder a positive contrast medium for use in IVP such as sodium diatrizoate 50% is to be preferred. If the main objective is to study changes within the urinary bladder, air is usually the preferred medium.

Case 48

Airedale terrier, female, 9 years old. About 6 weeks after a normal heat period this dog developed polydipsia, polyuria, and some vaginal discharge. It improved somewhat under treatment prescribed by a veterinarian. After another 3 weeks its condition suddenly deteriorated. It became febrile and vomited repeatedly. On admission to the clinic, it was very weak, its mucous membranes were pale, and its abdomen was enlarged. The vulva, from which there was a discharge, was swollen.

Radiographs revealed enlarged uterine horns. The diagnosis of pyometra was made. After transfusions, laparotomy was performed. The large uterus, which was filled with pus, and the ovaries were removed. When the surgical incision was closed the heart went into fibrillation. Resuscitation was unsuccessful and the dog expired.

Necropsy: Myocardial degeneration was found to be the cause of death.

Differential Diagnosis: As will be seen in Cases 50 and 51, there are conditions which can mimic in radiographic appearance that of an enlarged uterus. In case of uterine enlargement, pregnancy should always be considered. Fetal skeletons are not visible on radiographs until about 3 weeks prior to delivery. In the present case there was little question about the diagnosis. The fatal outcome was probably due to the delay in surgical treatment of the disease.

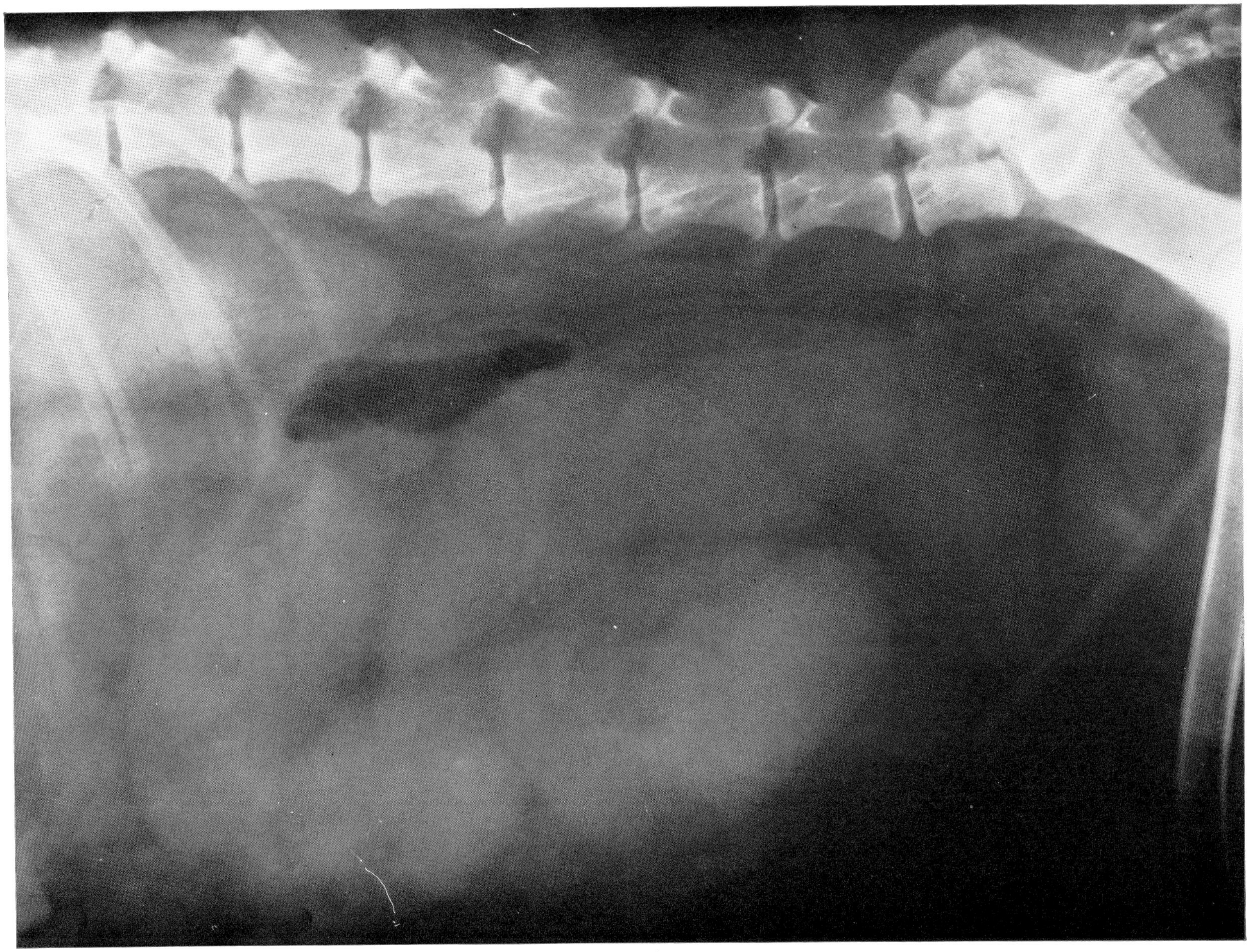

Case 48. On this lateral radiograph the abdomen is seen to contain large, thick, fluid-filled loops. There are no signs of fetal skeleton or gas in these loops. There is good outline of the contours.

Diagnosis: Uterine enlargement. Pyometra.

Case 49

German shepherd, female, 8 years old. About 2 weeks prior to admission to the clinic, after an apparently normal heat period this dog developed polydipsia, polyuria, and anorexia. It vomited after intake of water. At examination, vaginal discharge, enlargement of the vulva, and ecchymoses in the oral mucosa were noted. The dog was pale and very weak. It groaned when the abdomen was palpated. A large mass was felt in the mid abdomen.

Radiographs revealed large fluid-filled loops which occupied most of the abdominal cavity. There was a slight, patchy density blurring the contours of the abdominal organs especially in the mid abdomen.

The diagnosis was that of perforated pyometra with complicating peritonitis. Antibiotics and transfusions were given and laparotomy was scheduled. The owner, however, refused to have the dog operated upon and the animal was euthanatized at his request.

Necropsy: The diagnosis of pyometra and peritonitis was confirmed. The wall of the uterus was perforated by an abscess.

Differential Diagnosis: Pyometra was the obvious diagnosis in this case. Peritonitis also was apparent. The mottled or patchy density blurring the contours of the abdominal organs was typical of peritonitis.

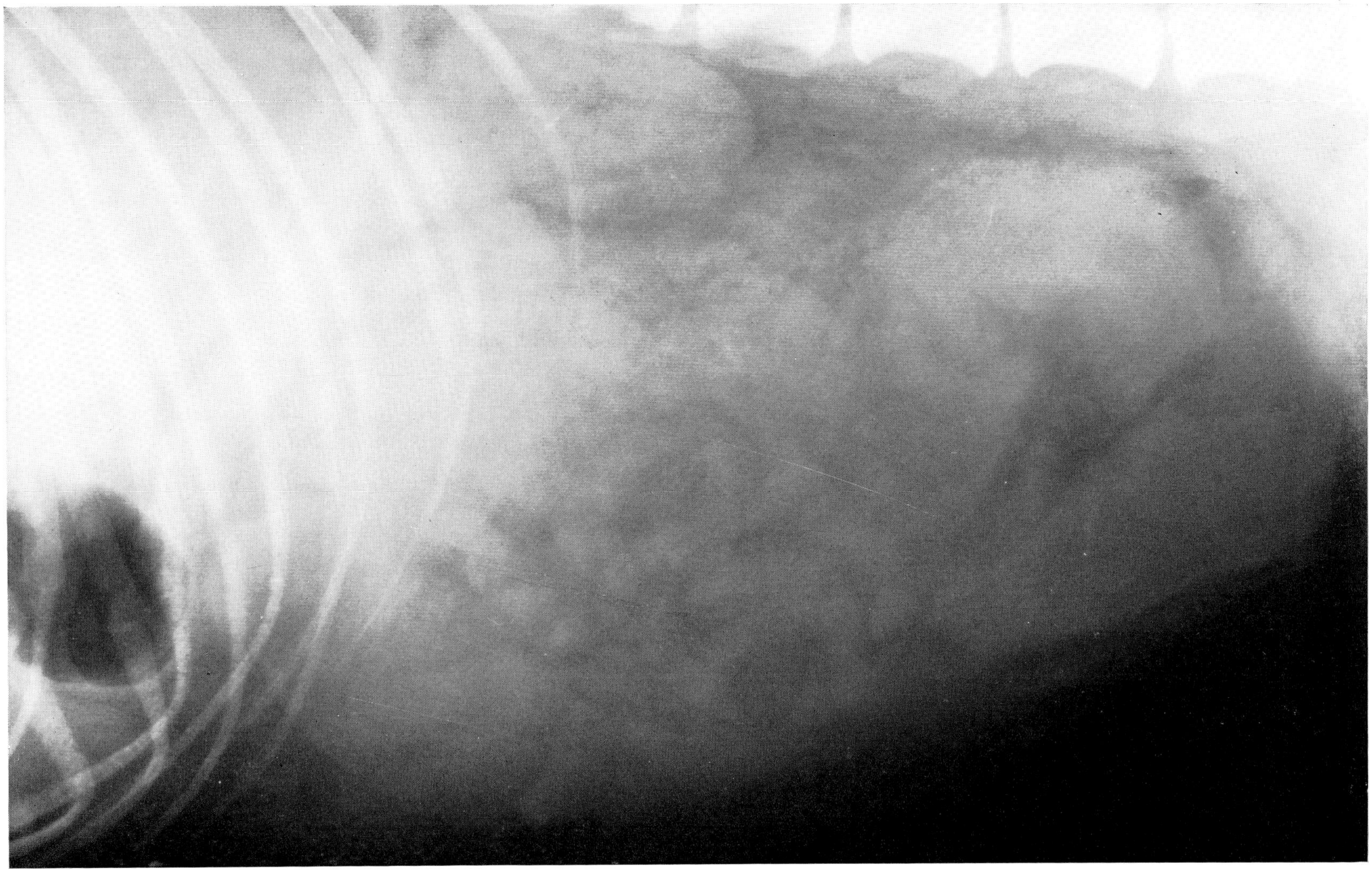

Case 49. On this lateral radiograph the enlarged uterus can easily be seen, but it is obvious that the contours of the abdominal organs are less well delineated than those in the radiograph of Case 48. There is a slight patchy density especially in the mid abdomen.

Diagnosis: Enlargement of the uterus. Pyometra. Peritonitis.

Case 50

Kerry blue terrier, female, 6 years old. This dog had vomited and had showed increased thirst for a couple of days. The clinical history was rather vague as the dog was brought to the clinic by a person who knew little about it. Radiographs revealed large fluid-filled loops in the abdomen. A diagnosis of pyometra was made. At operation, performed on the day of admission, an intestinal foreign body, instead of pyometra, was found. The foreign body was removed. The dog made a rapid recovery.

Differential Diagnosis: In retrospect, it is not difficult to make the differential diagnosis in this case. A number of circumstances contributed to the erroneous diagnosis. An inadequate clinical history and a superficial clinical examination paved the way. The fact that there was gas in the distended loops was overlooked. If this had been noticed and a compression device had been used the correct diagnosis should have been made prior to the operation.

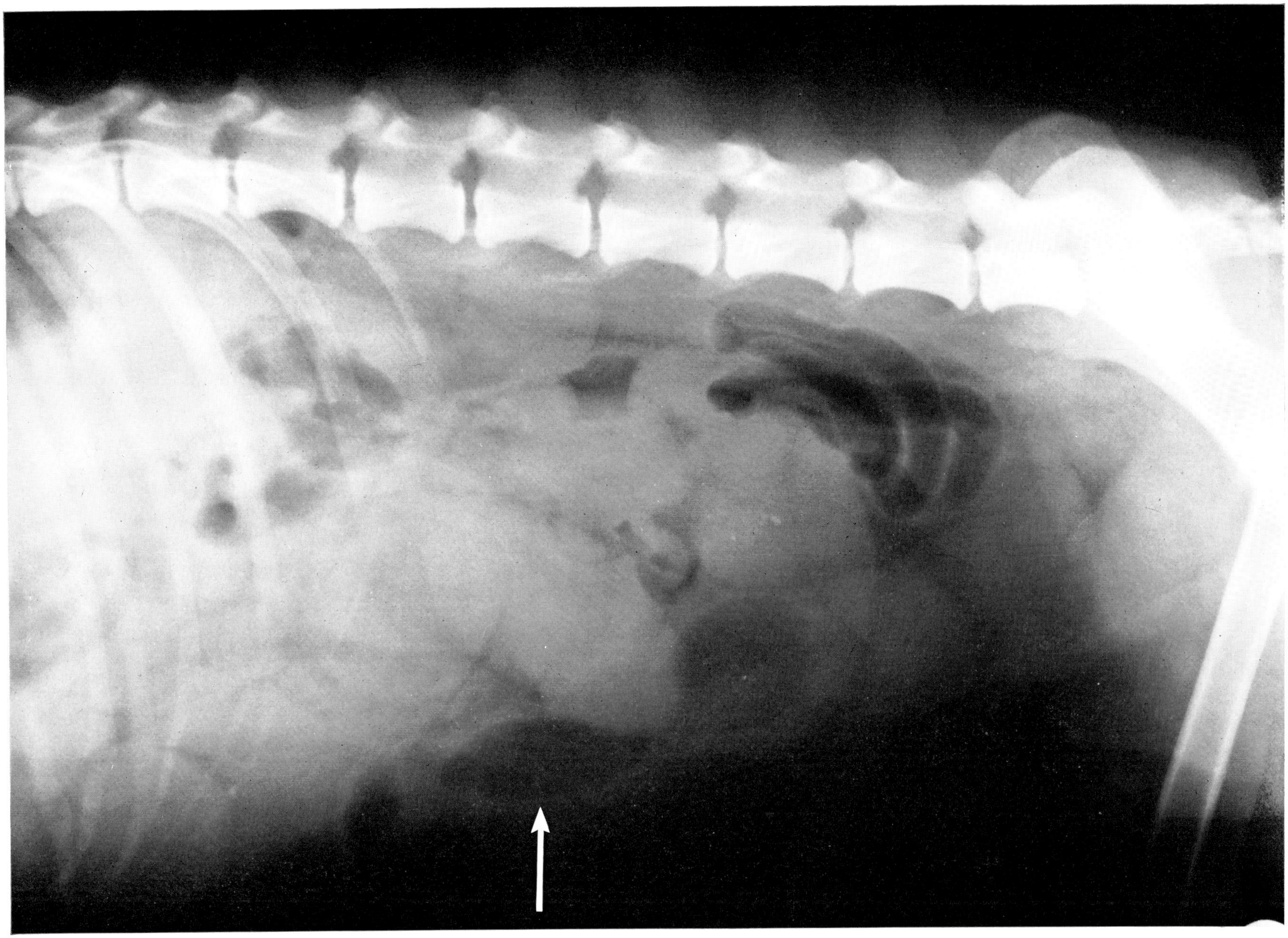

Case 50. The lateral radiograph of the abdomen is dominated by large predominantly fluid-filled but also gas-filled loops (arrow).

Diagnosis: Ileus, erroneosuly diagnosed as pyometra.

Case 51

Collie, female, 10 years old. This dog had a hysterectomy because of pyometra 3 weeks prior to admission to the clinic. Its general condition improved after the hysterectomy, but during the 10 days prior to admission it became listless and developed marked polydipsia. On the day of admission its condition had rapidly deteriorated. At examination the abdominal wall was found to be rather rigid, and the abdomen was painful on palpation. An oblong mass could be palpated.

Radiographs revealed an elongated mass similar to a fluid-filled enlarged uterine horn in the abdomen. The diagnosis of pyometra could be excluded as the dog had already undergone hysterectomy. The diagnosis of splenomegaly was made. As the density of the enlarged spleen was rather uneven, tumors were suspected to have invaded the spleen.

Splenectomy was performed. The spleen was extremely large, and was full of tumors of varying size. There were tumors also in the liver. The owner refused to let the dog be euthanatized. The surgical incision healed nicely, but the animal's condition remained poor. It was returned home 10 days after the splenectomy. About 6 weeks later it was brought back to the clinic in a very poor condition. This time the owner requested that the dog be put to sleep. Necropsy was not performed.

Differential Diagnosis: With the knowledge that the dog had undergone hysterectomy, splenomegaly appeared to be the logical diagnosis. The rounded uneven densities within the spleen indicated tumors.

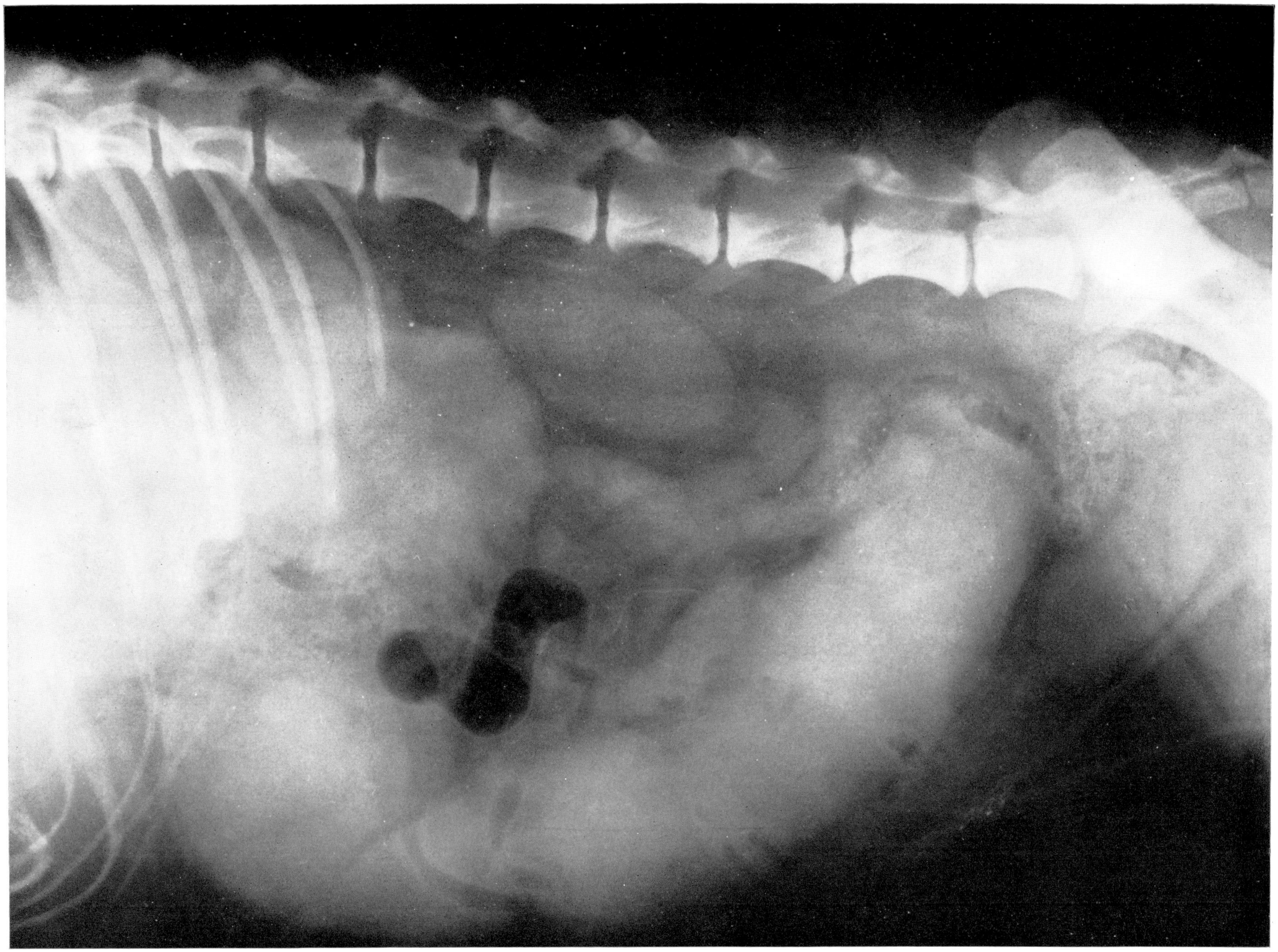

Case 51. There is a very thick, sausage-like mass in the abdomen on this lateral radiograph. Pyometra would have been a possible diagnosis since the mass could have been a fluid-filled distended uterine horn. However, the dog had undergone hysterectomy. The most likely alternative diagnosis was that of an enlarged spleen, apparently invaded by tumors.

Diagnosis: Splenomegaly, caused by invasion of tumors.

Case 52

Poodle, female, 10 years old. This dog had previously been healthy and had always had regular heat periods of normal length. At 2 years of age it had a normal pregnancy and gave birth to a litter of 5 puppies. Its latest heat period had started about 14 days prior to admission to the clinic. Since about a week it had been anorectic, had vomited occasionally, and had polydipsia. On the day of admission its condition had deteriorated rapidly. At examination it was listless, experienced pain on palpation of the abdomen, and had a bloody discharge from the vulva. On radiographs of the abdomen the contours of the abdominal organs were obscured by a fuzzy, mottled haze. The uterus seemed to be slightly enlarged. The diagnosis of peritonitis and/or diffuse hemorrhage was made. A perforated pyometra was suspected as the cause of peritonitis. Laparotomy was performed. The abdomen was found to be full of blood with the peritoneum showing signs of an acute inflammatory reaction. The uterus was moderately enlarged, and there were ecchymoses in its wall. Vitamin K_1 was administered intramuscularly as Dicumarol poisoning was suspected. The dog died on the operating table. The owner refused necropsy.

Differential Diagnosis: The mottled, patchy density which involved the entire abdomen indicated that there was either a widespread diffuse hemorrhage, or a diffuse peritonitis. It was found during laparotomy that there was blood in the abdomen, but there seemed to be an inflammatory reaction in the peritoneum as well. Because the dog died during the operation, and the owner refused necropsy it was not possible to demonstrate conclusively whether or not there was an inflammation of the uterus, which was only moderately enlarged.

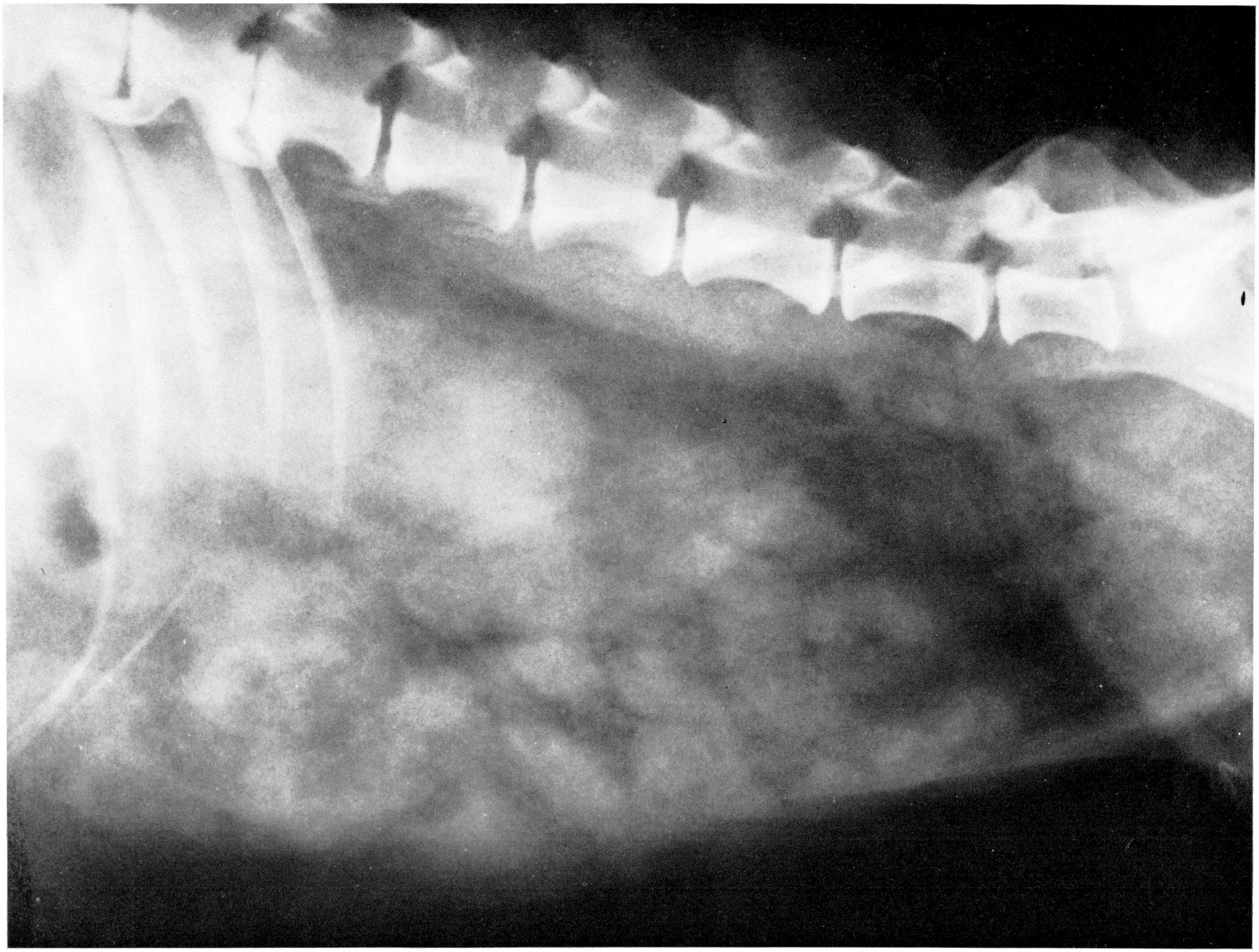

Case 52. **A,** Lateral radiograph. Almost the entire abdomen is fuzzy in appearance because of a mottled density covering the abdominal field. The uterus seems to be slightly enlarged.

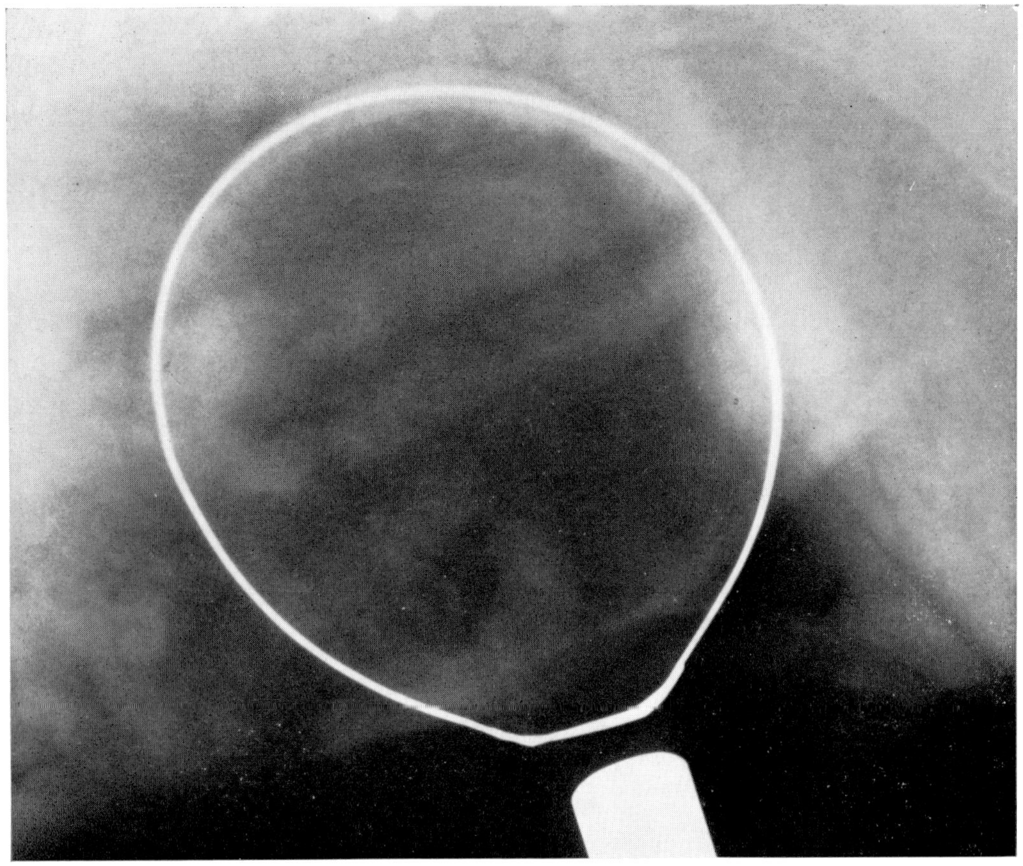

Case 52. **B,** Lateral radiograph. For a clearer demonstration of the uterus a wooden spoon framed by a metal wire was pressed against the caudal portion of the abdomen during exposure. The bowel loops and the urinary bladder have been pushed aside, making it possible to demonstrate the bifurcation of the uterus and the actual size of the uterine horns.

Diagnosis: Intraabdominal hemorrhage and peritonitis of undetermined origin. Enlargement of the uterus.

Case 53

Collie, female, 9 years old. On admission to the clinic, this dog had had anorexia and polydipsia for more than 2 weeks. Its condition had deteriorated rapidly. At examination, purulent discharge was seen coming from the vulva and the mucous membranes were pale. The abdomen was enlarged and flaccid but tender on palpation.

A mass could be palpated in the mid abdomen. Radiographs revealed a large mass in the left and mid abdomen. This mass had diffuse contours. There was also an irregular and diffuse density caudal, slightly dorsal, and to the right of the mass.

Barium was administered orally to outline the stomach and the liver and to determine to what extent the bowel was involved in the mass. The dog vomited immediately after the barium swallow, just before the radiographs were made. On these radiographs there was only a small amount of contrast medium in the stomach and duodenum. The bowel did not seem to be involved in the tumor. A tentative diagnosis of enlargement of the uterus and a tumor in the left ovary was made. A perforation or rupture of a pyometra was suspected. The possibility of a splenic tumor could not be completely ruled out. Operation was advised, but the owner refused to have it performed. Instead, he requested that the dog be euthanatized.

Necropsy: Multicystic adenocarcinoma of the left ovary with ascites. Pyometra.

Differential Diagnosis: The enlarged uterus was to a certain extent obscured by the fluid in the abdominal cavity. The areas of relatively low density in the caudal part of the abdomen could represent fat surrounded by fluid. (This was actually confirmed at necropsy.) There were rather large fat pads in the uterine ligaments. It was considered possible that the tumor was in the spleen, but it seemed less likely. Combined, as it was, with an enlargement of the uterus the tumor was believed to be in the left ovary.

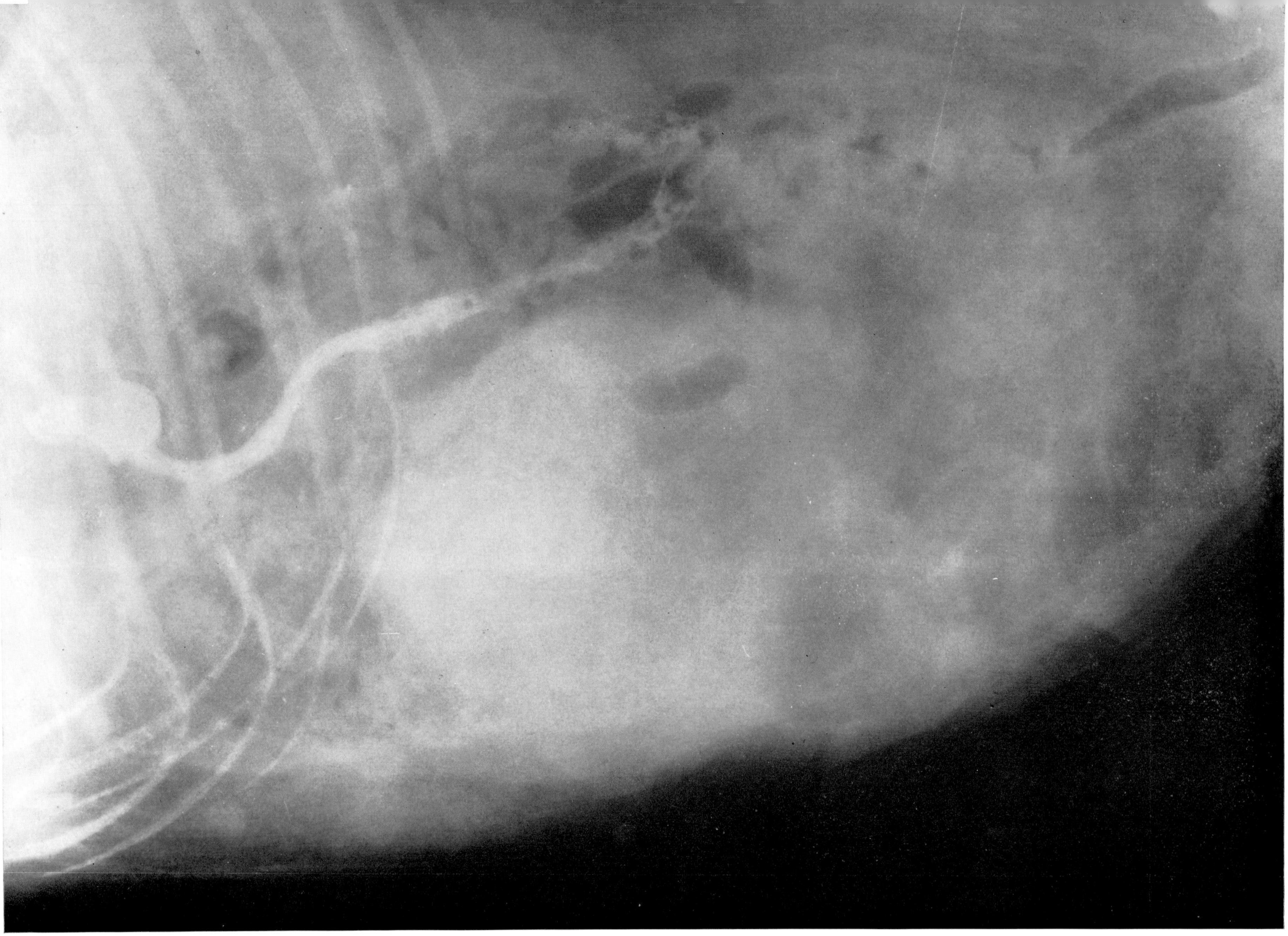

Case 53. **A,** Lateral radiograph made after a barium swallow. The dog vomited a few minutes after the barium was given, just before the radiograph was made. There are only traces of contrast medium in the stomach and the duodenum. In mid abdomen there is a rounded, rather ill-defined mass. Caudal and slightly dorsal to the mass there is a diffuse, irregular density; partly obscured by this density is a diffuse elongated mass. Ventral and somewhat cranial to the round mass is a formation, probably the ventral pool of the spleen, the borders of which are blurred by fluid.

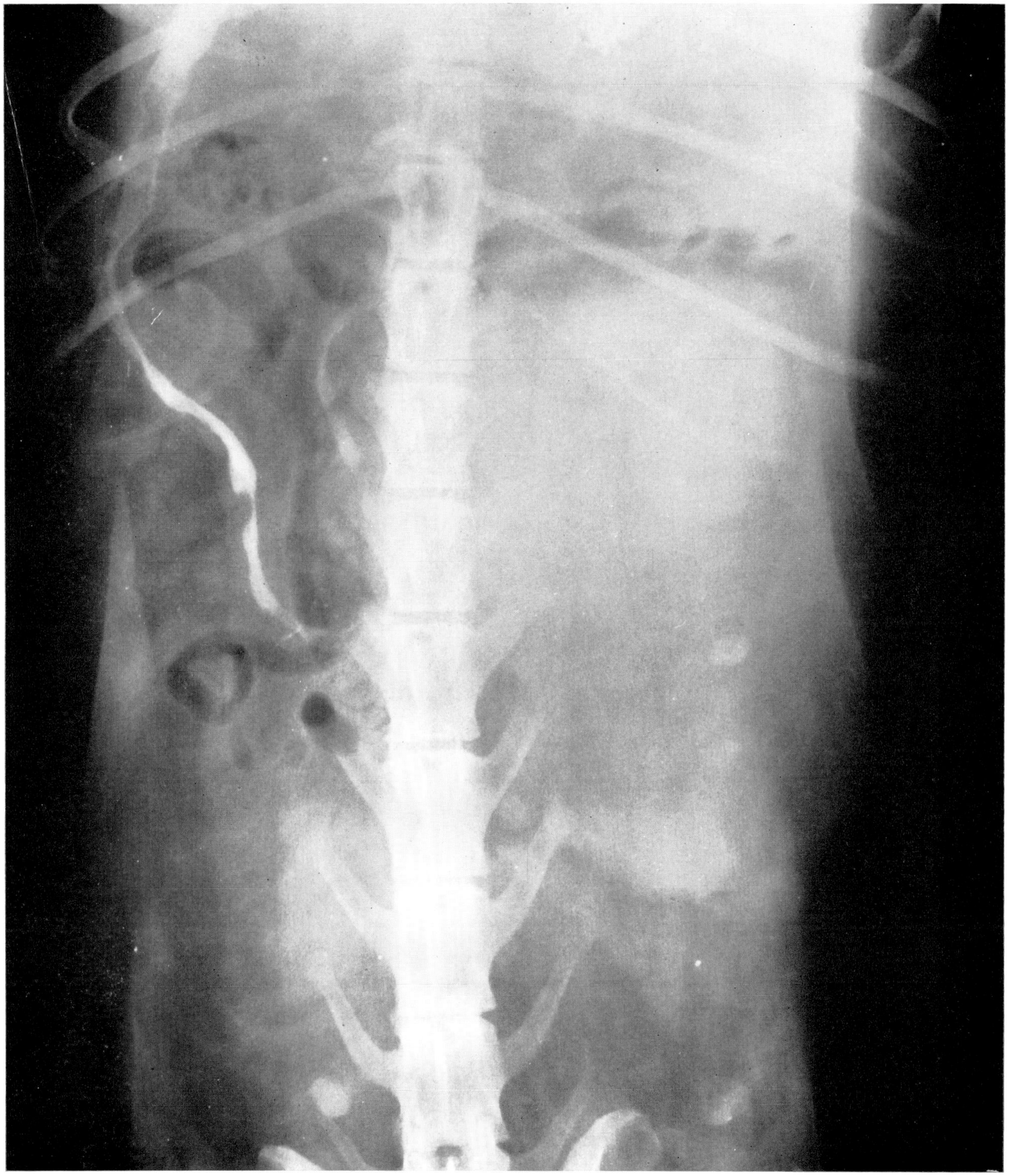

Case 53. **B,** Ventrodorsal radiograph. The rounded mass is to the left in the abdomen and appears larger than on the lateral radiograph. The entire caudal part of the abdomen has very diffuse contours.

Diagnosis: Multicystic adenocarcinoma of the left ovary with ascites. Pyometra.

Case 54

Scottish terrier, male, 12 years old. This dog had occasional hematuria for about 4 months. It also had had polydipsia and polyuria for some time and the last few days prior to admission to the clinic it refused food. It had vomited occasionally.

On examination the dog was listless, had pale mucous membranes, and had a slight elevation in temperature. Palpation of the abdomen revealed a rounded, hard, painful mass, the size of a tangerine, located cranial to the pubic bones. The prostate gland could not be palpated through the rectum. Radiographs showed a rather normal-looking abdomen. The dog was, however, poorly prepared for radiographic examination as there were ingesta in the stomach and the bowel. What seemed to be the urinary bladder was of fairly normal size and shape, with the exception of a dorsal bulge close to what was presumed to be the bladder's neck. As no other mass corresponding to what was found on palpation was detected, it was concluded that a bladder tumor was present. For this reason a retrograde urocystogram was made. This disclosed a different picture than that expected. What was interpreted as the urinary bladder on the first radiographs proved to be an enlarged prostate gland. Because of the ingesta-filled bowel loops, the bladder was obscured at the first radiographic examination. On the basis of the clinical examination, the laboratory tests, and the radiographic findings, the diagnosis of chronic nephritis, incipient uremia, and florid prostatitis was made. Because the owner wanted to bring the dog home with him it was released. The further fate of the dog is not known.

Differential Diagnosis: The present case is an excellent illustration of the hazards of interpreting changes in the bladder and prostate without the aid of a urocystogram. A retrograde urocystogram is easily made and should be secured in all cases in which there is a suspicion of cystitis, tumor of the bladder, or changes in the prostate gland.

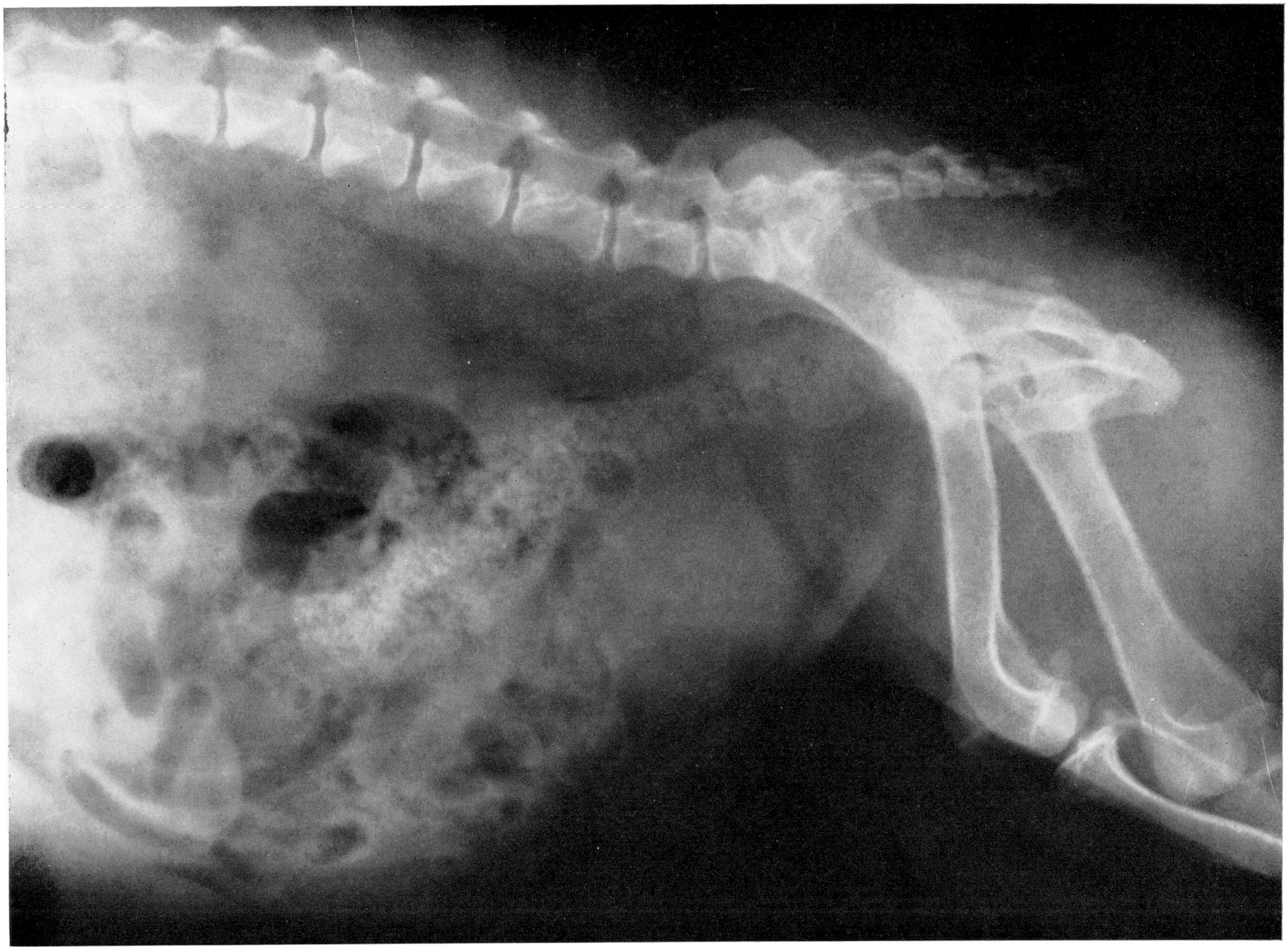

Case 54. **A,** Lateral radiograph in which there are no obvious pathologic changes in the abdomen. The dog has not been properly prepared for radiographic examination as there are ingesta in the bowel. What appears to be the urinary bladder has a dorsal bulge which impinges on the rectum. There are also some streaks of increased density in the cranial part of this formation interpreted as the bladder.

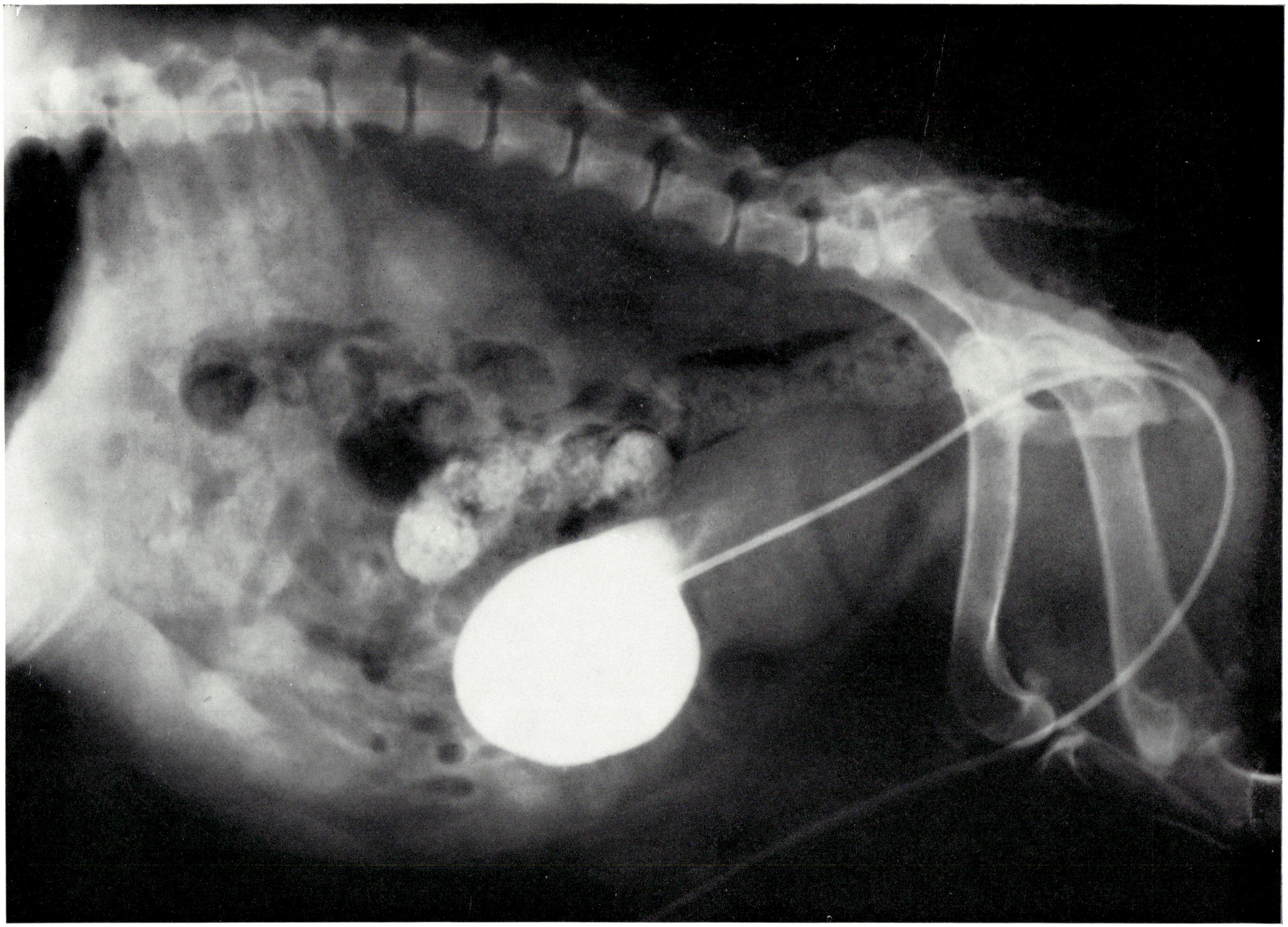

Case 54. **B,** Retrograde urocystogram made a few hours after the radiograph shown in **A.** The urinary bladder, which is displaced cranially by the very enlarged prostate gland, has a comparatively normal shape and a slightly thickened wall. There is a diffuse reflux of contrast medium into the enlarged prostate gland.

Diagnosis: Chronic nephritis and uremia. Prostatitis with enlargement of the prostate gland.

Case 55

Shetland sheep dog, male, 7 years old. This dog had been listless and anorectic and had vomited occasionally for about 4 days. When brought to the clinic it was febrile, stood with an arched back, and evidenced extreme pain on palpation of its abdomen. Rectal examination revealed no abnormality, and the caudal part of the prostate gland could be easily palpated. Radiographic examination showed a somewhat poorly delineated mass at the site of the urinary bladder. Caudal to this mass, which could be the bladder, there was another but smaller bladder-like formation, possibly a slightly enlarged prostate gland. There was a slight patchy density blurring the contours of the organs in the entire caudal portion of the abdomen. Since the dog had bilateral cryptorchidism it was suspected that the mass at the site of the bladder could be an enlarged testicle. A retrograde air cystogram revealed that the bladder-like formation caudal to the mass was the urinary bladder. This made the diagnosis of a torsion of an undescended testicle even more likely. Laparotomy was performed. The left testicle, which was in the abdomen, was very enlarged, edematous, and hemorrhagic. There was a 360-degree torsion of the funiculus causing strangulation of the testicle. Some fluid was present in the abdominal cavity and the peritoneum showed signs of inflammatory reaction. The right testicle, which was in the inguinal canal, was of less than half the normal size.

Both testicles were removed. The dog made a rapid recovery.

Differential Diagnosis: The presence of radiographic signs of peritonitis and the fact that the dog had cryptorchidism made it very possible that the mass seen on the radiograph was a retained, incarcerated, or tumor-infiltrated testicle. When it was shown by retrograde urocystogram that the urinary bladder was located caudal to the mass and that the bladder was not involved in the process, further evidence for this diagnosis was obtained. Only in extreme cases of prostatitis with abscesses, does the prostate gland extend cranial to the bladder, and in this case the mass could not be the prostate gland.

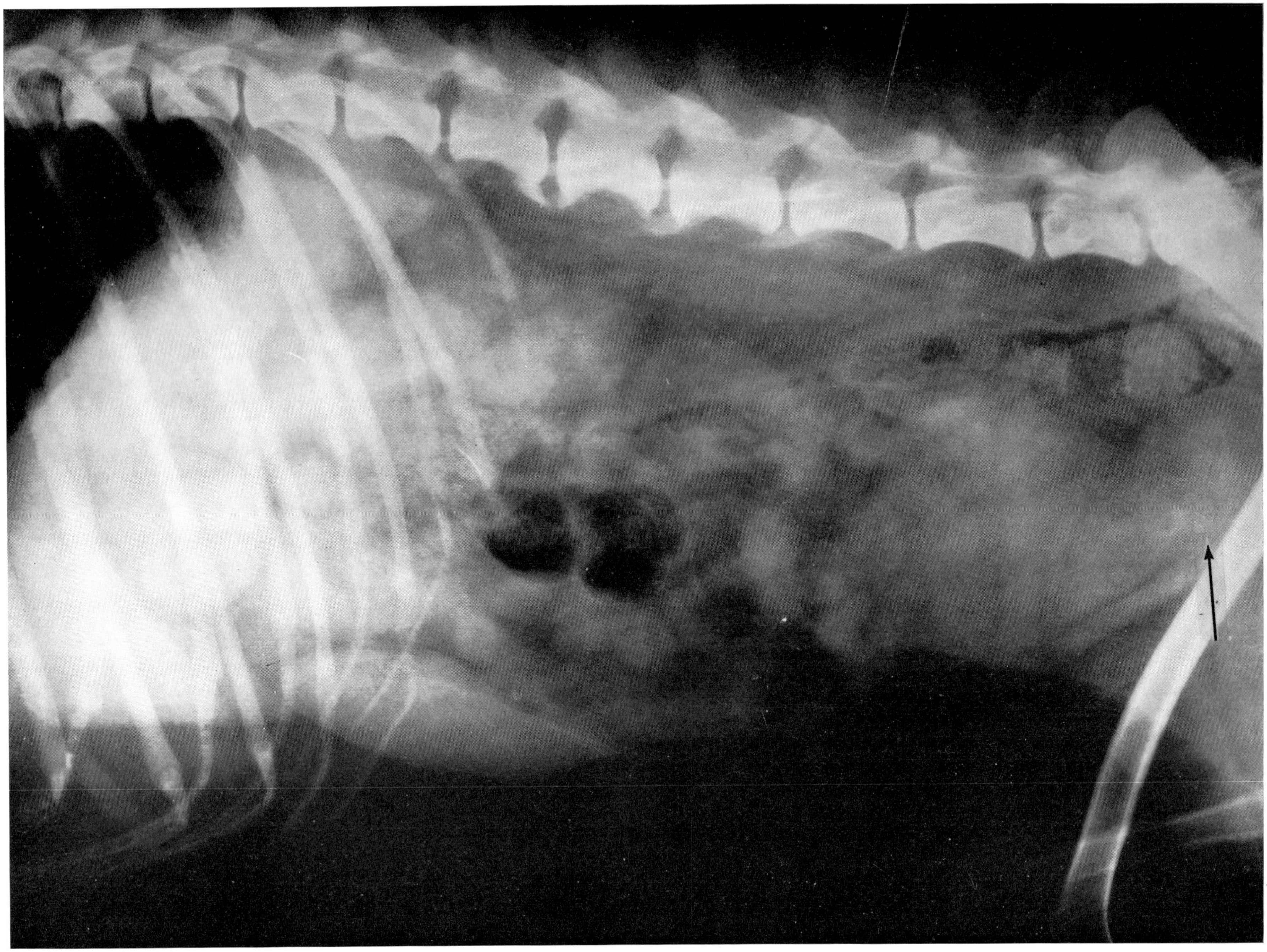

Case 55. **A,** Lateral radiograph. There is a mass, rather poorly delineated, in the caudal part of the abdomen. The mass is partly obscured and surrounded by an area of slight, patchy density. Just cranial to the pelvic inlet there is another bladder-like formation (arrow). Spondylosis at L2-L3 and L3-L4.

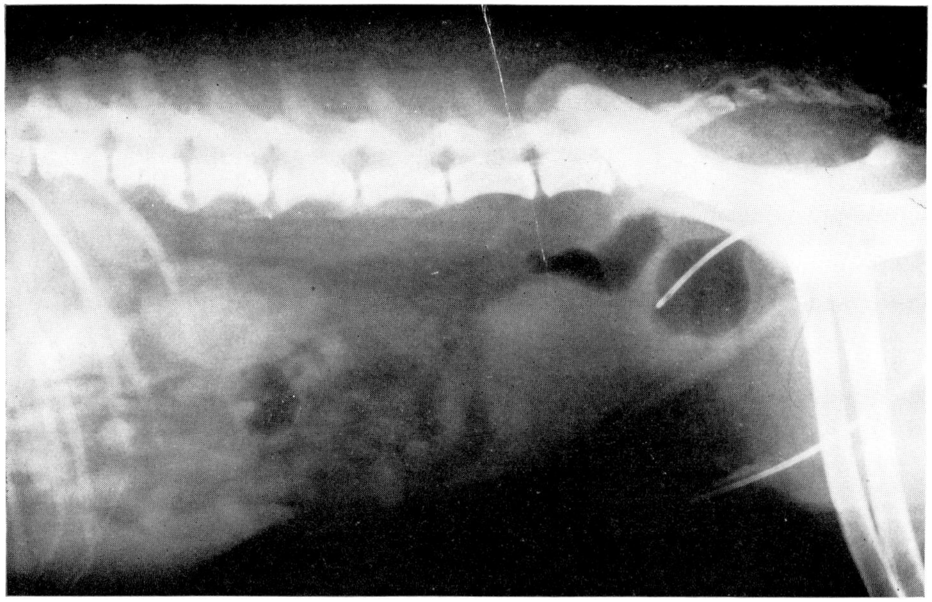

Case 55. **B,** This air cystogram shows that the previously described bladder-like formation actually is the urinary bladder. It is thus proven that the large mass easily seen on this radiograph is not within the bladder. It is also certain that it could not be the prostate gland as it is entirely positioned cranial to the bladder. It is to be remembered that the prostate gland also could be palpated through the rectum. There is gas in the descending colon on this radiograph.

Diagnosis: Funicular torsion and strangulation of a retained testicle.

Case 56

Cocker spaniel, male, 9 years old. This dog had had hematuria for some time. It suddenly became ill, was anorectic, vomited, and preferred to stand up with its back very arched. On admission to the clinic its abdomen was exceedingly painful and a mass was palpated cranial to the pubic bones.

Radiographs of the abdomen showed a mottled, flaky density blurring the contours of the abdominal organs. In spite of this blurring, the bladder, or what could be a mass at the site of the bladder, was seen. Air cystogram demonstrated that the mass was a markedly enlarged prostate gland. The bladder was displaced cranially. The enlarged prostate contained cavities which had become filled by air. A calculus of irregular shape was present in the largest cavity. The diagnosis of prostatitis with secondary peritonitis was established. The dog was euthanatized at the owner's request.

Necropsy: The radiographic diagnosis was confirmed.

Differential Diagnosis: There was little doubt that the flaky, mottled density seen over the entire abdominal field was a sign of peritonitis. The important point was to find the origin of the inflammation. Although there was no history of trauma, a rupture of the urinary bladder was considered possible, but not likely. Prostatitis was the more probable cause of peritonitis if it could be shown that the mass in the caudal part of the abdomen was the prostate gland.

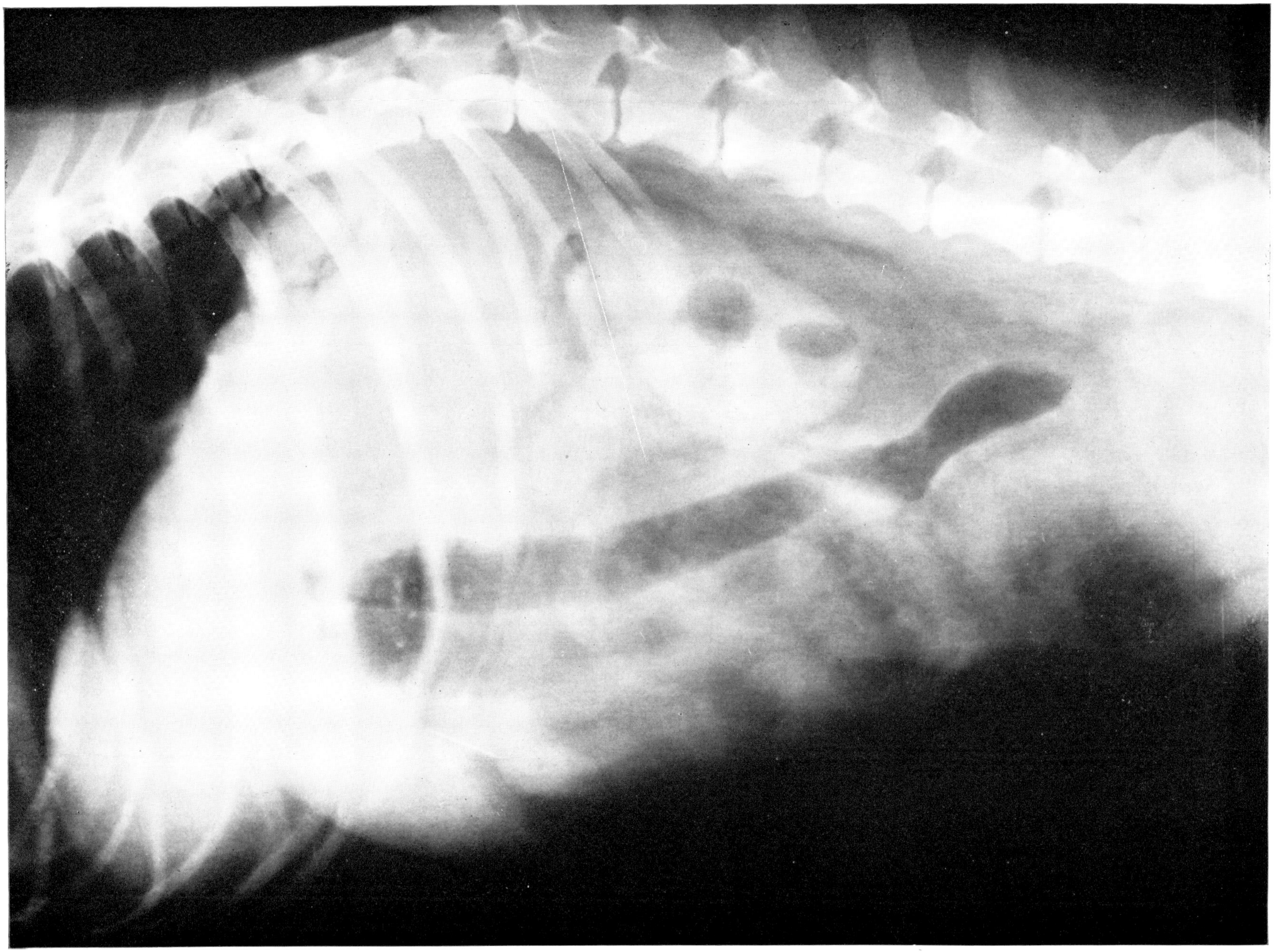

Case 56. **A,** Lateral radiograph. There is a mottled flaky density all over the abdomen. The contours of the abdominal organs, especially the bowel, are blurred by this density. In the caudal part of the abdomen there is an ill-defined, large, round mass of rather homogenous density. This seems to be an obstacle to the passage through the rectum as gas is being trapped in the descending colon.

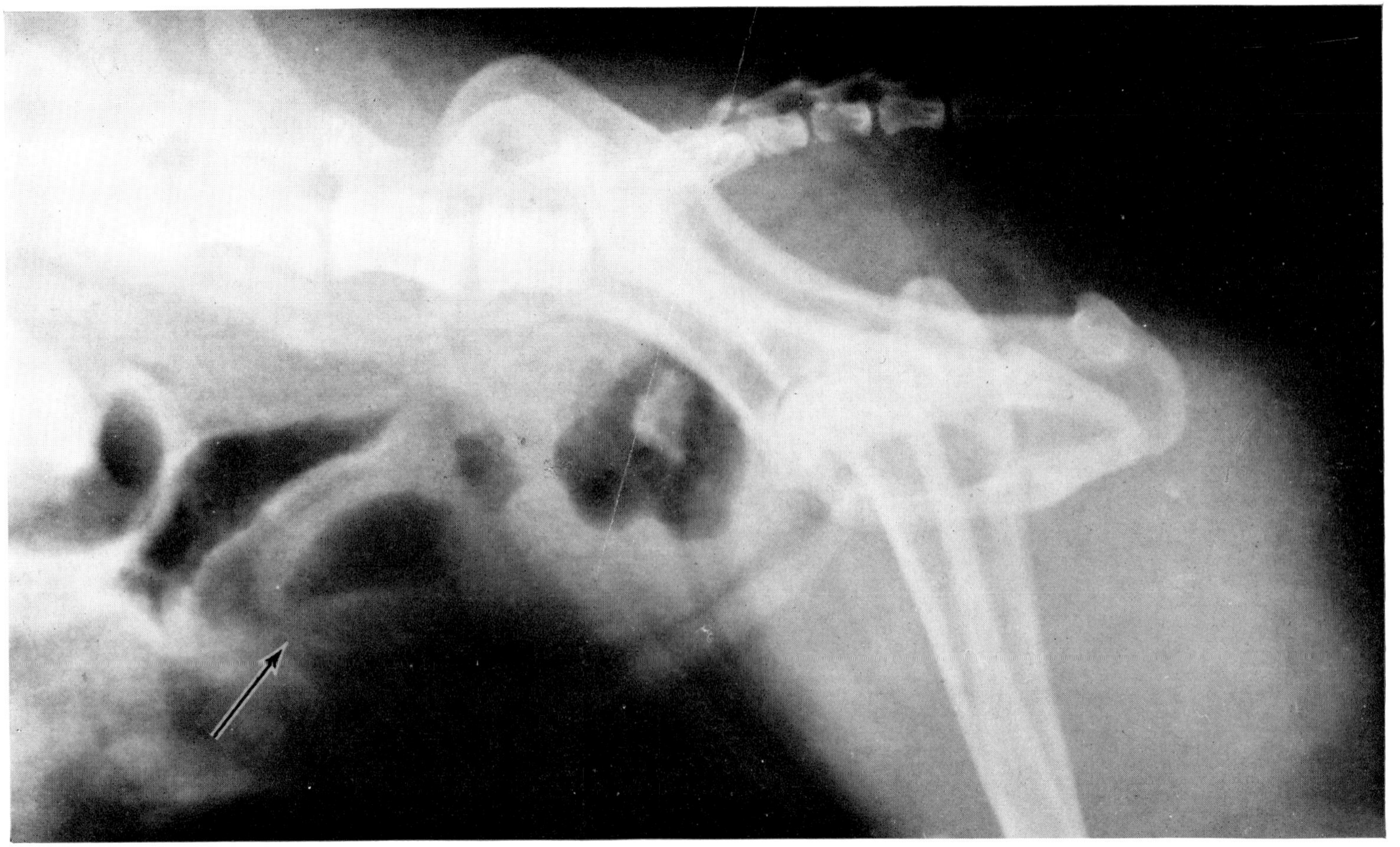

Case 56. **B,** Lateral air urocystogram. The urinary bladder (arrow), which has a thick wall, is displaced by the enlarged prostate gland. Within the prostate are cavities filled by air. The largest cavity is irregular in shape and contains a calculus which is also irregular in contour. Gas is seen trapped in the caudal part of the descending colon as on the previous radiograph. This could be an indication that the prostate is encroaching upon the rectum.

Diagnosis: Prostatitis with abscesses causing diffuse peritonitis.

Case 57

Miniature pinscher, female, 3 years old. This dog was brought to the clinic after having been hit by a car. At examination it was in a state of shock. There was no faculty of motion, or pain sensation in the left forelimb. This leg was lacerated and there was a hematoma on the medial side of the elbow. After receiving a blood transfusion the dog's general condition improved. It seemed to remain confused, however, and did not recognize its owner. The pupil of the right eye was wide and the pupillary reflex was slow and incomplete. On radiographs of the abdomen it was seen that the stomach was full of food. The bowel loops were gas-filled but not distended. There was no obvious sign of intraabdominal hemorrhage. The contour of the urinary bladder was not well delineated. For this reason a retrograde urocystogram was made using positive contrast medium (sodium diatrizoate). The contrast medium leaked out between the bowel loops, thus demonstrating a rupture of the bladder. At laparotomy a small rupture with a hematoma of the neck of the bladder was found. The rupture was sutured and the abdomen closed. The dog showed considerable improvement during the 10 days that it remained hospitalized. When it was released it had regained some faculty of motion and pain sensation of the left forelimb. It appeared normal mentally.

Differential Diagnosis: On the original radiograph the only indication of rupture of the bladder was the absence of a distinct contour of the urinary bladder. It is wise to remember that even with a normal contour of the urinary bladder with no signs of hemorrhage and with a history that the dog has urinated after an accident, the bladder may still be ruptured. Urocystogram is the only reliable means, except laparotomy, of demonstrating a rupture of the bladder. This does not necessarily imply that every animal that has been involved in an accident must undergo urocystography. If the bladder is of a normal contour, no evidence of fluid or hemorrhage is seen in the abdomen, no hematuria is noted, and the animal can empty its bladder spontaneously, there is little reason for an immediate urocystogram. If there is the slightest suspicion of trauma to the abdomen, the animal should, however, be carefully watched and radiographs should be repeated whenever necessary. If there is a rupture, of any size, of an organ, blood will show up as a diffuse density on the abdominal radiograph. If there is a rupture anywhere in the urinary or biliary tract, fluid can be demonstrated on the radiographs within 12 hours.

For demonstration of a rupture of the urinary tract, a water-soluble contrast medium is to be preferred over air as the contrast medium. Air that leaks from a ruptured bladder is more difficult to distinguish from gas in the bowel than is a water-soluble iodinated compound. On the other hand, for demonstration of tumors of the urinary bladder, air is the preferred medium.

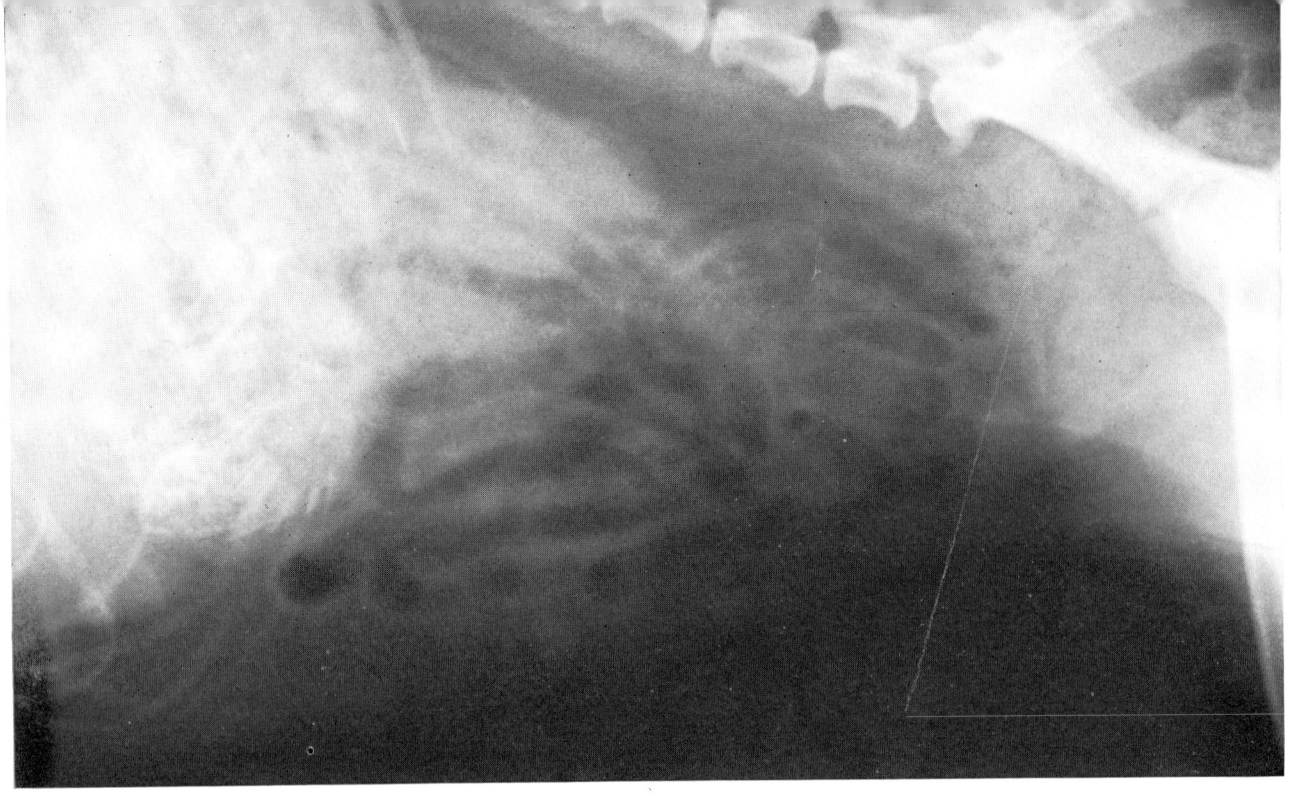

Case 57. **A,** Lateral radiograph. The stomach is full of food and the bowel is gas-filled. There is a very slight increase of density in the abdomen and the contour of the urinary bladder cannot be clearly seen.

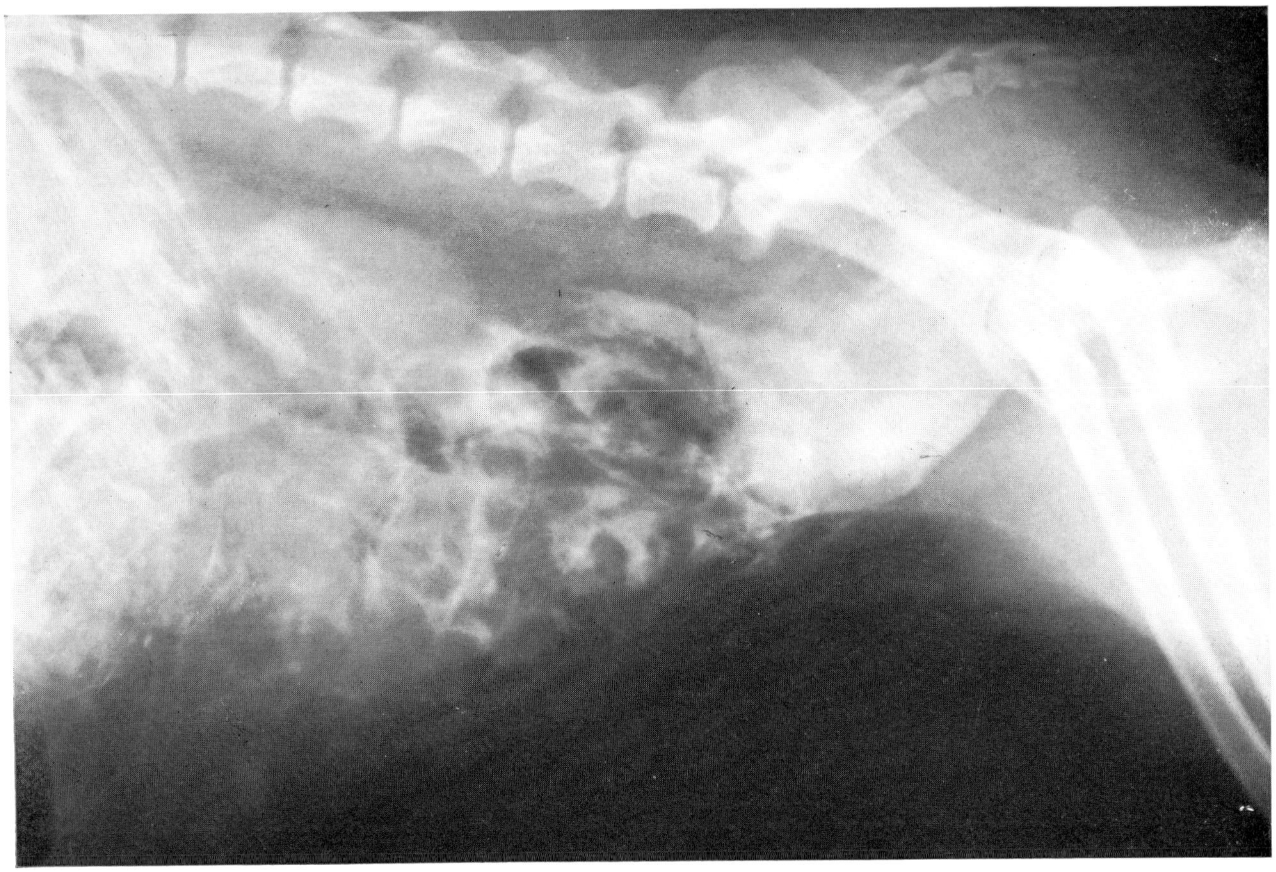

Case 57. **B,** Lateral urocystogram made with a water-soluble contrast medium. There is contrast medium in the bladder, which has diffuse contours. Contrast medium is also found between the bowel loops, proving the presence of a rupture of the bladder.

Diagnosis: Traumatic rupture of the urinary bladder, cerebral concussion, and injury to the left brachial nerve plexus.

Case 58

Pekinese, male, 8 years old. This dog was hit by a car. When brought to the clinic during the night it could walk on all four legs. Blood dripped from its penis. Radiographs revealed fractures of the pubic and ischiatic bones. A retrograde urocystogram showed evidence of rupture of the urinary bladder. At laparotomy a complete rupture of the bladder could not be detected. Small rifts, edema, and hemorrhage in the wall of the bladder only were noted. There was also some blood in the abdominal cavity. Two small superficial tears in the bladder wall were sutured and the abdominal incision was closed. Radiographs made the following morning revealed that there was contrast medium in the bladder as well as in the pelvis of the kidneys and in the ureters. A second urocystogram disclosed the true diagnosis—rupture of the urethra.

When the abdomen was reopened a rupture of the urethra just caudal to the prostate gland was found. The urethra was repaired and a catheter, sutured to the penis, was left in the urethra. The dog made a slow but complete recovery.

Differential Diagnosis: The diagnosis of rupture was correct, but its location was missed. One explanation for this was that the catheter was inserted too far. Nevertheless it should have been possible to determine the diagnosis. There was leakage of contrast medium into the soft tissues of the pelvic cavity; this is never seen in uncomplicated cases of a ruptured bladder.

When it became evident that the bladder was dislocated cranially and that it contained almost all of the contrast medium, the diagnosis of rupture of the urethra was easily made. In order to confirm the diagnosis, contrast medium was injected through a catheter with its tip well below the ischiatic arch. The injection was made during exposure of the radiograph. (This technique is preferable when pubic and ischiatic bones have been fractured and a rupture of the urethra is suspected.)

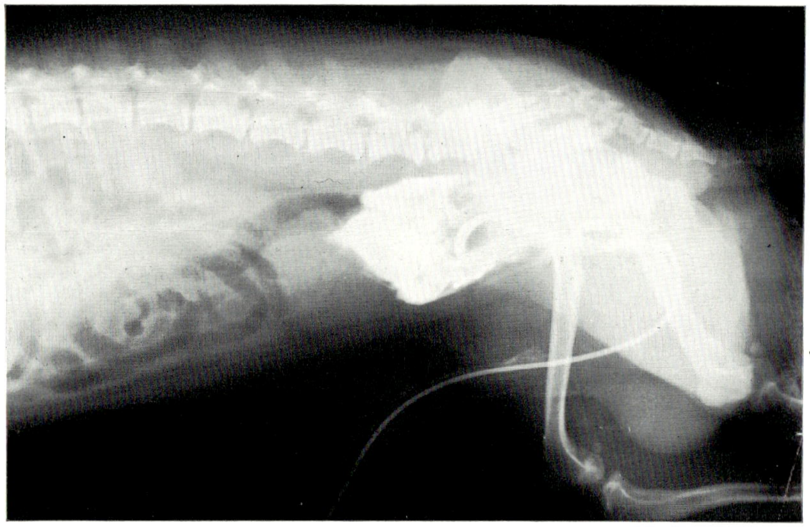

Case 58. **A,** Lateral "urocystogram." The catheter makes several loops cranial to the pubic bones. Contrast medium is unevenly distributed in the caudal part of the abdomen and in the pelvic cavity, indicating rupture of the urethra.

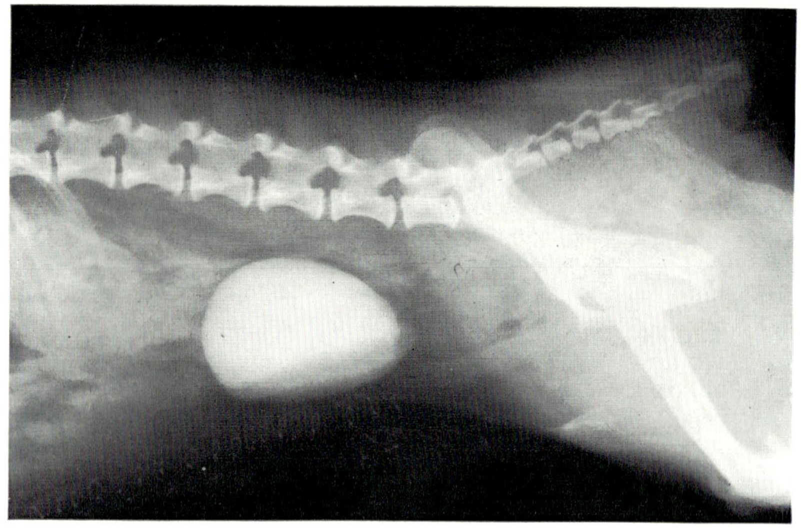

Case 58. **B,** Lateral radiograph made the following morning. The previously injected contrast medium is now in the urinary bladder. It has arrived there by means of resorption by the peritoneum and other tissues and through excretion by the kidneys. A minimal amount of contrast medium can be seen in the pelvis of the kidneys and in the ureters. The bladder and the prostate gland (the latter can barely be seen) are both displaced cranially because of the rupture of the urethra.

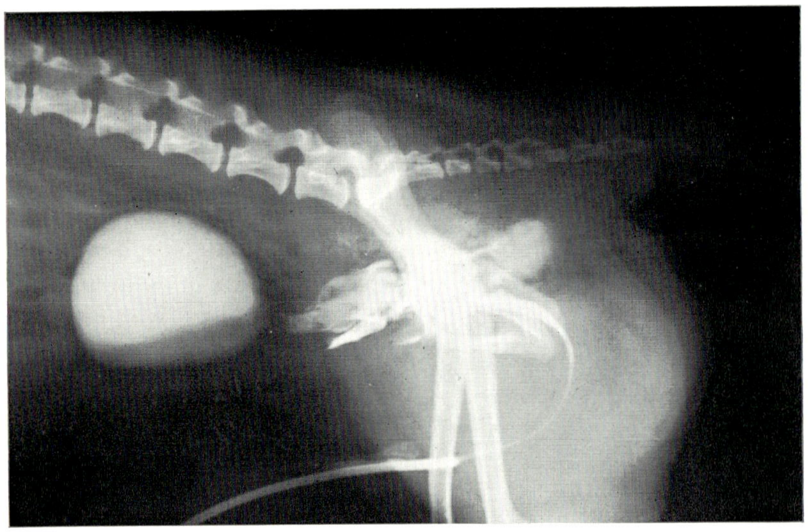

Case 58. **C,** Lateral radiograph made during injection of contrast medium through a catheter with its tip in the urethra just caudal to the penile bone. There is leakage of contrast medium from the urethra at the level of the pubic bones.

Diagnosis: Fracture of the pubic and ischiatic bones. Rupture of the urethra caudal to the prostate.

Case 59

Bernese mountain dog, female, 10 months old. This dog vomited the day prior to admission to the clinic. The owner found its temperature to be elevated (40° C). Penicillin was prescribed by a veterinarian, but the following day the temperature reached 41° C. The only remarkable findings at examination were the fever and pain on deep palpation of the abdomen just caudal to the costal arch. The dog was hospitalized. Radiographs of the lungs showed no abnormality. Blood tests showed a high white blood cell count (30,000) and a high percentage of immature white blood cells. Radiographs revealed a somewhat diffuse abdomen. There was a round radiopaque structure twice the size of a pea in the mid abdomen. This could be demonstrated at the same location on several radiographs made subsequently. It was interpreted as a calculus in one of the ureters.

An intravenous pyelogram revealed an enlarged left kidney with a dilated renal pelvis and a distended ureter filled with contrast medium down to a point where the calculus was lodged. The diagnosis of an obstructing urethral calculus was thus confirmed.

At operation an abscess was found between the enlarged left kidney and its capsule. There was a calculus in the winding, enlarged ureter about 14 cm from the kidney. The kidney and its ureter were removed. The dog made a rapid recovery.

Differential Diagnosis: Calculi in the ureters are not frequently found in dogs. They seem to be as unusual in this location as urinary bladder calculi are common.

Urinary calculi in the dog are, with few exceptions, radiopaque and they should therefore not be difficult to find provided the digestive tract is properly emptied prior to the radiographic examination. An intravenous pyelogram is useful for confirmation of the diagnosis, as seen in this case.

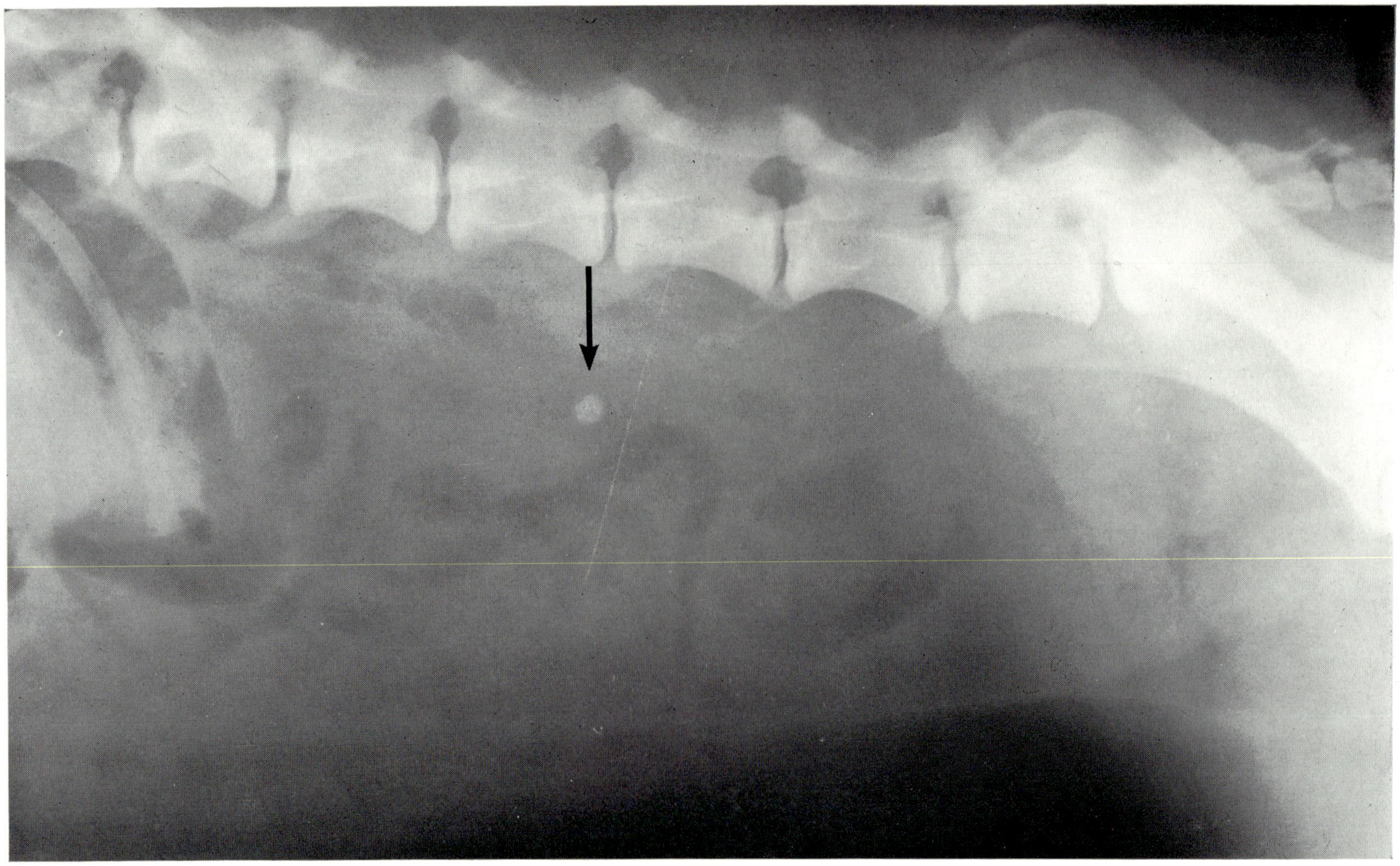

Case 59. **A,** Lateral radiograph shows a slightly diffuse abdominal field and poorly delineated abdominal organs. In mid abdomen, ventral to the disc L4-L5, is a round object larger than a pea (arrow).

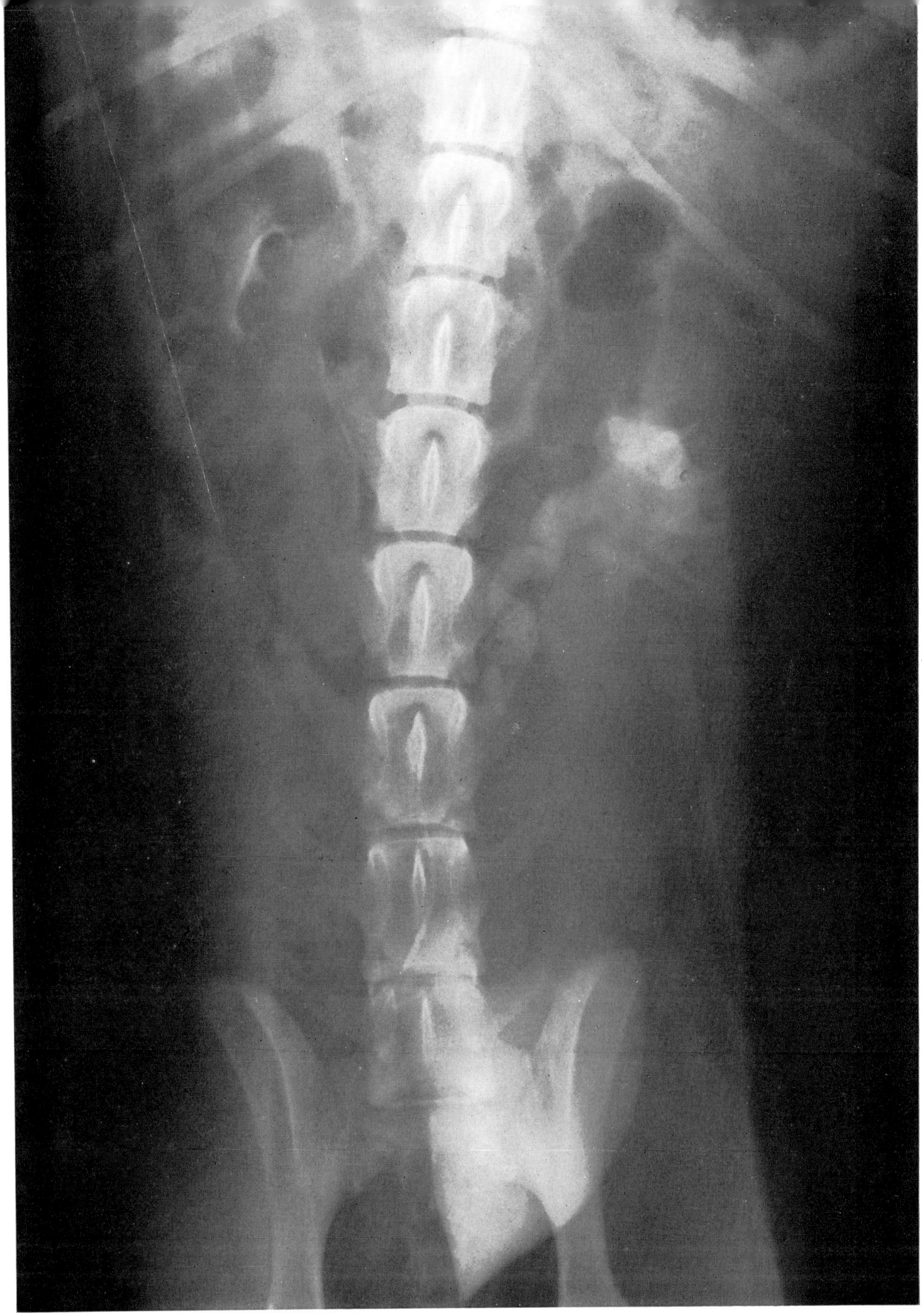

Case 59. **B,** Ventrodorsal radiograph made 15 minutes after intravenous injection of 20 ml of sodium diatrizoate 50%. Abdominal compression was first applied and the film was exposed about 2 minutes after release of this pressure. The right renal pelvis only contains a small amount of contrast medium and its ureter is very thin. Most of the contrast medium passing from the right kidney has already gone into the bladder. The left kidney is enlarged; its pelvis and first part of its ureter are distended and filled with contrast medium to the point where the calculus is lodged.

Diagnosis: Calculus in the left ureter causing urinary stasis with hydronephrosis and pyelonephritis. Subcapsular renal abscess.

Case 60

Dachshund, male, 10 years old. For 6 months the dog had had several episodes of hematuria. About 1 month prior to the first examination at the clinic it had experienced transient episodes of difficulties in urinating. The day after such an episode of about 6 hours' duration, the owner brought the dog to the clinic. He reported that the dog had urinated just before entering the clinic.

At examination the dog appeared to be in good condition. Radiographs revealed that it must have had a bone meal quite recently. There were large pieces of bone in the stomach and the entire bowel was filled with ingesta. No calculi were seen in the urinary bladder, the kidneys, or the urethra. The owner was advised to bring the dog back after a few days, this time with the dog better prepared for radiographic examination.

Six days later, late in the evening, the dog was brought to the clinic as an emergency case. It had tried to urinate several times but had been unable to do so for 24 hours. On admission it was noticed that its abdomen was distended and a very large urinary bladder could be palpated. Radiographic examination revealed a solitary calculus larger than a pea in the urethra about 5 cm caudal to the os penis. The dog was operated on and made a rapid recovery.

Differential Diagnosis: This case demonstrates the importance of emptying the intestines before making radiographs of the urinary tract.

In retrospect it is easy to understand why the prostate gland was mistaken for the bladder. On the radiograph the bladder, containing the calculus and very little urine, is obscured by bowel loops containing ingesta.

It would have been easy to find the calculus and to differentiate between bladder and prostate if an air urocystogram had been made.

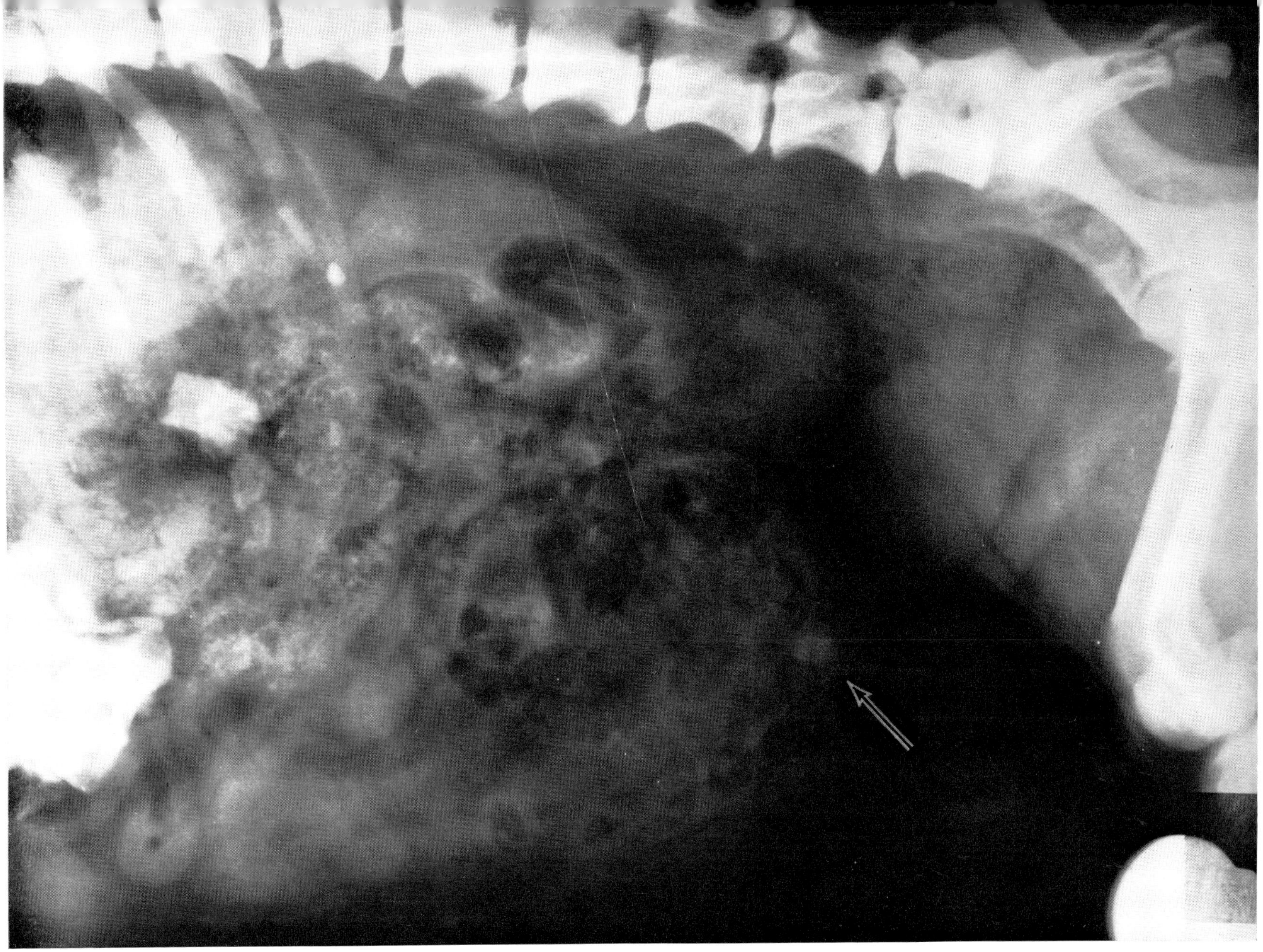

Case 60. **A,** Lateral radiograph made at the first admission to the clinic. The entire digestive tract is filled with ingesta. The stomach contains large pieces of bone and the bowel harbors particles of ingesta of varying size and density. A bladder-like structure is seen at the usual site of the urinary bladder. Cranial to this there is another small bladder-like structure which can hardly be seen because of the ingesta-filled bowel loops superimposed on it. Within this formation, or superimposed on it, is a round radiopaque structure which later proved to be a urinary calculus (arrow).

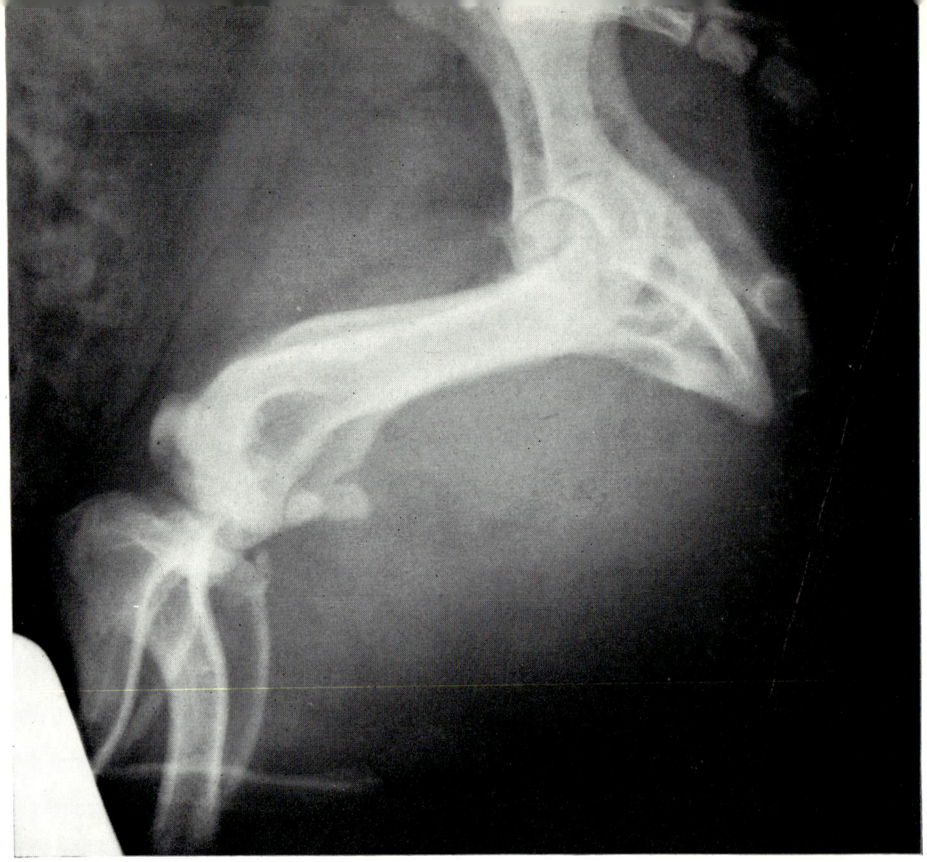

Case 60. **B,** Lateral radiograph for demonstration of calculus in the urethra. The hind legs are extended cranially to get them out of the way of the urethra. No calculus can be seen. The prostate gland, which was erroneously mistaken for urinary bladder, is well delineated.

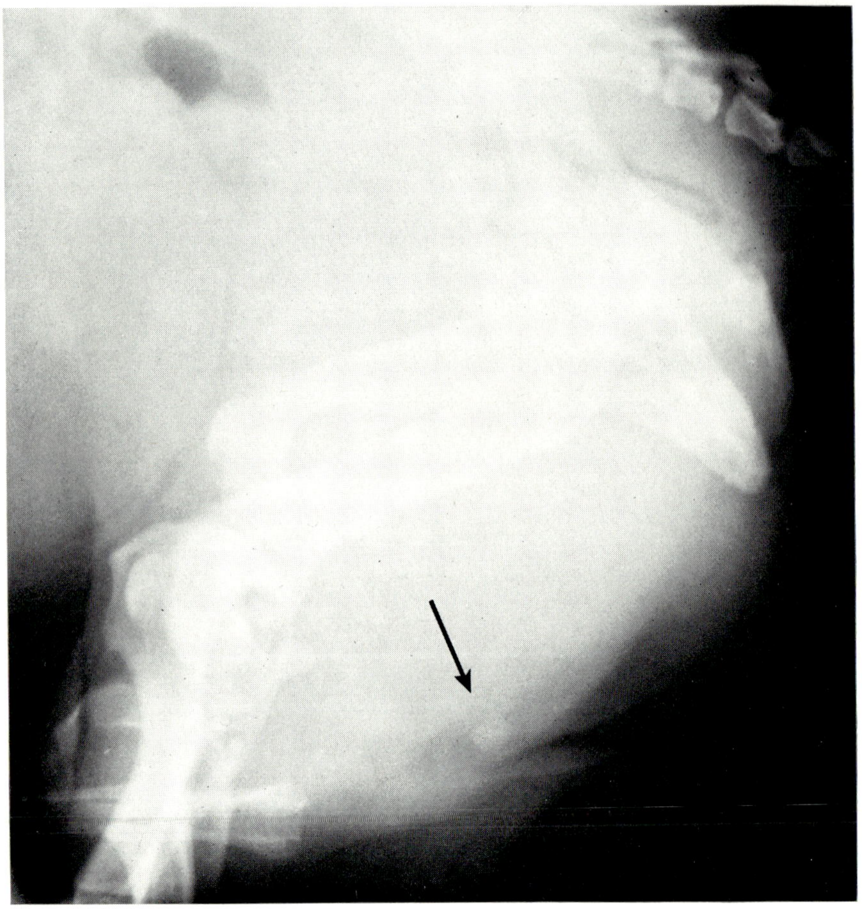

Case 60. **C,** Radiograph of the urethra on the second admission to the clinic. The urinary calculus, which on the first admission was in the bladder, is now in the urethra (arrow) about 5 cm caudal to the os penis. It apparently obstructs the urethra since the urinary bladder is very much enlarged.

Diagnosis: Urolithiasis. A calculus which initially was in the urinary bladder later obstructed the urethra.

Case 61

Dachshund, male, 9 years old. For about a year this dog had had a swelling on the left side of the anus. The swelling had slowly increased in size and for about a month there had also been a smaller swelling on the right side. Defecation had become increasingly more difficult. The dog was brought to the clinic because of constipation of 3 days' duration. The diagnosis of perineal hernia with a large diverticulum of the rectum on the left side was made. The diverticulum, which was packed with dried feces, was emptied manually. The dog was put on the waiting list for surgical treatment.

Two days later, in an attempt to defecate, the dog suddenly cried out in pain and the owner discovered that the perineal hernia on the left side had suddenly doubled in size. The dog became restless and tried to urinate repeatedly. It was brought to the clinic the same day.

On admission, a fluctuating mass was found in the perineal hernia, and retroflexion of the urinary bladder with prolapse into the hernia was suspected. Radiographic examination, including a urocystogram, confirmed the diagnosis. The dog was operated on, the bladder reduced, and the perineal hernia reefed. The dog made an uneventful recovery, but later had a relapse of its perineal hernia.

Differential Diagnosis: The diagnosis was easily made. No differential diagnostic problem was presented.

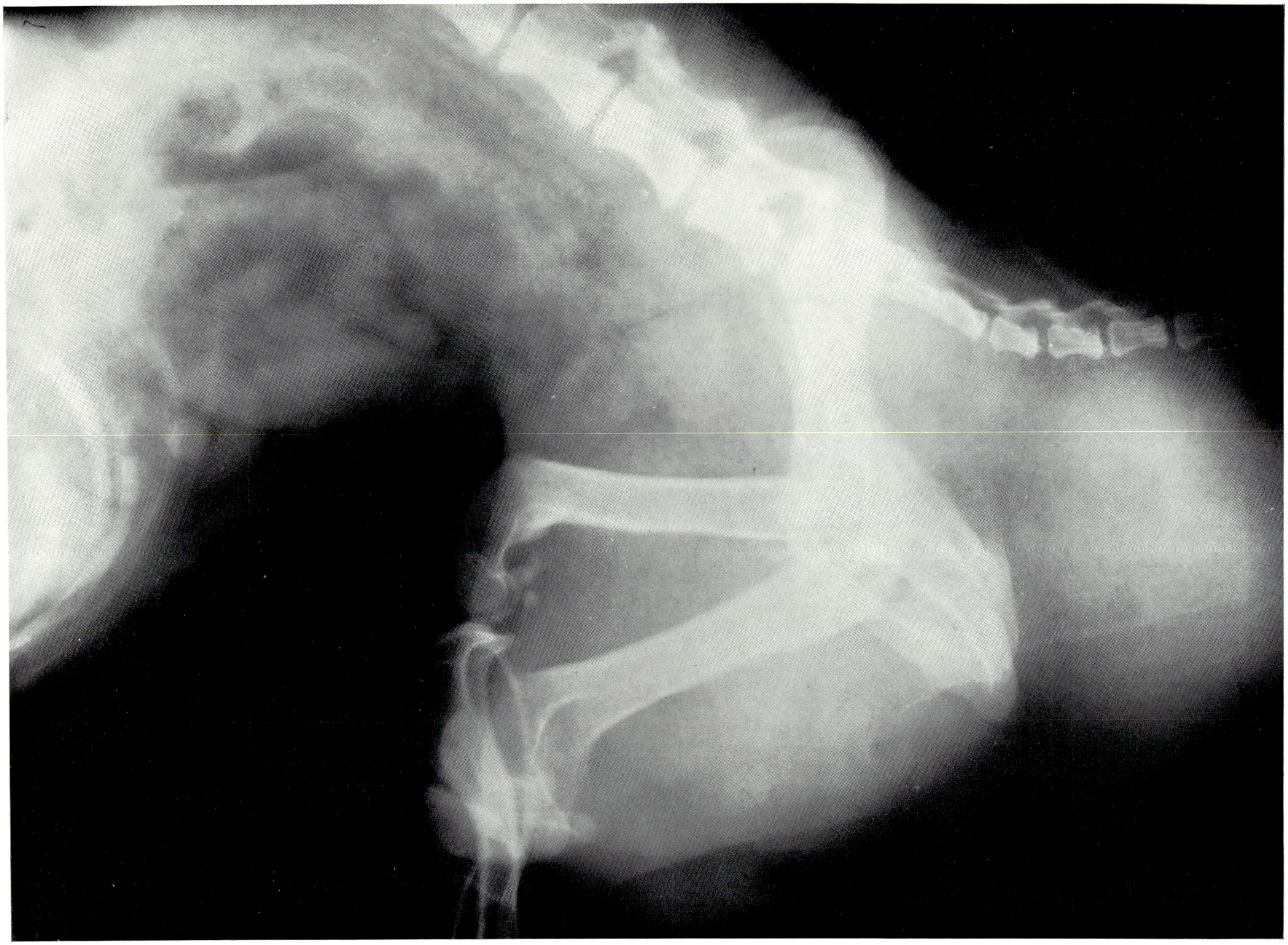

Case 61. **A,** Lateral radiograph demonstrating a diffuse, rather dense, soft-tissue mass in the perineal hernia. It is noteworthy that no contour of the urinary bladder is seen in the caudal part of the abdomen.

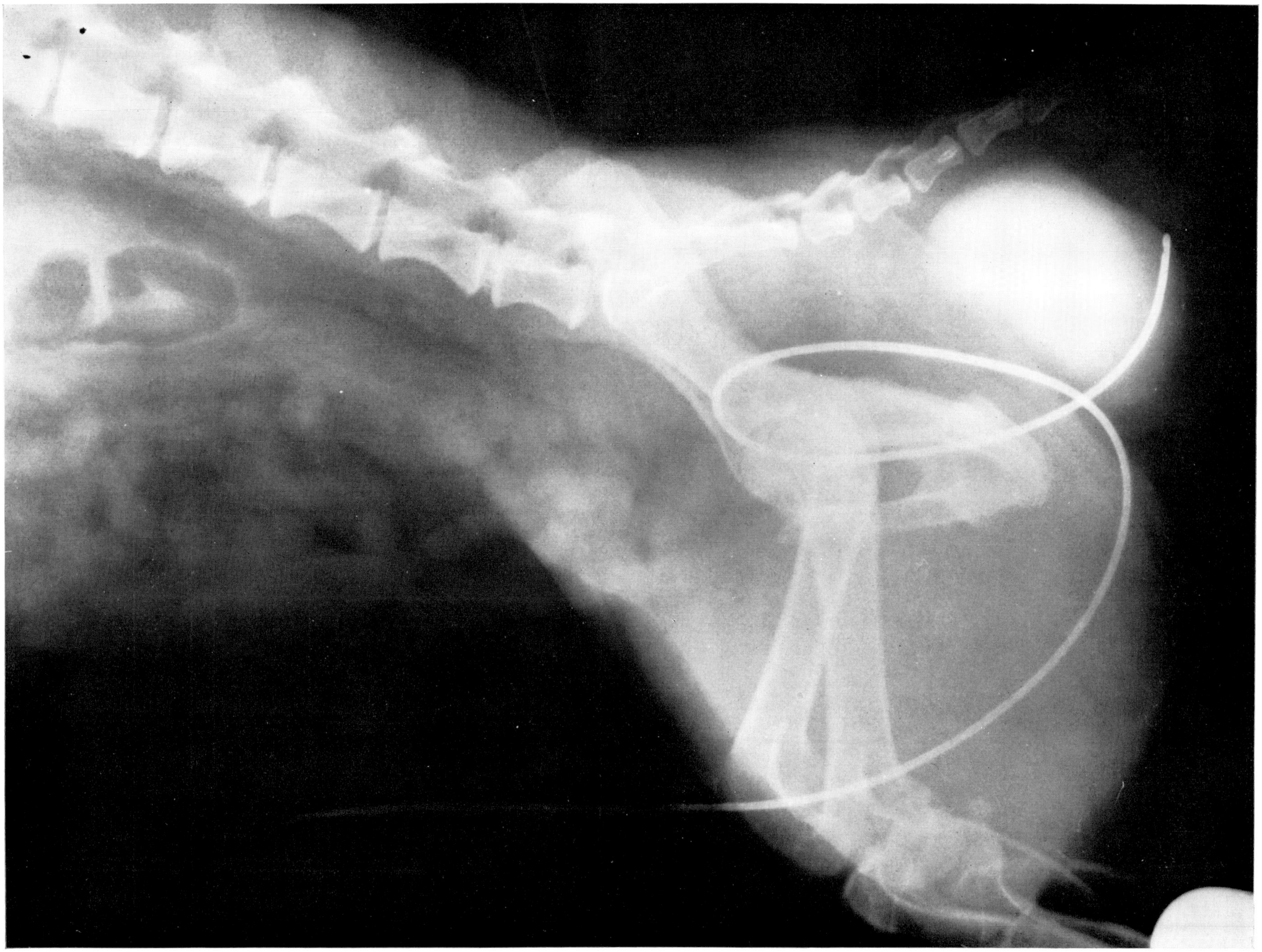

Case 61. **B,** Lateral retrograde urocystogram. The catheter in the urethra makes a turn at the pelvic inlet and is then directed caudally. The tip of the catheter is in the urinary bladder which contains contrast medium. The bladder is lodged in the perineal hernia.

Diagnosis: Retroflexion and protrusion of the urinary bladder into a perineal hernia.

Case 62

Cat, female, 1 year old. This cat delivered one dead kitten. Labor continued but no more kittens were born. After a day the owner brought the cat to the clinic. A fetus could be palpated in the abdomen. Radiographs revealed it to be in a position that made delivery impossible. Its head and one foreleg were in one uterine horn while the other part of the body was in the other uterine horn. One forelimb was in the cervix. Cesarean section was performed, a dead kitten was removed, and the cat made a rapid recovery.

Differential Diagnosis: The position of the fetus constituted an absolute obstacle for normal delivery. Radiographic examination is of value in dystocia. In this case it provided evidence that a normal delivery could not be expected.

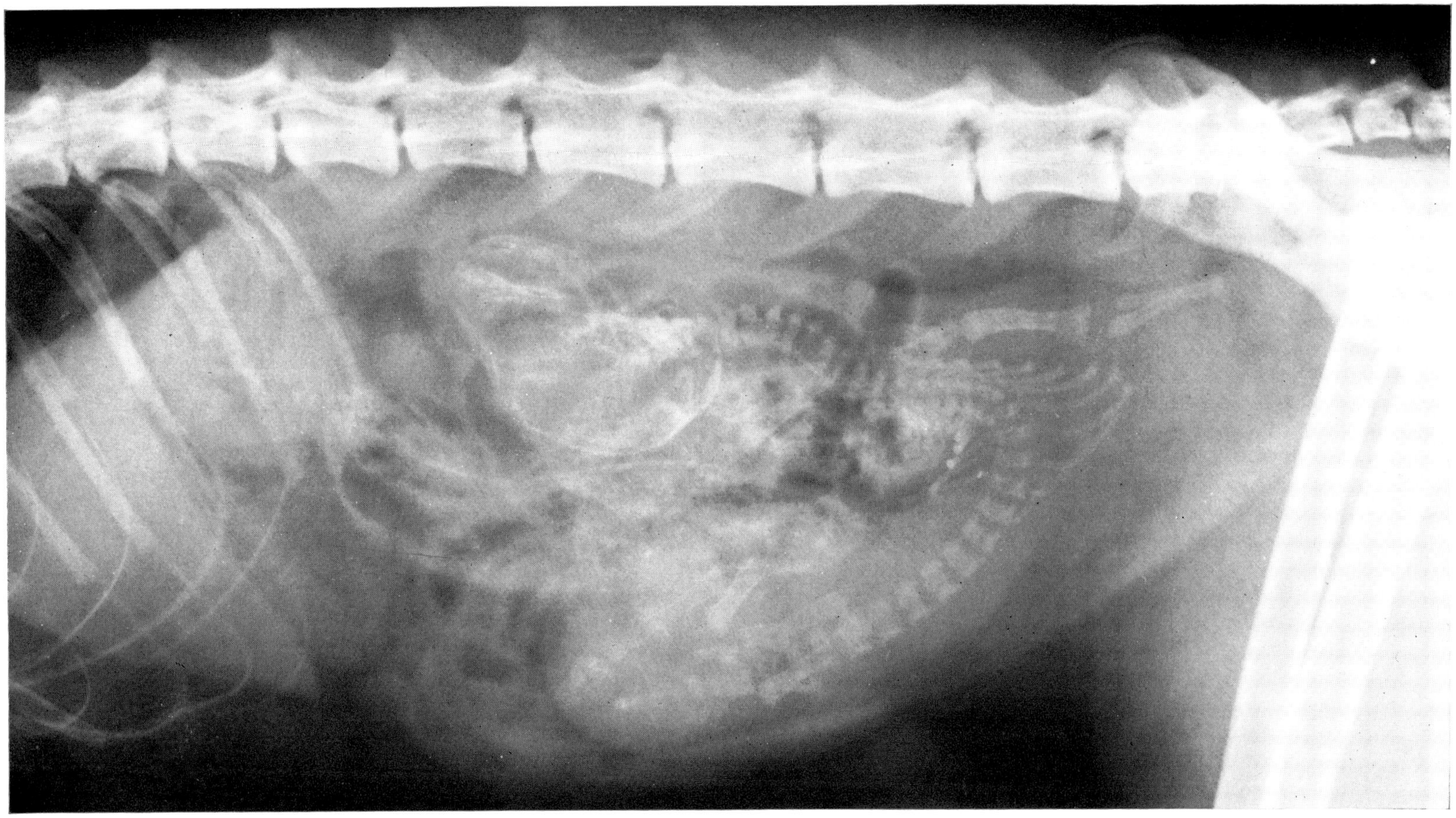

Case 62. Lateral radiograph. There is one fetus in the uterus. Its position with the head, neck, and one foreleg in one uterine horn, the other in the cervix, and the rest of the body in the other uterine horn is incompatible with normal delivery.

Diagnosis: Dystocia due to transverse position of a fetus.

Case 63

Cat, female, age unknown. The owner had observed that this cat was pregnant. Labor had begun 2 days prior to admission, but had subsided after about 4 hours. On admission the cat was listless and had a voluminous abdomen which was painful on palpation. Several fetuses could be palpated. There was a reddish, purulent, malodorous discharge from the vulva and the cat was febrile. Radiographic examination revealed the uterus to be full of emphysematous disintegrating fetuses. The cat recovered following hysterectomy.

Differential Diagnosis: Gas in the otherwise fluid-filled uterus and advanced disintegration of the fetuses signaled severe inflammation of the uterus. The classical radiographic sign of fetal death, gas beneath the cranial vault, could be demonstrated in one fetus.

The only differential diagnostic problem was whether or not the uterus was ruptured. Due to the severe changes in the uterus, this was not possible to determine.

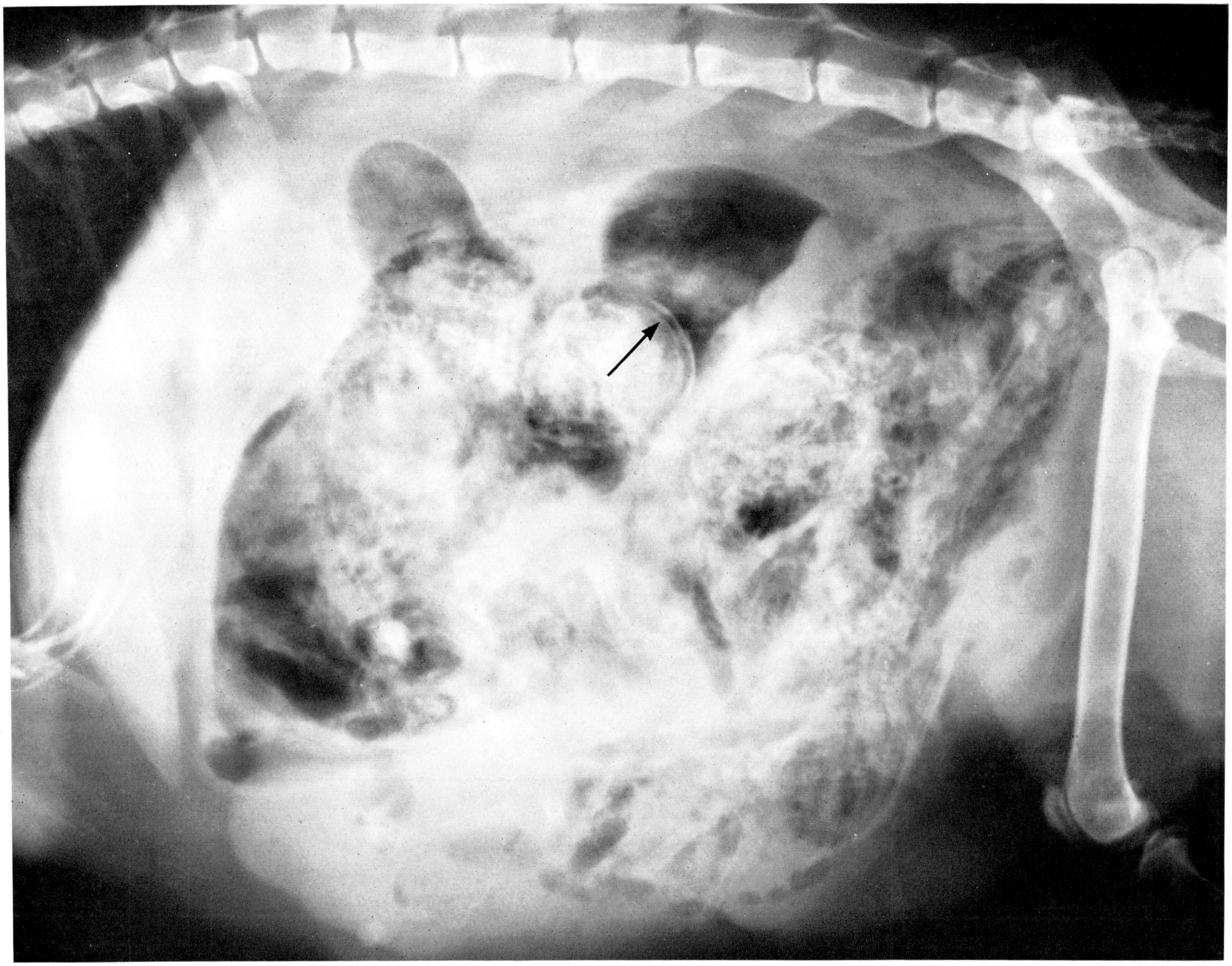

Case 63. Lateral radiograph. A greatly enlarged abdomen containing a uterus filled with fetuses which are disintegrating is noted. There is a great amount of air in the uterus as well as within the fetuses. In one fetal skull there is gas beneath the cranial vault (arrow).

Diagnosis: Full-term pregnancy. Endometritis, probably caused by gas-forming bacteria. Emphysematous fetuses.

Case 64

Cat, female, 7 years old. Three weeks prior to admission this cat had been in heat for about 2 weeks. It seemed normal at first, but gradually became ill. It had been very listless and anorectic for a few days when it was brought to the clinic. At examination it showed an enlarged abdomen which was painful on palpation. There was a purulent discharge from the vulva. Radiographs revealed the presence in the abdomen of a large loop distended by gas. The loop was interpreted as being a uterine horn filled with gas. To the left and located ventrally in the abdomen, a radiopaque mass, probably a collapsed mummified fetus, was seen. It was apparently lodged outside the gas-filled uterine horn. The digestive tract was empty. There were no obvious signs of peritonitis.

The diagnosis of physometra (gas in the uterus) was confirmed at laparotomy. The left uterine horn, which was gas-filled and distended, had ruptured. The rupture was sealed off by the omentum which adhered to the uterus around the rupture. Encapsulated by the omentum was a mummified mass of bone.

The cat made a slow but complete recovery.

Differential Diagnosis: The possibility of foreign-body ileus can be excluded. The gas-filled structure shows little resemblance to bowel and the "foreign body" seems to be outside the gas-filled loop. In combination with the clinical history the radiographs provided the diagnosis.

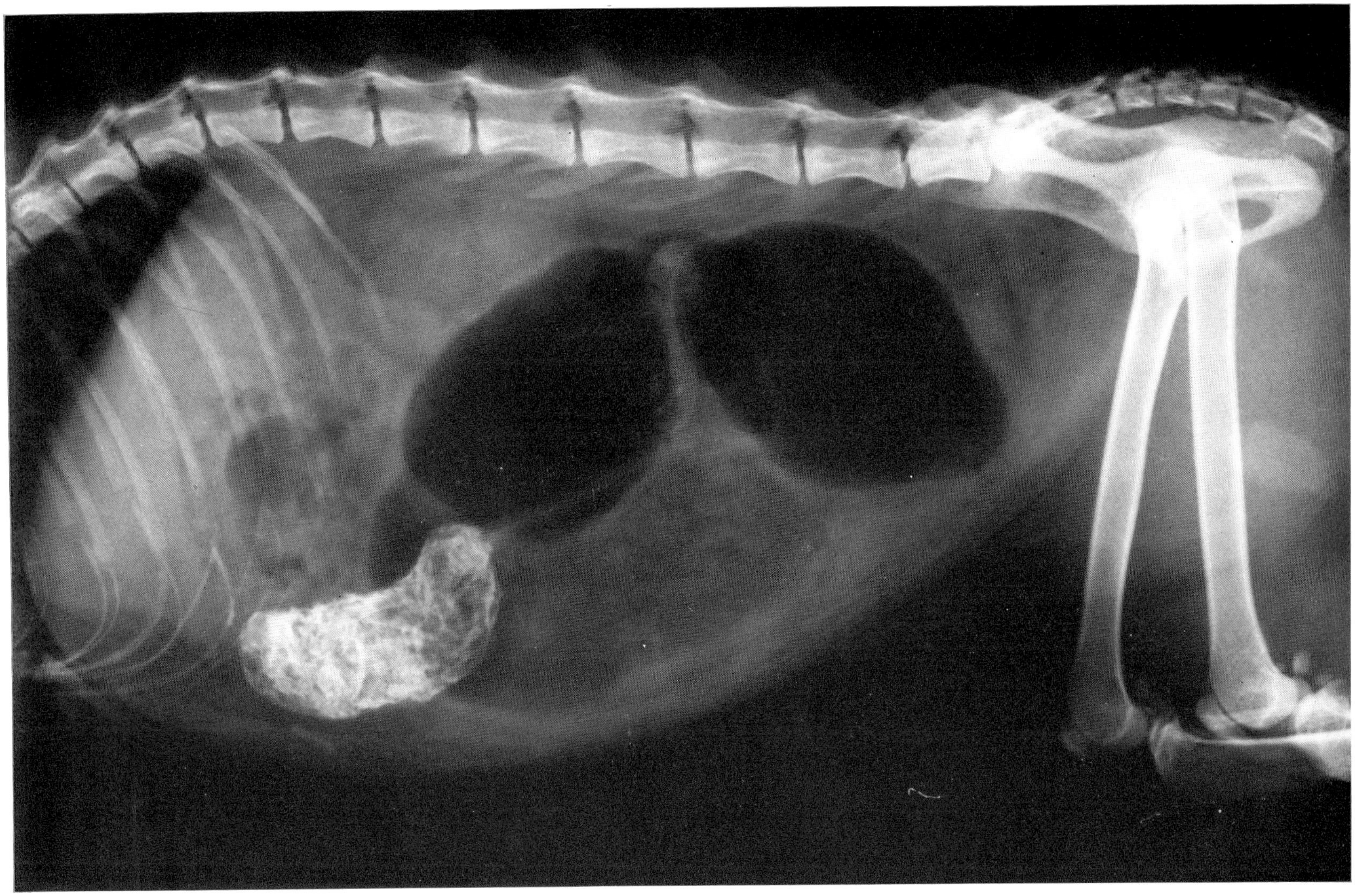

Case 64. **A,** Lateral radiograph. There are three rather distinct compartments in the gas-filled loop which occupies most of the space in the abdomen. Cranial to the loop is a very radiopaque object similar to feces containing bone. Dorsal to this mass is an area with a slightly mottled appearance.

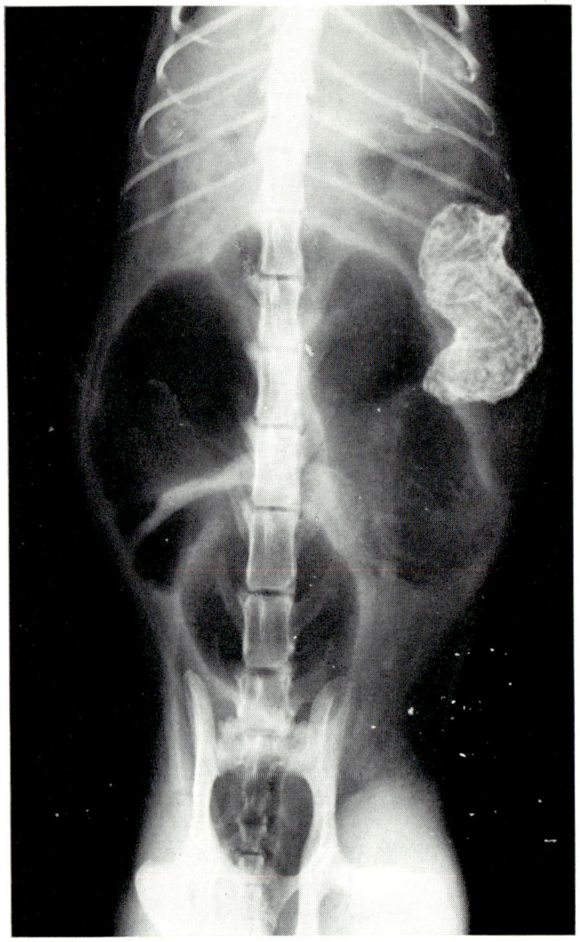

Case 64. **B,** Ventrodorsal radiograph. In this projection it is obvious that the radiopaque mass lies outside the gas-filled loop. The compartmental structure of the loop is easily recognized.

Diagnosis: Physometra. Sealed uterine rupture. Extrauterine mummified fetus.

Case 65

Dachshund, female, 4 years old. This dog gave birth to eleven puppies 48 hours prior to admission. Five of these puppies were alive when the dog was admitted because of illness, with high fever and listlessness, that had been manifest since delivery.

At examination the abdomen was found to be very painful on palpation and the mammary glands were swollen, painful, bluish-red, and very warm. The dog's temperature was 39.8° C. There was a brownish discharge from the vulva. Radiographs revealed the uterus to be moderately enlarged, containing fluid and some gas. The diagnosis of postpartum endometritis was made and the dog was treated with streptomycin and penicillin. The owner reported later that the dog recovered within 3 days.

Differential Diagnosis: The differential diagnosis between ileus and pyometra has been discussed previously (Case 50). It was pointed out that the enlarged uterine horns of a pyometra contain fluid but usually not gas, in contrast to distended bowel loops in ileus which usually contain both fluid and gas.

The present case is an illustration of the fact that an enlarged uterus may contain both fluid and gas. The uterine horns are wider than expected 2 days following parturition. Involution had thus been slow. This may in itself not be pathologic after a pregnancy with eleven fetuses, which is an unusually large number for a dachshund. It is obvious that the mastitis in itself could give the high temperature and poor general condition found in this dog. However, the presence of gas in the uterus indicates that there are also inflammatory changes in this organ.

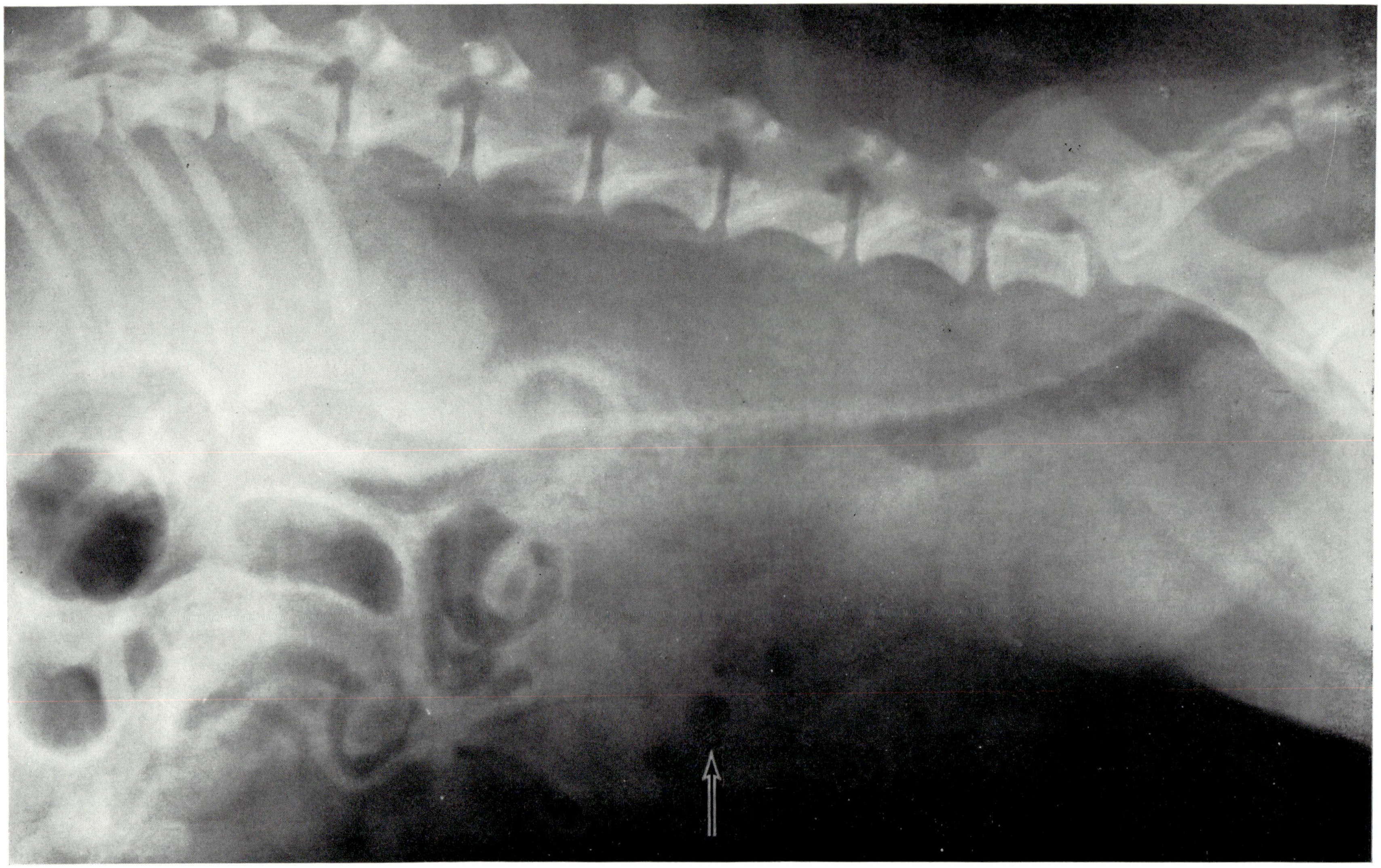

Case 65. **A,** Lateral radiograph. In the caudal half of the abdomen there are some large fluid-filled loops also containing a few bubbles of gas (arrow).

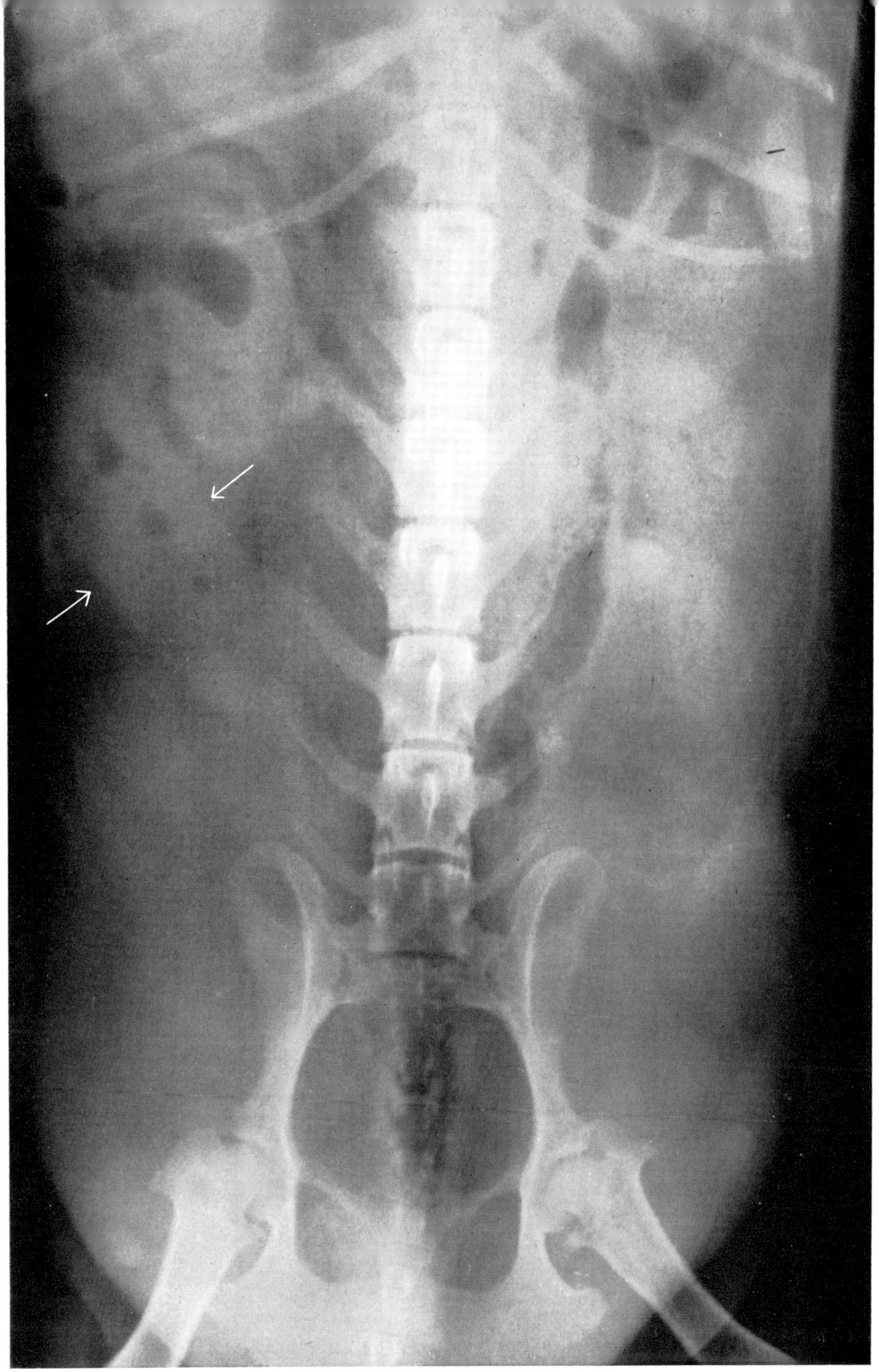

Case 65. **B,** Ventrodorsal radiograph. The entire caudal portion of the abdomen has a somewhat diffuse, slightly dense appearance. To the right of the animal is a fluid-filled loop of the uterus with a few gas bubbles (arrows).

Diagnosis: Postpartum endometritis. Mastitis.

Case 66

Collie, female, 12 years old. When this dog was first brought to the clinic it showed all the classical signs of pyometra. Radiographs confirmed the diagnosis and ovariohysterectomy was performed. Two days after the operation the dog had signs of rhinitis and conjunctivitis. After another 2 days, diarrhea complicated the picture. The following day the dog could barely stand on its legs. Antibiotics and daily transfusions were given from the second postoperative day until the dog was released on the owner's request. Medication with streptomycin and penicillin was prescribed.

The dog was returned to the clinic 6 days later with a very high temperature and a history of anorexia and vomiting of several days' duration. The surgical wound was well healed and the sutures were removed. At examination the dog appeared to be in very poor condition. It had dyspnea and tachycardia. Its mucous membranes were pale. The respiratory sounds were increased on the left side and decreased on the right side. Nothing remarkable could be felt on palpation of the abdomen. Abdominal radiographs showed no abnormality. No sign of peritonitis was found. The outline of the liver, however, was somewhat diffuse.

Radiographs of the thorax revealed the presence of fluid in the right pleural cavity with a marked cranial (elevated) position of the right side of the diaphragm. The heart was slightly shifted toward the right side. On fluoroscopic examination it was shown that the right side of the diaphragm moved less than the left side. On the basis of these findings a diagnosis of peritonitis localized to the right and to the most cranial part of the abdomen was made. The changes seen in the right side of the thorax were interpreted as due to sympathetic pleuritis caused by changes beneath the diaphragm on this side. Laparotomy was performed, but the dog expired during the operation. A localized peritonitis was found on the right side close to the diaphragm. Also a subphrenic abscess was present closer to the midline. There was pleuritis on the right side of the thorax.

Necropsy: The diagnosis made at operation was confirmed.

Differential Diagnosis: The site of localized peritonitis in this case is unusual. Because of the density of the liver, the abscess and the adhesions which were mainly subphrenic could not be seen. The fact that there was pleural effusion only on the right side led one to consider the possibility of a subphrenic abscess even in the absence of demonstrable changes in the abdominal cavity.

Case 66. **A,** Lateral radiograph of the cranial part of the abdomen. The cardia, part of the fundus, and the pyloric antrum of the stomach as well as part of the spleen and some bowel loops can be seen clearly. Their contours are not blurred by any density. The borders of the liver are, however, diffuse and the density of the liver is uneven.

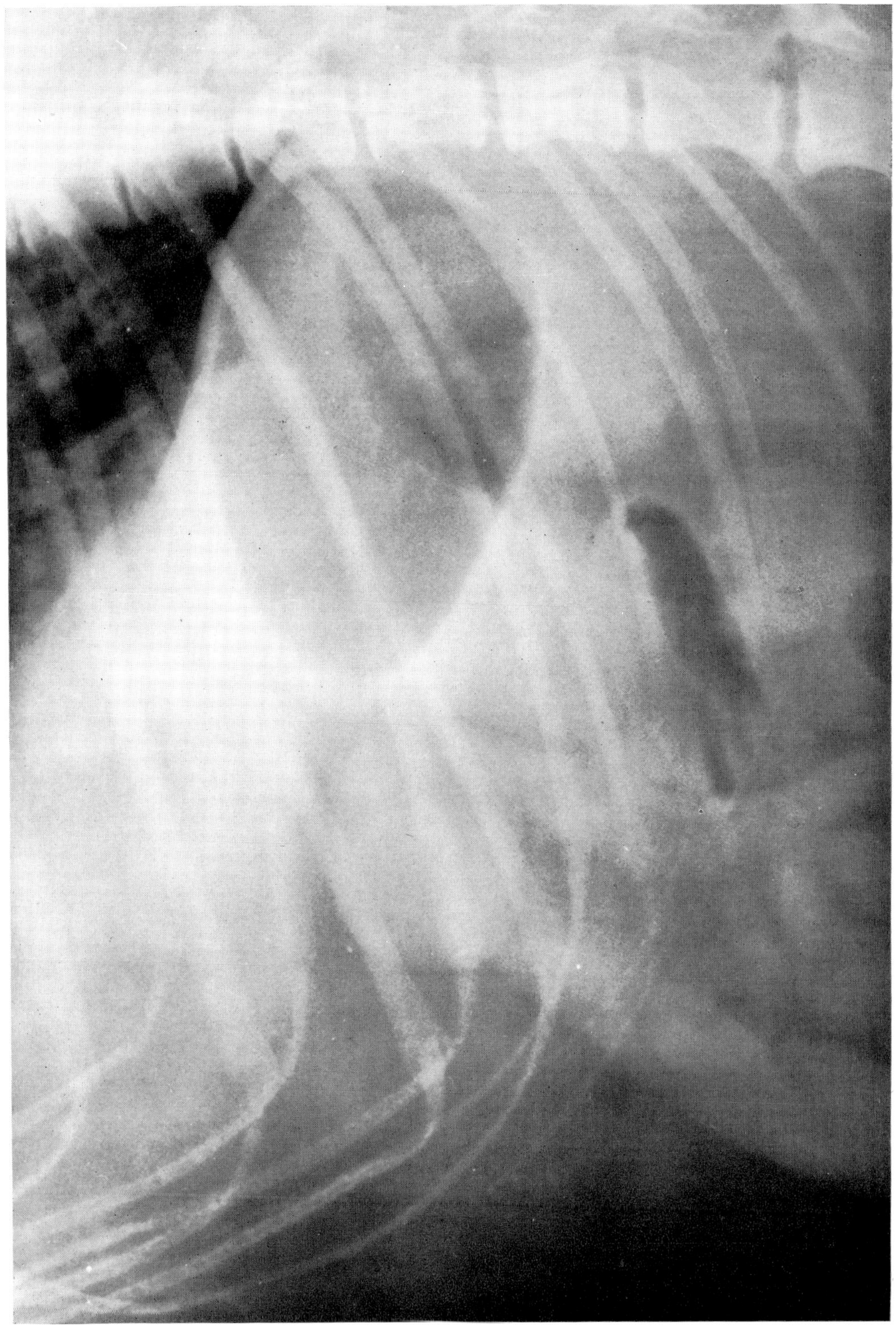

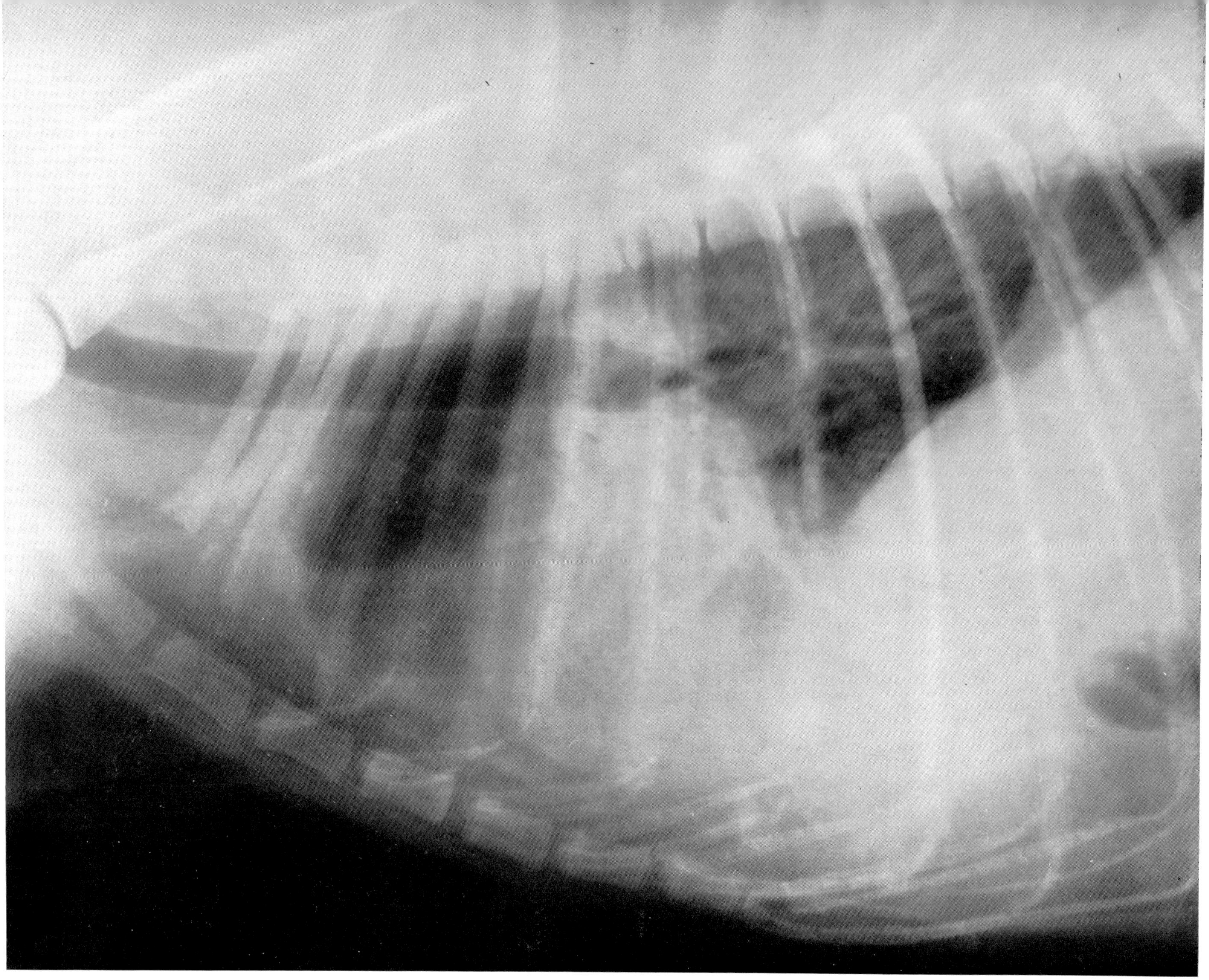

Case 66. **B,** Lateral radiograph. There is an increased density, especially in the ventral portion of the thorax. The heart shadow is partly obscured by this density and there is no clear border between the heart and the diaphragm. There is an increase in the pulmonary vascular and bronchial markings dorsocaudal to the heart, which is slightly elevated from the sternum. The diaphragm is bulging cranially.

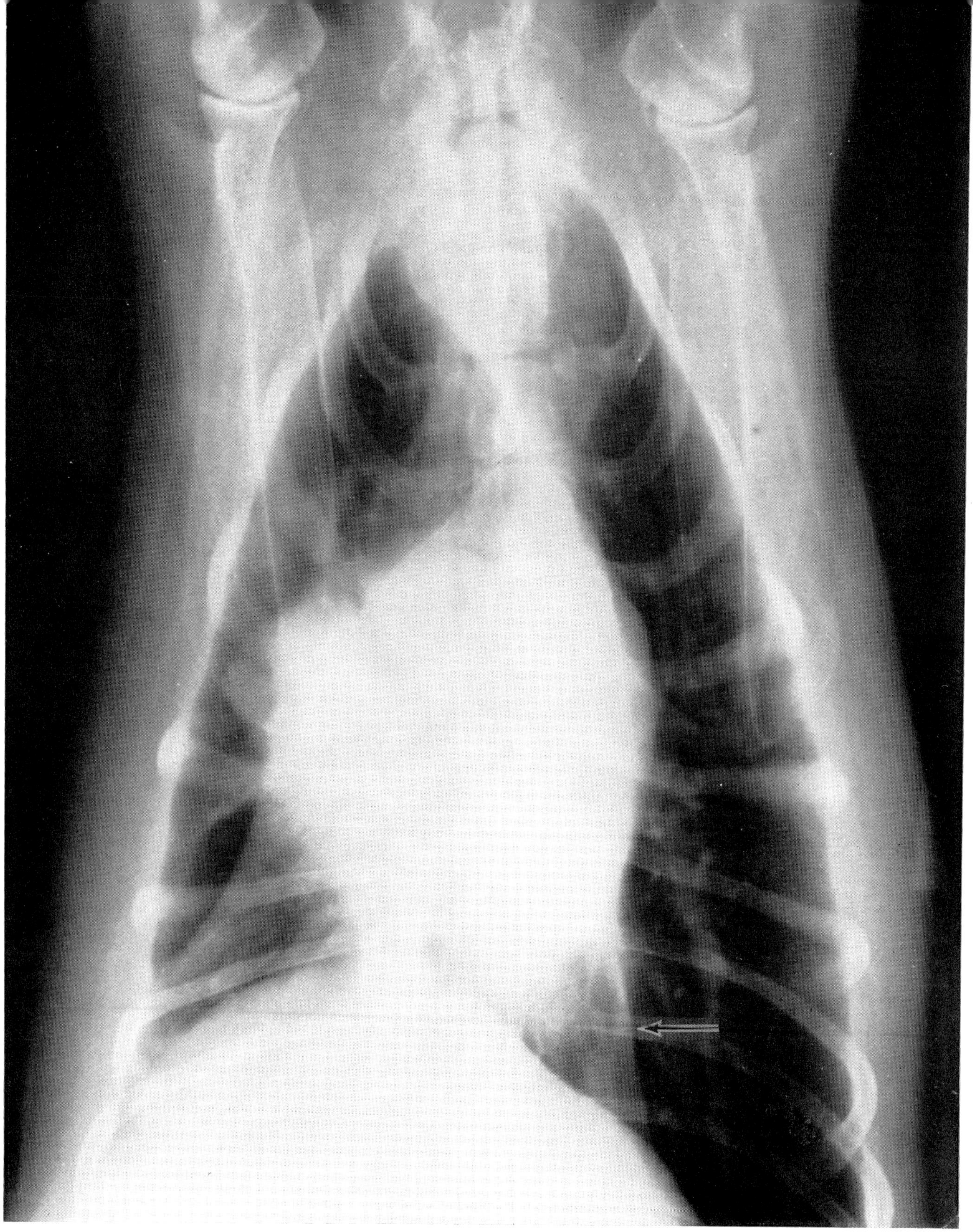

Case 66. **C,** Ventrodorsal radiograph. The heart is slightly shifted to the right and the right part of the diaphragm is elevated. There are some distinct interlobar borders. One of the most distinct is that between the intermediate lobe and the left diaphragmatic lobe (arrow). There is an increased density of the intermediate lobe and the right diaphragmatic lobe. Signs of fluid between the cardiac and diaphragmatic lobe on the right side are noted. Fluid is present between the right apical and cardiac lobes and in the phrenicocostal sinus.

Diagnosis: Peritonitis, subphrenic abscess, sympathetic pleuritis, and pulmonary atelectasis.

Case 67

Welsh corgi, female, 3 years old. This dog underwent cesarean section because of dystocia. The surgical wound healed well and the dog was in good condition for 6 days. It then developed anorexia and fever. Penicillin was prescribed by a veterinarian, but no improvement was noted. After 4 days of illness the dog was referred to the clinic. At examination the abdomen was painful and a mass could be palpated in the mid abdomen. The mass and a diffuse peritonitis were identified on radiographs. The diagnosis of foreign-body peritonitis was made. There was evidence that the foreign object was a piece of cloth, probably left in the abdomen when the dog had the cesarean section. At laparotomy an abscess containing a cloth was found. Many adhesions were present. The dog made an uneventful recovery.

Differential Diagnosis: The diagnosis of peritonitis was obvious. The mass in the mid abdomen had a center with a structure indicative of a textile foreign body.

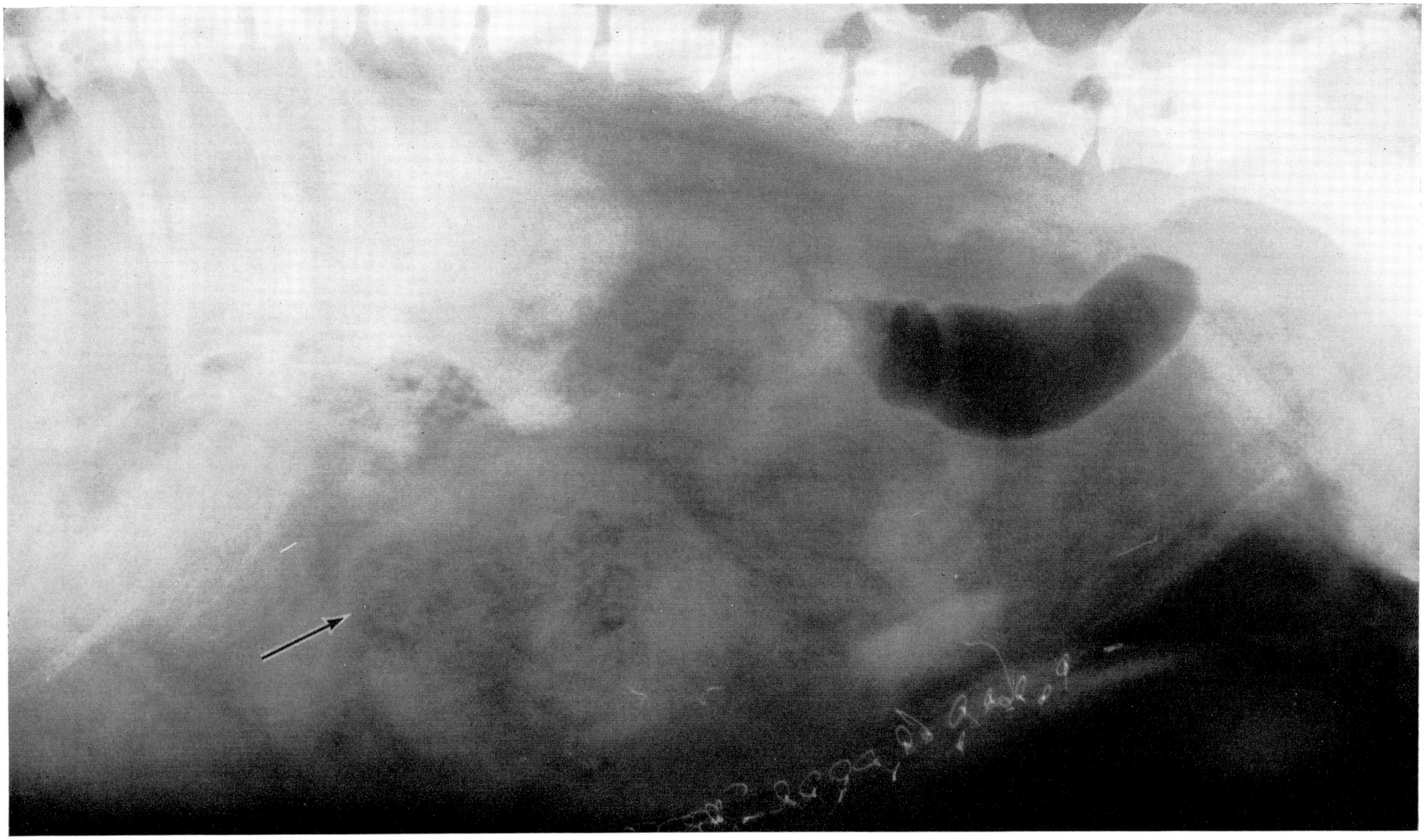

Case 67. On this lateral radiograph there is an increased abdominal density which is partly mottled in appearance. It obscures many details, but a round mass with a "textile" center can be seen in the mid abdomen (arrow). Some fecal material and gas are present in the descending colon. There are metal sutures in the abdominal wall.

Diagnosis: Foreign-body peritonitis (piece of cloth left in the abdomen during cesarean section performed 10 days previously).

Index

Note: The numbers following the entries refer to case numbers, rather than folios.

The Radiological Diagnosis in Canine and Feline Emergencies

An Atlas of Thoracic and Abdominal Changes